CBS—Quick Medical Examination Review Series

PHYSIOLOGY

FIFTEENTH EDITION

Edited by :

DR. M.S. BHATIA (MD, Dip. WPA, MNAMS)
Professor & Head, Department of Psychiatry
University College of Medical Sciences
&
Guru Teg Bahadur Hospital,
Dilshad Garden, Delhi - 110095.

Previously at :
Maulana Azad Medical College and Associated Hospitals, New Delhi.
&
Lady Hardinge Medical College and Associated Hospitals, New Delhi

Contributing Editor :
DR. NIRMALJIT KAUR (MD)
Senior Specialist, Department of Microbiology
Dr. R.M.L. Hospital
New Delhi - 110001

Previously at :
LHMC &Smt. S.K. Hospital , New Delhi

CBS

CBS Publishers & Distributors Pvt. Ltd.

NEW DELHI • BANGALORE • PUNE • CHENNAI • COCHIN (INDIA)

DEDICATED TO READERS WHO READ, UNDERSTAND & RECIPROCATE

ISBN : 978-81-239-1816-7

First Edition : 1992
Second Edition : 1993
Third Edition : 1994
Fourth Edition : 1995
Fifth Edition : 1996
Sixth Edition : 1997
Seventh Edition : 1998
Eighth Edition : 1999
Ninth Edition : 2000
Tenth Edition : 2001
Eleventh Edition : 2002
Twelveth Edition : 2003
Thirteenth Edition : 2004
Fourteenth Edition : 2005
Fifteenth Edition : 2010

Published by Satish Kumar Jain and produced by V.K. Jain for
CBS Publishers & Distributors Pvt. Ltd.,
4819/XI Prahlad Street, 24 Ansari Road, Daryaganj, New Delhi - 110002, India.
e-mail: cbspubs@vsnl.com, cbspubs@airtelmail.in
Website: www.cbspd.com

Branches:

- ***Bangalore:*** 2975, 17th Cross, K.R. Road, Bansankari 2nd Stage, Bangalore - 560070 Fax: 080-26771680 • e-mail: cbsbng@dataone.in
- ***Pune:*** Shaan Brahmha Complex, Basement, Appa Balwant Chowk, Budhwar Peth, Next to Ratan Talkies, Pune - 411002 Fax: 020-24464059 • e-mail: pune@cbspd.com
- ***Cochin:*** 36/14, Kalluvilakam, Lissie Hospital Road, Cochin - 682018, Kerala • e-mail: cochin@cbspd.com
- ***Chennai:*** 20, West Park Road, Shenoy Nagar, Chennai - 600030 • e-mail: chennai@cbspd.com

Printed at : Somya Printers, Delhi-110053

PREFACE

Life is a continuous learning process. Human beings are born to learn and gain knowledge. Education is a means to acquire knowledge and skills that an individual desires to practise. Examinations are the means to evaluate that knowledge. Though no method of evaluation is without flaw, the process of standardization has resulted in a multiple choice system of examination. This system satisfies the basic qualities of a measuring instrument viz., validity, reliability and objectivity.

Recently, a number of books have been published about these examinations but the **best book still remains that which covers the maximum number of questions, which had been asked in that particular examination,** because the chance of repetition of these questions from so-called **"Question Bank"** remains very high. Recently, it has been observed that many **"Question Banks"** have overlapped. So, it is best to do a book which is complete and covers the **"Question Banks"** of maximum number of examinations. This book is being forwarded in this direction.

This book is designed as a supplement to the standard textbooks. It includes the **Referenced - MCQ's** (of previous years papers) of various PG Medical Entrance and Services Examinations **speciality-wise and Chapter-wise** arranged. The students while preparing the text or just before the examination can quickly go through this book. This will help in detecting the areas of weakness in understanding the text and thus, will improve the skills with multiple choice system of examination. It is a favourite book for **"Paper-setters".**

The importance of doing MCQ's alongwith text has increased tremendously because recently, it has become a tendency to frame MCQ's usually not covered by the standard textbooks followed at undergraduate level. **"Quick Medical Text Review Series"** can be a useful adjuant to this book.

Beware of the **Fraudulent Books** available in the market, which covers a part of copied '**Question Bank**' from this book, and also, based on '**Constructed**' rather than '**Original**' Question Book. It is suggested not to waste time on these books. Every MCQ matters a lot in a highly competitive exams.

I request the readers not to forget to send their opinions, as also suggestions and contributions if any, about all aspects of this book. It will be of invaluable help in enhancing the utility of the book in future.

All suggestions are welcome and will be duly acknowledged in future editions.

— Editors

A book of the Readers, for the Readers, by the Readers

NOTE

The MCQ's of multiple response type (i.e. with **more than one correct answer** have been omitted in this Edition. Kindly refer to separate books (PGI MD Entrance Exam & DNB Entrance Exam.Part-I) by the same author and Publishers.

ADVICE

Read carefully the suggestions in the beginning of this book.

Prepare text from books suggested in the beginning of each chapter and go through **Referenced MCQ's** of this book. Don't waste time in inexperienced, **incomplete and Fraudulent courses conducted for PG Entrance Medical Examinations.**

ABOUT THE BOOK

This book has been compiled with the main aim to help the students to **quickly revise the Chapter-wise up-to-date referenced questions** asked in various entrance examinations (Years indicated in the brackets).

Quick Medical Examinations Review Series contain Speciality-wise 45,000 MCQ's based on up-to-date papers from 1978 onwards.

The important examinations covered in this book (with code word in the bracket) are :

	Examinations	*Code used*
(A)	***All India level***	
1.	All India Postgraduate Entrance Examination	(AI)
2.	AIIMS MD Entrance Examination	(AIIMS)
3.	PGI MD Entrance Examination	(PGI)
4.	Combined Medical Services Examination by UPSC	(UPSC)
5.	Civil Services Entrance Examination, Part-I (Medicine)	(CS)
6.	Army Medical Corps Entrance Examination	(AMC)
7.	Diplomate of National Board Entrance Examination	(DNB)
8.	NIMHANS PG Entrance Examination	(NIMHANS)
9.	Sanjay Gandhi PG Institute Entrance Examination	(SGPGI)
10.	CIP Ranchi PG Entrance Examination	(CIP)
11.	Manipal Academy of Higher Education PG Entrance	(Manipal/MAHE)
12.	Sree Chitra Tirunal Institute for Medical Science & Technology	(SCTIMST)
13.	Command Hospital, Bangalore	(CH)
14.	Bhabha Atomic Research Centre	(BARC)
15.	Institute of Aerospace Medicine	(IAM)
(B)	***State level***	
16.	Delhi MD Entrance Examination	(Delhi)
17.	Bihar MD Entrance Examination	(Bihar)
18.	JIPMER PG Entrance Examination	(JIPMER)
19.	CMC PG Entrance Examination	(CMC)
20.	Rohtak PG Entrance Examination	(Rohtak)
21.	MP State PG Entrance Examination	(MP)
22.	AP State MD Entrance Examination	(AP)
23.	TN State MD Entrance Examination	(TN)
24.	Karnataka Postgraduate Medical Examination	(Karnataka)
25.	Maharashtra PG Entrance Examination	(Maharashtra)
26.	Kerala State MD Entrance Examination	(Kerala)
27.	Rajasthan Postgraduate Entrance Examination	(Rajasthan)
28.	PG Entrance Examination, Varanasi	(BHU)
29.	Burdwan University	(BU)
30.	Combined Entrance Examination for PG Courses, U.P.	(UP)
31.	Punjab State PG Entrance Examination	(Punjab)
32.	Aligarh Muslim University PG Entrance Examination	(AMU)
33.	Nizam's Institute Entrance Examination, Hyderabad	(Nizam's)
34.	Postgraduate Admission Test, Orissa	(Orissa)
35.	Calcutta University Public Service Commission	(CUPSC)
36.	TN Public Service Commission	(TNPSC)
37.	Calcutta PG Entrance Examination	(Calcutta)
(C)	***Foreign Examinations***	
	PLAB, FCGP, GMC, FLEX, USMLE, MRCP, FRCS, MRCOG, etc.	

Source of Errors (Physiology)

Example 1 : **Juxtamedullary nephrons in kidney constitute what percentage of total nephrons :** **Delhi 1993**

a) 15%
b) 50%
c) 70%
d) 80%

Answer : None of the above is correct. Answer is 90%.

Example 2 : **Gastric secretion is not influenced by :** **Delhi 1986**

a) Diet
b) Gastrin
c) Secretin
d) Cholecystokinin

Answer : a,b & d are stimulants whereas c is inhibitory. Question should have been "Gastric secretion is not ***stimulated*** by"

Example 3 : **Adrenaline insufficiency causes :** **AIIMS 1989**

a) A rise in plasma sodium/potassium ratio
b) Low B.P.
c) Increased breakdown of protein
d) A fall in extracellular fluid volume

Answer : Both "b" and "d".

Example 4 : **Brown -Sequard syndrome involves all of the following except :** **Delhi 1994**

a) Pain
b) Temperature
c) Proprioception
d) Crude touch

Answer : "None of the above" (i.e. All of the above choices are seen)

ADVICE

Questions with inaccurate language or wrong choices should better be left unattempted.

IMPORTANT PHYSIOLOGY TEXT FOR MCQ's

CNS	:	Physiologic anatomy of synapse, Sensory receptors, Motor functions of spinal cord and Postural reflexes, Functional areas of brain, Important tracts
CVS	:	Rhythmic excitation of heart, Normal ECG (Values of different components), Cardiac output, venous return and their regulation, Coronary circulation, Jugular pulse
Lungs	:	Pulmonary function tests (various capacities) and effect of common diseases on them, Transport of Gases (O2, CO2), Regulation of Respiration
Kidney	:	Structure and Physiology of a nephron, Kidney function tests
GIT	:	Functional types of movements, digestion of food, important local hormones and enzymes
Circulation	:	Hemodynamics of blood flow (especially to heart, lungs, kidney etc.), Dynamics of shock
Endocrinology	:	Hypothalamus, Pituitary, Thyroid, Parathyroid, Pancreas, Sexual function, Adrenal
Blood	:	Production and function of important blood components, Haemostasis and Blood coagulation (factors, mechanism, disorders)
Special senses	:	Optics of vision, Receptor functions of the retina, Mechanism of hearing and smell
Miscellaneous	:	Metabolism of carbohydrate, fat, protein and vitamins. Temperature regulation. All factual data, Named laws, principles, signs and tests

IMPORTANT TIPS OF PHYSIOLOGY

Read

* Concentration of substances in the Glomerular filtrate from Bhatia **Quick Medical Text Review Series, Physiology.**

* About Jugular venous pulse from **Ganong's Review of Medical Physiology.**

* About Pituitary hormones from Bhatia's **Quick Medical Text Review Series, Physiology.**

* About Pulmonary function Tests from Ganong's **Review of Medical Physiology,** or Bhatia **Quick Medical Text Review Series, Physiology.**

* About normal distribution of ions in body from Ganong's **Review of Medical Physiology**.

* Exercise induced changes from R.K. Marya's **Medical Physiology.**

* About various Named Laws from Bhatia's **Quick Medical Text Review Series, Physiology.**

* About blood flow to different organs from Bhatia's **Quick Medical Text Review Series, Physiology.**

* About various hemodynamic indices from Table in Bhatia's **Quick Medical Text Review Series, Physiology.**

* About Functional Areas of Cerebral Cortex from Bhatia's **Quick Medical Text Review Series, Physiology.**

* Ageing related changes from R.K. Marya's **Medical Physiology**.

* One must know important points from Bhatia's **Quick Medical Text Review Series, Physiology.**

CONTENTS

COMBINED MEDICAL SERVICES EXAMINATION
(Conducted by UPSC)

- It contains original solved papers from **1983 onwards**
- All papers are **Subjectwise & Yearwise** arranged
- Answers are given at the foot and **detailed explanations** are given at the end.
- Detailed **instructions** about this examination are given
- Important **references** to be read are also given
- Each year's paper is classified into two separate parts arranged subjectwise
- Book is suited for Quick revision before the examination and also to know its pattern
- High chance of repetition in this exam as well as in other UPSC conducted Exams
- Read the papers before undertaking preparation (to know the pattern), then read text and again check your knowledge by doing papers
- Also useful for **Civil Services Examination, Part I** (Medical Sciences) as the question Bank is same
- Also read book on **Civil Services Examination, Part I (Medical Sciences)** (by same author and publishers) as the **Question Bank** of two exams may overlap.
- All suggestions and Contributions are welcome and write to the Editor : **Dr. M.S. Bhatia,** D-1, Naraina Vihar, New Delhi-110028

1

IMPORTANT TEXT OF CNS

NERVE FIBER TYPES IN MAMMALIAN NERVE

Fiber Type		Function	Fiber Diameter (mm)	Conduction Velocity (m/sec)	Spike Duration (m/sec)	Absolute Refractory Period (m/sec)
A	α	Proprioception; somatic motor	12-20	70-120		
	β	Touch, pressure	5-12	30-70	0.4-0.5	0.4-1
	γ	Motor to muscle spindles	3-6	15-30		
	δ	Pain, Temperature, touch	2-5	12-30		
B		Preganglionic autonomic	<3	3-15	1.2	1.2
C	dorsal root	Pain, reflex responses	0.4-1.2	0.5-2	1.2	2
	sympathetic	Postganglionic sympathetics	0.3-1.3	0.7-2.3	2	2

RELATIVE SUSCEPTIBILITY OF MAMMALIAN, A, B, AND C NERVE FIBERS TO CONDUCTION BLOCK PRODUCED BY VARIOUS AGENTS

	Most Susceptible	Intermediate	Least Susceptible
Sensitivity to hypoxia	B	A	C
Sensitivity to pressure	A	B	C
Sensitivity to cocaine and local anaesthetics	C	B	A

SENSORY RECEPTORS

Sensation	Receptors
Touch	Meissner's corpuscles
	Menkel's discs, Hair bulb endings
Pain	Free Nerve endings
Heat	Ruffini end organ
Cold	Krause's end bulb
Pressure	Pacinian lamellated corpuscles
	Golgi-Mazzoni body

NUMERICAL CLASSIFICATION SOMETIMES USED FOR SENSORY NEURONS.

Number		*Origin*	*Fiber Type*
I	α	Muscle spindle, annulospiral ending	A α
	β	Golgi tendon organ	A α
II		Muscle spindle, flower-spray ending; touch, pressure	A ß
III		Pain and temperature receptors; some touch receptors	A δ
IV		Pain and other receptors	Dorsal root C

SEQUENCE OF EVENTS IN CONTRACTION AND RELAXATION OF SKELETAL MUSCLE.

Steps in contraction

1. Discharge of motor neuron.
2. Release of transmitter (acetylcholine) at motor end plate.
3. Generation of end-plate potential.
4. Generation of action potential in muscle fibers.
5. Inward spread of depolarization along T tubules.
6. Release of Ca^{++} from lateral sacs of sarcoplasmic reticulum and diffusion of thick and thin filaments.
7. Binding of Ca^{++} to troponin C, uncovering myosin binding sites on actin.
8. Formation of cross-linkages between actin and myosin and sliding of thin or thick filaments, producing shortening.

Steps in relaxation

1. Ca^{++} pumped back into sarcoplasmic reticulum.
2. Release of Ca^{++} from troponin.
3. Cessation of interaction between actin and myosin.

CONCENTRATION OF VARIOUS SUBSTANCES IN HUMAN CSF AND PLASMA

	Substance	*CSF*	*Plasma*	*Ratio CSF/Plasma*
Na^+	($mEq/kg\,H_2O$)	147.0	150.0	0.98
K^+	($mEq/kg\,H_2O$)	2.9	4.6	0.62
Mg^{++}	($mEq/kg\,H_2O$)	2.2	1.6	1.39
Ca^{++}	($mEq/kg\,H_2O$)	2.3	4.7	0.49
Cl^-	($mEq/kg\,H_2O$)	113.0	99.0	1.14
HCO_3	(mEq/liter)	25.1	24.8	1.01
PCO_2	(mm Hg)	50.2	39.5	1.28
pH		7.33	7.40	...
Osmolality	($mOsm/kg\,H_2O$)	289.0	289.0	1.00
Protein	(mg/dl)	20.0	6000.0	0.003
Glucose	(mg/dl)	64.0	100.0	0.64
Inorganic P	(mg/dl)	3.4	4.7	0.73
Urea	(mg/dl)	12.0	15.0	0.80
Creatinine	(mg/dl)	1.5	1.2	1.25
Uric acid	(mg/dl)	1.5	5.0	0.30
Lactic acid	(mg/dl)	18.0	21.0	0.86
Cholesterol	(mg/dl)	0.2	175.0	0.001

MCQ's OF CNS

What is important in CNS

Physiologic anatomy of synapse, Sensory receptors, Motor functions of spinal cord and Postural reflexes, Functional areas of brain, Important tracts.

1. Increase in the threshold level if the stimulus is slowly allowed to increase is termed as : AIIMS 2006, 2007
A. Adaptation B. Accommodation
C. Electrotonus D. Refractoriness

2. Adrenaline, dopamine, serotonin works by which of the following channels? AIIMS 2006
A. One pass gated B. Four pass gated
C. Seven pass gated D. Ligand gated

3. The main difference between REM sleep and wakefullness is : AIIMS 2006
A. EEG desynchronization
B. Rapid eye movements
C. Decreased muscle tone
D. Penile erection

4. On electromyography, all of the following features suggest denervation, except : AIIMS 2006
A. Unregulated firing of individual muscle fibres
B. Small short-duration polyphasic action potentials
C. Presence of positive sharp waves
D. Spontaneous firing of motor units

5. Cushing's Triad include all except : AIIMS 2006, AI 2007
A. Hypertension B. Bradycardia
C. Hypothernia D. Irregular respiration

6. An anterolateral cordotomy relieving pain in right leg is effective because it interrupts the : AIIMS 2005
A. Left dorsal column
B. Left ventral spinothalmic tract
C. Left lateral spinothalmic tract
D. Right lateral spinothalmic tract

7. Beta waveforms in electroencephalogram designate which of the following states of the patient : AIIMS 2005
A. Deep Anaesthesia
B. Surgical Anaesthesia
C. Light Anaesthesia, eyes closed, relaxed
D. Awake/alert state

8. Group-A nerve fibers are most susceptible to : AIIMS 2005
A. Pressure B. Hypoxia
C. Local anaesthetics D. Temperature

9. Synaptic potentials can be recorded by : AIIMS 2005
A. Patch clamp technique
B. Voltage clamp technique
C. Microelectrode
D. EEG

10. Which of the following methods is not used for measurement of body fluid volumes ? AIIMS 2005
A. Antipyrine for total body water
B. Inulin for extracellular fluid
C. Evans blue for plasma volume
D. ^{125}I-albumin for blood volume

11. Muscarinic receptors are located in : AP 1990, 96
A. Membrane of effector structures innervated by post. ganglionic parasympathetic nerve endings.
B. At neuromuscular junction on the muscle membrane
C. Membrane of parasympathetic ganglia.
D. Membrane of the sympathetic ganglia.

12. The reticular formation is a diffuse collection of : Bihar 1999, 2001
A. Only sensory neurons
B. Only motor neurons
C. Only autonomic centres
D. All of the above

13. Which of the following statements is not true : AP 1991, 98
A. Decorticate rigidity is greater than decerebrate rigidity.
B. Righting reflexes are absent in the decerebrate animal.
C. Visual righting reflex is present in a thalamic animal.
D. Decorticate rigidity is seen only when the animal is at rest.

Ans. 1. B 2. C 3. C 4. B 5. C 6. C 7. D 8. A 9. C 10. D
11. A 12. D 13. A

14. The following statements about nystagmus are true except : TN 1992

A. It is present in cerebellar lesion.
B. It is a symptom of vestibular lesion.
C. The direction of nystagmus is in the same direction of rotation.
D. Direction of nystagmus is in the same direction as that of during rotation.

15. The neurons in the substantia nigra, which project to the globus pallidus and which are inhibitory in nature secrete at their endings : TN 1992

A. Acetyl choline B. Dopamine
C. GABA D. Glycine

16. The following are signs and symptoms associated with Parkinson's disease except : AP 1991

A. Muscle rigidity B. Intention tremor
C. Akinesia D. Tremor at rest

17. Hemiballismus occurring in one of the left extremities generally results from lesion in right : TN 1991

A. Caudate nucleus B. Putamen
C. Amygdaloid body D. Subthalamic nucleus

18. In what part of the brain do most of the signals from the Golgi tendon apparatus and muscle spindles go? PGI 1992

A. The somesthetic cortex
B. The thalamus
C. The basal ganglia
D. The motor cortex
E. The cerebellum

19. In what part of the central nervous system to the signals probably originate to provide most of the support of the body against gravity? PGI 1992

A. The bulboreticular facilitatory area
B. The basal gangila
C. The motor cortex
D. The cerebellum

20. Damage to which area of the cerebral cortex is likely to cause the greatest degree of loss of intellectual capabilities in a right-handed person? AMC 1998

A. The frontal lobes.
B. The left somesthetic sensory and sensory association areas.
C. The right somesthetic sensory and sensory association areas.
D. The left posterior superior temporal gyrus.

21. Decerebrate animal results from following experimental procedure : Bihar 1999

A. Cerebrum removal
B. Transection of upper border of midbrain
C. Inter-collicular transection
D. Section above thalamus

22. Integration of temperature information by the nervous system occurs mainly in the : AIIMS 1996

A. Spinal cord B. Hypothalamus
C. Amygdala D. Peripheral receptors

23. Which of the following cortical layers is stimulated most by the diffuse thalamocortical system? PGI 1982, 94

A. Layer 2 B. Layer 3
C. Layer 4 D. Layer 5

24. If the connections are cut between the cortex and the thalamus, which one of the following types of brain waves can still be recorded in the cortex? PGI 1993

A. Alpha waves B. Beta waves
C. Theta waves D. Delta waves

25. Almost all of the cerebral cortex has direct two-way communication with which one of the following subcortical structures? Delhi 1990

A. Cerebellum
B. Thalamus
C. Hypothalamus
D. Bulboreticular facilitatory area

26. The percentage of sensory fibres in a motor nerve is : JIPMER 1992

A. 0% B. 10%
C. 20% D. 40%

27. In which type of nerve fibres is conduction blocked maximally by pressure? JIPMER 1992

A. C B. A-alpha
C. A-beta D. A-gamma

28. Increased Gamma efferent discharge is seen in all except : JIPMER 1993

A. Anxiety
B. Stimulation of skin
C. Jendrassik's maneuver
D. Rapid shallow breathing

29. In cerebellar disease, all the statements are correct except : Delhi 1997

A. The Romberg's sign is positive
B. There is Adiadokokinesia
C. There is Pendular knee jerk
D. There is involuntary tremor

30. In a person with a history of alcohol abuse which of the following aspects of memory is most likely to be impaired? DNB 1991

A. Accurate perception of stimuli
B. Immediate recall of new information
C. Recall of events occurring a few weeks previously
D. Recall of events in the remote past
E. Recognition of familiar objects

Ans.									
14. C	15. B	16. B	17. D	18. E	19. C	20. D	21. C	22. B	23. C
24. B	25. B	26. D	27. C	28. D	29. D	30. C			

31. **Vomiting centre is located in : AMC 1995**
A. Cervical spinal cord
B. Thalamus
C. Hypothalamus
D. Medulla oblongata

32. **Sensory impulses originating in the periphery : DNB 1990**
A. Ascend by unknown pathways to cortex
B. Never pass through reticular formation
C. Must all pass through reticular formation
D. Pass in part through reticular formation and in part bypass it

33. **The prime regulator of blood flow through exercising muscles is : Kerala 1990**
A. Venous tone
B. Systemic BP
C. Vasodilator metabolites
D. Sympathetic control

34. **The excitatory postsynaptic potential (EPSP) differs from the end plate potential in that the EPSP is : Kerala 1999**
A. Propagated
B. A reversal of charge
C. Not associated with an increased permeability to both potassium and sodium ions
D. Not decreased by curare

35. **A stimulus event is called a reinforcer only if it can be shown to : AIIMS 1999**
A. Produce reduction of a homeostatic need.
B. Lead to a increased probability of response.
C. Serve as an unconditioned response for operant behavior.
D. Elicit the response that follows it.
E. Lead to generalization of response strength .

36. **The normal amount of C.S.F in man is about : Delhi 1988, 97**
A. 50 cc B. 100 cc
C. 150 cc D. 200 cc

37. **A patient complains of muscle weakness. On administration of neostigmine, it disappears. What is its mechanism of action ? AP 1989, 96**
A. It blocks action of acetyl choline.
B. It interferes with the action of amineoxidase.
C. It interferes with the action of carbonic anhydrase.
D. It interferes with the action of acetyl-choline esterase.

38. **A unilateral upper motor neuron lesion in the internal capsule is best characterized by : NIMHANS 1989, 95**
A. Diminished use of contralateral appendages below the lesion.
B. Muscle fasciculations.
C. Ipsilateral hypotonicity.
D. Flexion of the leg.

39. **The cerebellum : NIMHANS 1989, 96**
A. Has a totally inhibitory output from its cortex.
B. Has only excitatory signal output from its deep nuclear layers.
C. Has a conscious interpretation of motor activity.
D. Has inhibitory influence on muscle tone in humans.

40. **Hyperkinetic syndromes such as chorea and athetosis are usually associated with pathological changes in : AP 1991**
A. Motor areas of cerebral cortex.
B. Anterior hypothalamus.
C. Pathways for recurrent collateral inhibition in the spinal cord.
D. Basal ganglia complex.

41. **Aqueous humor differs from CSF in that the former : AIIMS 1986, 92**
A. Has protein content similar to plasma
B. Is an ultrafiltrate of plasma
C. Serves no important nutritive function
D. Contains a higher concentration of ascorbic acid

42. **Interneurons are : TN 1993**
A. Essential part of withdrawal reflex
B. Essential part of stretch reflex
C. Essential part of all reflexes
D. Always excitatory

43. **Non-myelinated axons differ from myelinated in that they : Bihar 1989, 96**
A. Are more excitable
B. Lack nodes of Ranvier
C. Are not capable of regeneration
D. Are not associated with Schwann cells

44. **What is true regarding the gamma efferent neuron? Rohtak 1985, 93**
A. A group of motor neuron with a smaller diameter than that of alpha effernt neurons.
B. Innervates intrafusal fibres.
C. Innervates muscle fibres that stretch annulospital endings.
D. All of the above.

45. **Which of the following reflexes disappear in the absence of functional connections between the spinal cord and the brain? DNB 1992**
A. Swallowing reflex B. Sweating reflex
C. Withdrawal reflex D. Erection of penis
E. All of the above

Ans.									
31. D	32. D	33. C	34. D	35. B	36. C	37. D	38. A	39. A	40. D
41. D	42. A	43. B	44. D	45. A					

46. A patient with loss of function of posterior columns of spinal cord will exhibit all, except : NIMHANS 1988, 97

A. Diminished vibration sense
B. Some loss of pain sensation
C. Normal plantar response
D. A clumsy gait made worse on closure of eyes

47. The speed at which an axon conducts an action potential is directly related to : AMU 1986, 99

A. The diameter of dendrites
B. The diameter of axon
C. The length of axon
D. The amount of axonal branching

48. A neuron which exhibits saltatory conduction differs from one which does not, in that the former: AIIMS 1986, 91

A. Produces its action potential through sodium ion influx.
B. Produces its action potential through potassium ion influx.
C. Exhibits continuous conduction.
D. Conducts from one node of Ranvier to the next.
E. Conducts impulses more slowly.

49. First relay station of pain is : Delhi 1995

A. Spinal cord B. Medulla
C. Pons D. Thalamus

50. Vasomotor reflexes may be mediated through special areas of the : Delhi 1993

A. Medulla B. Spinal cord
C. Cerebrum D. Hypothalamus
E. All of the above

51. Resting membrane potential of nerve is equal to equilibrium potential of : AI 1990, 93

A. Na+ B. K+
C. Cl- D. Ca+

52. The Spinothalamic tract does not contain fibres for: AI 1993

A. Touch sensation
B. Pressure
C. Pain
D. Discriminatory sensation

53. Vessels not under sympathetic control are : Delhi 1993

A. Cerebral B. Splanchnic
C. Cardiac D. Cutaneous

54. CSF in comparison to blood contains all except : AMU 1990, Delhi 1993

A. Lower calcium B. Lower chloride
C. Lower sodium D. Lower cells

55. Motor area of Brodmann is : Delhi 1993

A. 1 B. 4
C. 5 D. 7

56. Relation between nerve thickness and conduction velocity is : Delhi 1990, 92

A. Linear B. Parabolic
C. Hyperbolic D. No relation

57. Upto what systolic pressure is the brain capable of autoregulation : Delhi 1992

A. 65 mm of Hg B. 55 mm of Hg
C. 45 mm of Hg D. 75 mm of Hg

58. Satiety centre in hypothalamus is regulated by : Delhi 1992

A. Gastric dilatation B. Blood glucose levels
C. Blood insulin levels D. All of the above

59. Delta waves in EEG are seen in : JIPMER 1992

A. REM sleep
B. Deep sleep
C. Awake with eyes open
D. Awake with eyes closed

60. The cerebellum is important in all of the following except : CSE 1996

A. Enabling the CNS to predict future positions of moving parts of the body.
B. Initiation of muscular movements.
C. Co-ordination and damping of muscular movements.
D. Maintaining smooth progression of the movement.

61. Where is motor activity probably initiated in the brain ? UPSC 1982, 94

A. Motor cortex B. Premotor cortex
C. Basal ganglia D. Cerebellum

62. The rigidity seen in Parkinson's disease is due to : CSE 1996

A. Excessive stimulation of alpha motor neurons of all the muscles
B. Hypofunction of motor cortex
C. Absence of cerebellar inhibition
D. Increased sensitivity of stretch reflex

63. Face is represented by area : Delhi 1990

A. I B. II
C. III D. IV

64. Which of the following are true of median eminence : AIIMS 1985; AI 1998

A. Portion of ventral hypothalamus
B. Hypothalamus hypophyseal vessels arise here
C. Outside the blood-brain barrier
D. All are correct

65. In a child , nerve conduction velocity reaches the adult level by : DNB 1993

A. Birth B. 1-2 years
C. 3-4 years D. 6-8 years

Ans.										
	46. B	47. B	48. D	49. A	50. E	51. C	52. D	53. A	54. B	55. B
	56. A	57. A	58. B	59. B	60. B	61. A	62. A	63. C	64. D	65. C

66. Unconscious kinesthetic sensations are carried by **PGI 1984, Delhi 1990, 96**

A. Anterior spinal horns
B. Spinal ganglion
C. Nucleus pulposus
D. Posterior columns

67. Genu of internal capsule has : **Delhi 1990**

A. Sensory fibres from thalamus to brain
B. Motor fibres from lower limb
C. Motor fibres from upper limb
D. Motor fibres from trunk

68. Sensory area-I of the cerebral cortex carries : **AIIMS 1996**

A. Pain fibres
B. Touch fibres
C. Fibres for fine movement
D. Tactile discrimination and two point discrimination

69. The primary function of basal ganglia is : **CSE 1997**

A. Sensory integration
B. Short term memory
C. Pre-programming of voluntary activity
D. Control of equilibrium

70. Tremors associated with cerebellar disease are : **AIIMS 1986, 95**

A. Present at rest
B. Present with action
C. Restricted to hands and trunk
D. Associated with fine movements only

71. Wallerian degeneration of ruptured nerve starts in : **Delhi 1981, 85. 93**

A. 6 hours B. 12 hours
C. 24 hours D. 6 weeks

72. First synapse for peripheral sensation is : **Delhi 1984, 92**

A. Cerebellum B. Anterior horn cells
C. Posterior horn cells D. Midbrain

73. For each 1°F rise of temperature, cerebral blood flow falls by : **Delhi 1984, 94**

A. 1% B. 2%
C. 4% D. 7%

74. Buerger waves (α-waves) of EEG have the rhythm per sec as : **PGI 1984; Delhi 1984, 89, 93**

A. 0-4 B. 4-7
C. 8-13 D. 13-30

75. Broca's area of speech lies at : **Delhi 1985, 90**

A. Superior border of frontal lobe
B. Inferior border of frontal lobe
C. Posterior border of frontal lobe
D. Superior temporal gyrus

76. The frequency of β-waves (per sec) in EEG is : **Delhi 1987, 93**

A. 0-4 B. 4-7
C. 7-13 D. 13-30

77. First neurotransmitter discovered was : **AIIMS 1984, 95**

A. Dopamine B. Norepinephrine
C. 5-HT D. Acetylcholine

78. True visceral pain arises from : **DNB 1998**

A. Compression B. Irritation
C. Distension D. Chemical stimulation

79. The fibre which is the thickest in human nerve is : **Delhi 1999**

A. Touch B. Pain
C. Temperature D. Proprioception

80. Pain carrying fibres are : **JIPMER 1997**

A. Aα Aβ B. Aα, C
C. Aδ, C D. Aδ, Aα

81. Bitemporal hemianopia is seen in lesions of : **Delhi 1990, 94; UPSC 1991**

A. Optic tract B. Optic chiasma
C. Optic nerve D. Occipital lobe

82. Destruction of pneumotoxic centre in pons causes : **Delhi 1986, 94**

A. Apnoea
B. Forceful respiration
C. Apneustic respiration
D. Accelerated respiration

83. Isometric relaxation phase lasts for —— sec. : **AIIMS 1985, 92**

A. 0.04 B. 0.08
C. 0.12 D. 0.14

84. During light sleep, the sleep spindles that appear have the frequency of : **Delhi 1984, 94**

A. 1-2/sec B. 6-12/sec
C. 14-16/sec D. 21-26/sec

85. Renshaw cell inhibition is a typical example of : **AIIMS 1984, 97**

A. Presynaptic inhibition
B. Direct inhibition
C. Recurrent inhibition
D. Recurrent excitation

86. The maximum rate of axonal transport is : **AMC 1985, 99**

A. 200 mm/day B. 400 mm/day
C. 600 mm/day D. 800 mm/day

87. Preganglionic sympathetic neurons stimulation causes all except : **Delhi 1984, 96**

A. Secretion of saliva
B. Dilatation of pupils
C. Hepatic glycogenolysis
D. None of the above

Ans. 66. D 67. A 68. D 69. C 70. B 71. A 72. C 73. D 74. C 75. B
76. D 77. D 78. C 79. D 80. C 81. B 82. C 83. B 84. C 85. C
86. B 87. D

88. Bilateral lesions in lateral hypothalamic area produce : PGI 1984, 92

A. Anorexia B. Polyphagia
C. Omniphagia D. Any of the above

89. All or none law refers to : AIIMS 1984; PGI 1995

A. Resting potential
B. Spike potential
C. Excitatory postsynaptic potentials
D. Strength of contraction

90. Vagotomy does not prevent the increase in gastric secretion which normally occurs in response to : AIIMS 1993

A. Injection of insulin
B. Injection of histamine
C. Sight and smell of food
D. Emotional disturbance

91. The percentage of pyramidal fibres making direct synaptic connection with motor neurons : PGI 1983, 96

A. 5 B. 10
C. 30 D. 40

92. Lowest level of integration of stretch reflex is at : AMC 1987, 94

A. Cerebral corte B. Upper medulla
C. Lower medulla D. Spinal cord

93. Weber Fechner law deals with : PGI 1983

A. Frequency discrimination
B. Receptive field organization
C. Intensity discrimination
D. Two point discrimination

94. Which structures in the body are normally devoid of blood capillaries : AMC 1984, 92

A. Cartilaginous plates of long bones
B. Corneas
C. Dermis of skin
D. The cartilaginous plates and the lens

95. No matter where a particular sensory pathway is stimulated along its course to the cortex, the conscious sensation produced is referred to the location. This is : Delhi 1986, 94

A. Law of projection B. Muller's law
C. Hardy Wien's law D. Bell Magendie's law

96. Interneurones are not functioning in ——— reflex: AIIMS 1982, 94

A. Swallowing B. Stretch
C. Flexion D. Visual

97. An important facilitatory neurotransmitter mediating coitus induced ovulation is : PGI 1993

A. Dopamine B. Serotonin
C. Adrenaline D. Noradrenaline

98. The muscles typically exhibiting isometric contractions are : AIIMS 1996

A. Extraocular B. Respiratory
C. Antigravity D. Masticatory

99. The receptor portion of the muscle spindle is innervated by : PGI 1996

A. Type-I fibre B. Type-II fibre
C. a + b D. None of the above

100. Painful stimuli are conveyed by : AIIMS 1994

A. A alpha and C fibres
B. B and C fibres
C. A delta and B fibres
D. A delta and C fibres

101. The most important factor for regulating cerebral blood flow under normal conditions is the : AMC 1984, 93

A. Rate of cerebral carbon dioxide formation.
B. Rate of cerebral oxygen consumption.
C. Degree of sympathetic stimulation of peripheral vasculature.
D. Rate of release of potassium from the cerebrum.

102. Right and left vagus respectively go to: PGI 1994

A. SA node, AV node
B. AV node, SA node
C. AV node, bundle of His
D. SA node, bundle of His

103. The part which is electrically silent in an anaesthesized preparation : PGI 1997

A. Cerebellum B. Motor area
C. Parietal area D. Hypothalamus

104. Blood brain-barrier is made-up of : AIIMS 1996

A. Astrocytes B. Oligodendrocytes
C. Oligodendroglia D. Microglia

105. Bathmotropic effect is produced by : PGI 1998

A. Stimulation vagus
B. Nerves other than vagus
C. Atropine
D. Sectioned vagus

106. Koniocortex refers to : AIIMS 1990

A. Agranular cortex
B. Granular cortex
C. Cortex of long vertical columns
D. All of the above

107. Chronaxie is longer in : AIIMS 1990

A. Less excitable tissue B. More excitable tissue
C. Unexcitable tissue D. Skeletal muscles

108. GABA (an inhibitory neurotransmitter) acts by : AIIMS 1983, 93

A. Increasing the permeability of a neuron to K+
B. Increasing the permeability of a neuron to Na+
C. Increasing the permeability to Ca++
D. Decreasing the permeability of the cell to Ca++

Ans.										
	88. A	89. B	90. B	91. B	92. D	93. C	94. D	95. A	96. B	97. B
	98. C	99. C	100. D	101. A	102. A	103. B	104. A	105. A	106. A	107. A
	108. A									

109. The excitatory neurotransmitter in CNS is : AMC 1984, 92

A. Serotonin B. Histamine
C. GABA D. Melatonin

110. Which of the following is present in high concentration in the putamen and caudate nucleus : AIIMS 1986, 95

A. Acetylcholine B. GABA
C. Dopamine D. Histamine

111. Gag reflex is mediated by cranial nerve : Rohtak 1995

A. VII B. IX
C. X D. XII

112. All are true about brain except : AI 1996

A. Energy stored
B. Can utilize fatty acids
C. Dependent on glucose
D. Sensitive to hypoxia

113. Sleep spindles are characterized by : Rohtak 1996

	Voltage	Frequency
A.	High	High
B.	High	Low
C.	Low	High
D.	Low	Low

114. Uvular reflex has afferents from cranial : Delhi 1993

A. V B. IX
C. X D. XII

115. The root value of patellar reflex is : Rajasthan 99

A. L1, 2, 3 B. L3, 4
C. L2, 3, 4 D. L3, 4, 5

116. Light reflex has its center located in : DNB 1998

A. Occipital cortex B. Midbrain
C. Pons D. Medulla

117. The fiber with maximum diameter is : PGI 1992

A. A-alpha B. A-beta
C. B D. C

118. Spike duration is maximum in nerve fibre : AMU 1984, 91

A. A-alpha B. A-beta
C. A-delta D. C

119. Which of the following may show antidromic conduction : Rohtak 1985

A. Synapse B. Axons
C. Both a+b D. None

120. The following substances are not utilized or produced in fed state of brain : DNB 1990

A. Lactic acid B. Pyruvic acid
C. Alpha ketoglutarate D. All of the above

121. Extensor muscle hyperreflexia in a case of injury to midbrain between inferior and superior colliculi is due to : PGI 1982, 88, 91

A. Generalized loss of facilitation.
B. Generalized loss of inhibition.
C. Decreased stretch of annulospiral endings in muscle.
D. Loss of inhibition delivered to gamma efferent neurons.
E. Decreased alpha efferent neuron activity.

122. The effect of sex hormones on cerebral blood flow is that it : PGI 1982, 94

A. Increases B. Decreases
C. Variable D. None of the above

123. What can be the most likely mechanism responsible for the abrupt cessation of skeletal muscle contraction in a normal subject attempting to lift a heavy load? AMU 1984, 92

A. Activation of stretch receptors in Golgi tendon organ.
B. Activation of stretch receptors in annulospiral endings.
C. Skeletal muscle ischaemia.
D. Inactivation of stretch receptors in Golgi tendon organ.

124. The Golgi tendon organ differs in function from annulospital endings in the tendon organ : AIIMS 1982, 94

A. Is more sensitive to distending force.
B. Causes reflex inhibition of ipsilateral heteronymous, antagonistic, alpha neurons.
C. Causes a reflex inhibition of homonymous alpha, efferent neurons.
D. All of the above.

125. Pons contains : Delhi 1986, 97

A. Apneustic center B. Pneumotaxic center
C. Carotid bodies D. a+b

126. The oxygen consumption of human brain is : TN 1982, 91

A. 1.0ml/100g brain/min
B. 1.5 ml/100g brain/min
C. 3.5 ml/100g brain/min
D. 5.0 ml/100g brain/min

127. Oxygen consumption of whole human brain in ml/min is about : DNB 1990

A. 29 B. 35
C. 49 D. 61

128. In brain ischaemia, systemic blood pressure rises. This is called : AIIMS 1986, 92

A. Monro Kellie doctrine
B. Cushing reflex
C. Autoregulation
D. White reaction

129. The sequence of events i.e. red reaction (R) flare (F) and wheal (W) in triple response is : AMU 1997

A. R, F, W B. R, W, F
C. W, F, R D. W, R, F

Ans.									
109. A	110. C	111. B	112. A	113. C	114. B	115. C	116. B	117. A	118. D
119. B	120. D	121. D	122. C	123. A	124. C	125. D	126. C	127. C	128. B
129. B									

130. Which is an important reflex centre for authonomic nervous activity ? **AIIMS 1982, 91**
A. Cerebellum
B. Basal ganglia
C. Both cerebellum and basal ganglia
D. Hypothalamus

131. Which of the following is an example of an unmyelinated neuron? **AIIMS 1982,93**
A. Anterior horn cell
B. Preganglionic parasympathetic neuron
C. Preganglionic sympathetic neuron
D. Postganglionic parasympathetic neuron

132. In Spinal reflex, following are seen except : **AIIMS 1997**
A. Latency B. Fatiguability
C. Summation D. Memory

133. Athetoid movements are found in : **PGI 1980, 92**
A. Cerebellar lesion
B. Basal ganglia lesions
C. Thalamic lesion
D. Hypothalamic lesion

134. The band which disappears on muscle contraction is : **AIIMS 1981, 93**
A. I B. H
C. A D. Z

135. All of the following cross blood brain barrier readily except : **AMU 1983, 96**
A. Water B. CO_2
C. O_2 D. Na+

136. Broca' area is brain area :
A. 41 B. 42
C. 44 D. None of the above

137. Which of the following crosses the blood brain barrier most readily : **Delhi 86, Bihar 91**
A. O_2 B. K+
C. CO_2 D. HCO_3

138. CSF differs from plasma in having higher concentration of : **Bihar 1991**
A. Na+ B. K+
C. Cl- D. Glucose

139. Golgi tendon reflex to relax muscle is : **AIIMS 1986, 89, 91**
A. Monosynaptic involving medulla
B. Monosynaptic involving spinal cord
C. Polysynaptic involving spinal cord
D. None of the above

140. Rhomberg's sign is positive in lesion of : **AMC 1983, 84, 95**
A. Vestibulospinal tract
B. Spinocerebeller tract
C. Spinothalamic tract
D. Any of the above

141. The Purkinje fibres : **AIIMS 1995**
A. Are myelinated axons.
B. Have conduction velocity of about five times that seen in heart muscle.
C. Have action potentials about a tenth as long as those in heart muscle.
D. All of the above.

142. The motor unit is : **AMC 1985; AI 1990**
A. Muscle fibre and neurons supplying it.
B. Afferent fibre-centre-efferent fibre.
C. Motor neuron and its muscle fibres.
D. Single muscle fibre with it nerve.

143. Match List-I with List-II and select the correct answer using the codes given below the Lists : **CSE 1998**

List-I (EEG wave)	List-II (Characteristic)
A. α wave	1. Increased when eyes are opened
B. β wave	2. Occurs mainly in children
C. ϕ wave	3. Occurs in very deep sleep
D. δ wave	4. Disappears when eyes are opened

Codes :

	A	B	C	D
A.	1	4	2	3
B.	4	1	2	3
C.	4	1	3	2
D.	1	4	3	2

144. Anterior-spino cerebellar tract ends in cerebellum through which peduncle : **Kerala 1998**
A. Superior B. Middle
C. Inferior D. All

145. All of the following statements about the alpha rhythm of the electroencephalogram are true except : **Manipal 1995**
A. It has an amplitude of about 50 microvolts.
B. It has a frequency of 8-12 Hz.
C. Its frequency is higher than that of the delta rhythm.
D. It disappears when the subject closes his eyes.

146. Body posture and coarse movements are controlled mainly by : **PGI 1983; AIIMS 1993**
A. Cerebrum B. Cerebellum
C. Spinal cord D. Extrapyramidal system

147. Which of the following is concerned with conditioned reflexes : **AIIMS 1995**
A. Cerebral cortex B. Cerebral medulla
C. Cerebellum D. Hypothalamus

Ans. 130. D 131. D 132. D 133. B 134. B 135. D 136. C 137. C 138. C 139. C
140. B 141. B 142. C 143. A 144. A 145. D 146. D 147. A

148. Lowest level of integration of stretch reflex is : AIIMS 1987, 99
A. Cerebrum B. Cerebellum
C. Pons D. Spinal cord

149. Principal motor area is : AMC 1980; DNB 1999
A. 1 B. 2
C. 3 D. 4

150. Superficial reflexes are : PGI 1996; NIMHANS 1995
A. Corneal B. Jaw
C. Plantar D. Both a and c

151. Which one of the following statements is incorrect about impulses in right auditory nerve : AP 1991
A. Are initiated by distortion of hair cells in organ of corti.
B. Are carried to the cochlear nuclei of medulla.
C. Result in stimulation of 4th order neurons in medial geniculate body of thalamus.
D. Result in stimulation of auditory area in occipital cortex.

152. Circadian rhythm is controlled by : AIIMS 1984; Delhi 1987, 99
A. Suprachiasmatic nuclei
B. Raphe nuclei
C. Thalamus
D. Red nucleus

153. The term decerebration denotes : AIIMS 1994
A. Section of the whole cerebrum
B. Removal of one lobe of cerebral cortex
C. Removal of cerebellum from the rest of brain
D. A mild collicular section

154. Blood brain barrier is maximum permeable to : Delhi 1989, 90
A. Na+ B. K+
C. Chloride D. CO_2

155. For arousal response, important ascending pathway is : PGI 1996
A. Reticulocortica B. Corticogeniculate
C. Spinoreticular D. Limbal

156. Transection at the level of meduallry pyramids leads to : AIIMS 1996
A. Flacidity
B. Positive grasping reflex
C. Positive Babinski's sign
D. Hypotonia

157. Source of EEG is : AMC 1995
A. End plate potential of nerve cells
B. Polarity of nerve ganglions
C. Parietal cortex
D. EPSPs and IPSPs of cortical cells which behave like dipoles

158. The peripheral vasculature under the least control of the sympthetic nervous system is the : AIIMS 1996
A. Arterie B. Arterioles
C. Capillarie D. Venules

159. Which of the following factors has no direct stimulatory effect on the medullary respiratory center : Delhi 1997
A. Changes in arterial pCO2
B. Changes in arterial pH
C. Changes in arterial PO2
D. Changes in the nervous output from the joint proprioceptors

160. Temporal lobe lesion causes : AIIMS 1985, 99
A. Homonymus upper quadrantinopia
B. Homonymus lower quadrantinopia
C. Bitemporal hemianopia
D. Binasal hemianopia

161. The end plate potential is characterised by : AIIMS 1982, 95
A. Propagation B. All or none law
C. Depolarisation D. Hyperpolarisation

162. Damage to sensory area one of the cerebral cortex results in : AI 1998
A. Loss of perception of pain
B. Loss of tactile and two point discrimination
C. Loss of perception of touch
D. Loss of only tactile discrimination

163. Excitatory synaptic transmitter substances cause which ions preferentially to move through the postsynaptic membrane : AIIMS 1996
A. Calcium B. Potassium
C. Chloride D. Sodium

164. What transmitter substance is released by the spinal nerve ending of the neurons whose cell bodies are located in the raphe magnus nucleus : AIIMS 1996
A. Endorpin B. Substance P
C. Glycine D. Serotonin

165. What type of neuronal circuit is typified by the nervous control of muscular activity : AIIMS 1994
A. Diverging circuit` B. Converging circuit
C. Integrative circuit` D. Parallel circuit

166. The neuronal circuit with the greatest potential for producing a long-lasting output is the : AIIMS 1985
A. Diverging circuit with multiple inputs
B. Converging circuit with multiple outputs
C. Reverbrating circuit
D. Integrative circuit

Ans.									
148. D	149. D	150. D	151. D	152. A	153. D	154. D	155. A	156. C	157. D
158. C	159. C	160. A	161. C	162. B	163. D	164. D	165. A	166. C	

167. Pressure on the footpads of an animal with a transected spinal cord causes the foot to : PGI 1996

A. Move anteriorly B. Move posteriorly
C. Be withdraw D. Thrust downward

168. Which sensory system might be more important for maintaining a persons's balance when he is running against the wind than when he is running with the wind : PGI 1996

A. Vestibular apparatus
B. Proprioceptors of the neck
C. Exterioceptive system
D. Ears

169. Which of the following transmitter substances probably always or almost tend to inhibit the post-synaptic neuron : AIIMS 1994

A. Gamma-aminobutyric acid (GABA)
B. Dopamine
C. Glycine
D. Norepinephrine

170. Match List-I with List-II and select the correct answer using the codes given below the Lists : CSE 1998

List-I (Parts of basal ganglia and related areas)	List-II (Disorder)
A. Lentiform nucleus	1. Chorea
B. Subthalamic nucleus	2. Hemiballismus
C. Caudate nucleus	3. Athetosis
D. Substantia nigra	4. Parkinsonism

Codes :

	A	B	C	D
A.	3	1	2	4
B.	4	1	2	3
C.	4	3	1	2
D.	3	2	1	4

171. Skeletal muscle contraction is excited when the intracellular concentration of which ion rises above 10^{11} moles per liter in the sarcoplasm of the muscle cells : PGI 1980, 93

A. Na B. K
C. M D. Ca
E. Cl

172. The type of nerve fiber that has a conduct velocity of approximately one meter per second : Delhi 1984; UP 2003

A. Type-A alpha B. Type-A beta
C. Type-A gamma D. Type-C

173. In spinal shock, reflexes are : Delhi 1996

	Autonomic	Somatic
A.	Normal	↓
B.	Normal	↓
C.	↑	↓
D.	↓	↑

174. All of the following manifestations are seen in cases of cerebellar damage in human beings except : CSE 1998

A. Loss of non-declarative/reflexive memory
B. Loss of adjustment of vestibulo-ocular reflex
C. Static tremor and rigidity
D. Ataxia, atonia and asthenia

175. Parasympathetic system affects CVS mainly by altering : PGI 1986, 93

A. Vascular resistance
B. Vascular compliance
C. Force of contraction of heart
D. Heart rate

176. Baroreceptors mainly act through : AIIMS 1996

A. Sympathetic system
B. Parasympathetic system
C. Cerebral cortex
D. ↓ Blood volume

177. Human nervous system contains about——— neurons : Rohtak 1986, 95

A. 10^8 B. 10^{10}
C. 10^{12} D. 10^{16}

178. The Betz cells of the primary motor cortex are located in which layer of the cortex : PGI 1993

A. Layer-II B. Layer-III
C. Layer-IV D. Layer-V

179. Which primary cortical sensory area is located in the middle of the superior temporal gyrus : DNB 1999

A. Vision B. Hearing
C. Somatic sensation D. Taste

180. Damaging what area of the brain is likely to cause anterograde amnesia : AMU 1996

A. Prefrontal cortex B. Occipital cortex
C. The amygdala D. The hippocampus

181. When a person wishes to speak a certain thought, where does the thought originate : AIIMS 1997

A. In Broca's area
B. In the posterior part of the temporal cortex
C. In the supramarginal gyrus
D. In the facial region of the motor cortex

182. Inhibition of the spinal cord may be brought about by : PGI 1993

A. Glutamic acid B. Aspartic acid
C. Glycine D. Strychnine

Ans. 167. D 168. C 169. A 170. D 171. D 172. D 173. D 174. C 175. D 176. B 177. C 178. D 179. B 180. D 181. B 182. C

183. **CSF pressure in the lying down posture is : Delhi 1984, 86; UPSC 1984, 97**
A. 20-50 mm B. 50-150 mm
C. 150-200 mm D. 200-300 mm

184. **The neuromuscular transmitter is : AIIMS 1986; AI 1989; AP 1997**
A. Dopamine B. Epinephrine
C. Norepinephrine D. Acetylcholine

185. **Which one of the following pairs is not correctly matched? CSE 1998**

	Acid-base disturbance	S. bicarbonate, pCO2
A.	Compensated metabolic acidosis	↓ bicarbonate, ↓ pCO2
B.	Compensated metabolic alkalosis	↑ bicarbonate, ↑ pCO2
C.	Compensated respiratory acidosis	↑ bicarbonate, ↑ pCO2
D.	Compensated respiratory alkalosis	↑ bicarbonate, ↑ pCO2

186. **Osmoreceptors are present in : Delhi 1983; AI 1999**
A. Anterior hypothalamus
B. Internal carotid artery
C. Left atrium
D. Ventricle

187. **Stimulation of vagus nerve causes : AIIMS 1994**
A. Rise in blood pressure
B. Decreased intestinal secretion
C. Constriction of bronchial musculture
D. Relaxation of intestinal muscles

188. **Sham rage is produced when : AIIMS 1995**
A. Section is made at L2 vertebrae
B. Pons is removed
C. Medulla is removed
D. All the cortex is removed from the brain

189. **In experimental animal, ablation of flocculo nodular lobe leads to : AMC 1984; Delhi 1989, AI 1998**
A. Ataxia B. Cerebellar ataxia
C. Akinesis D. Cerebral palsy

190. **Which theory probably explains long term memory the best ? AIIMS 1980, 96**
A. The theory that it causes actual physical or chemical changes at the synapses.
B. The theory that there is change in RNA inside some of the neuron.
C. The theory that the glial cells arouse the neuron change.
D. The theory that the ionic composition of the neuron changes.

191. **The basic posture reflex is : AIIMS 1980,94**
A. Crossed extensor reflex
B. Golgi tendon reflex
C. Flexor reflex
D. Positive supporting reflex

192. **Each thin filament in muscle contains —— actin molecules and —— tropomyosin molecules : AIIMS 1992**
A. 100-200;20-30 B. 200-300; 30-40
C. 300-400; 40-60 D. 800-1000; 10-20

193. **The number of Na+ channels along axons of unmyelinated neurons are : AIIMS 1993**
A. 60 B. 70
C. 90 D. 110

194. **REM sleep is characterized by ______ waves on EEG :**
A. Delta B. Theta
C. Beta D. Alpha

195. **At which of the following site is blood brain barrier is least effective : Delhi 1998**
A. Cerebral cortex
B. Median eminence of hypothalamus
C. Caudate nucleus
D. Hippocampus

196. **End plate potential is characterized by : AIIMS 1994**
A. Hyperpolarization B. Normal polarity
C. Depolarization D. None of the above

197. **The term desynchronization indicates : Delhi 1998**
A. S-waves
B. Replacement of rhythmic wave with αwaves
C. Replacement of rhythmic EEG pattern with low voltage, irregular waves
D. All of the above

198. **Which of the following rhythm on EEG has minimum frequency : AIIMS 1992, 99; Delhi 1998**
A. Alpha B. Delta
C. Theta D. Beta

199. **Bilateral destruction of auditory cortex causes : AIIMS 1995**
A. Difficulty in interpretation of sound
B. Difficulty in hearing
C. Complete loss of hearing
D. Vertigo

200. **The existence of the 'axon reflex' proves that : CSE 1998**
A. It has separate sensory and motor pathways inside it.
B. The soma of the neuron acts as the reflex centre of the neuron.
C. It can conduct impulses both orthodromically and antidromically.
D. It has more than one type of neurotransmitters at its ending.

Ans.									
183. C	184. D	185. D	186. A	187. C	188. D	189. D	190. B	191. C	192. C
193. D	194. C	195. B	196. C	197. C	198. B	199. A	200. C		

201. Sympathetic cholinergic innervation is seen in : PGI 1995
A. Apocrine sweat glands
B. Eccrine sweat glands
C. Iris
D. Pancreas

202. EEG with spike and dome pattern is characteristic of —— epilepsy : AIIMS 1984, 97
A. Jocksonian B. Grandmal
C. Petitmal D. Temporal lobe

203. Lesions in —— lead to sensory ataxia : AIIMS 1964, 96
A. Posterior column
B. Vermis
C. Flocculo-nodular lobe
D. Vestibular apparatus

204. Which of the following effects in the heart would not be a result of increased vagal nerve activity : AMU 1996
A. Acetylcholine release at the nerve endings
B. Decreased ST interval
C. Bradycardia
D. Hyperpolarization of SA node

205. Baroreceptor impulses : AMU 1996
A. Inhibit the vagal centre
B. Decrease the arterial pressure
C. Result in decreased heart rate
D. Excite the vaso-constrictor centre

206. Development of myelin sheath in peripheral nervous system depends on : AMU 1996
A. Oligodendrocytes B. Astrocytes
C. Microglia D. Schwann cell

207. Cerebral blood flow begins to increase when venous blood PO2 falls below--------mm Hg : PGI 1995
A. 20 B. 30
C. 35 D. 40

208. Nociceptive stimuli are transmitted by : AIIMS 1997
A. Free nerve ending B. Pacinian corpuscles
C. Meckel's disc D. Ruffini and organ

209. Ultrasound refers to sound waves with a frequency of : Rajasthan 1992
A. 20/sec B. More than 20,000/sec
C. 200/sec D. 20-200/sec

210. All relay in sensory cortex except : Kerala 1994
A. Pain B. Touch
C. Temperature D. Olfaction

211. Destruction of lateral nucleus of thalamus causes : Kerala 1994
A. Hyperphagia B. Aphasia
C. Somnolence D. Restlessness

212. Which nerve does not have parasympathetic fibres: PGI 1993
A. 7th B. 9th
C. 10th D. 12th

213. Peripheral nerves can tolerate ischaemia up to : PGI 1994
A. 6 hours B. 12 hours
C. 24 hours D. 30 min

214. Which is amine neurotransmitter : AIIMS 1995
A. GABA B. Epinephrine
C. Acetylcholine D. Lignocaine

215. Intracranial fluid in body represents : Delhi 1995
A. 4 gm B. 100 gm
C. 40 gm D. 150 gm

216. Dysmetria is seen in : AP 1994
A. Extrapyramidal lesions
B. Cerebellar lesions
C. Pyramidal lesions
D. Cortical lesions

217. The theory of membrane potential was given by : Rajasthan 1989, 93
A. Bernstein B. Nernst
C. Newton D. Faraday

218. On an average, the number of muscle fibres is attached to one golgi tendon organ is : AIIMS 1991
A. 2-5 B. 5-10
C. 10-15 D. 20-30

219. The most ideal neurotransmitter is : UPSC 1990
A. 5-HT B. Substance-P
C. Acetylcholine D. All

220. The value of chronaxie is minimum in : PGI 1997
A. Type-A fibres
B. Type-C fibres
C. Skeletal muscle fibres
D. Cardiac muscle fibres

221. Which of the following has CSF/Plasma ratio as 1.00 : AIIMS 1980, 92
A. Na+ B. Mg++
C. Cl- D. Osmolality

222. Which of the following has minimum CSF/Plasma: Delhi 1985, 92; DNB 1997
A. Protein B. Cholesterol
C. Uric acid D. Lactic acid

223. Which of the following has the CSF concentration more than that of plasma : PGI 1991
A. Glucose B. Ca++
C. K+ D. Mg++

224. pH of CSF is : PGI 1992
A. 7.13 B. 7.23
C. 7.33 D. 7.40

Ans.									
201. B	202. C	203. A	204. B	205. B	206. D	207. B	208. A	209. B	210. D
211. A	212. D	213. B	214. A	215. A	216. B	217. B	218. C	219. C	220. D
221. D	222. B	223. D	224. C						

225. The fraction of intracellular ions normally exchanged during an action potential or amyelinated nerve fibre is : **Karnataka 1997**

A. $\frac{1}{100,000}$ to $\frac{1}{500,000}$

B. $\frac{1}{100}$ to $\frac{1}{500}$

C. $\frac{1}{10}$ to $\frac{1}{50}$

D. $\frac{1}{2}$ to $\frac{1}{5}$

226. Neurotransmitter implicated in Alzheimer's disease : **AMU 1988, 93**

A. Acetylcholine B. GABA
C. 5HT D. NE

227. Immediately following the transection of spinal cord in man there is : **Karnataka 1999**

A. A period of spinal shock that rarely lasts more than 24 hours.
B. General increase in skeletal muscle tone.
C. Retention of urine and faeces.
D. Retention of urine and faeces with increase in skeletal muscle tone.

228. Postero inferior cerebellar artery damage leads to loss of all of the following sensations except : **PGI 1993**

A. Pain B. Temp
C. Touch D. All sensations

229. Thirst is due to : **AIIMS 1993**

A. Loss of Na+ from the interstitial compartment
B. Loss of Na+ from extracellular compartment
C. Both
D. None

230. Which of the following is not true of the effects of trauma? **Karnataka 1994**

A. Hyperglycemia
B. Muscle catabolism
C. Decreased extracellular osmolarity
D. Elevation of plasma ftom free fatty acids

231. Brown Sequard syndrome, sensation lost on same side is : **AIIMS 1993**

A. Pain B. Temp.
C. Touch D. Proprioception

W.232. Brown sequard syndrome involves all of the following fibres except : **Delhi 1994**

A. Pain B. Temperature
C. Proprioception D. Crude touch

233. Slow muscle fibres have : **Delhi 1994**

A. ↓ endoplasmic retinaculum
B. ↓ Calcium stores
C. ↓ Glycogen
D. ↑ Mitochondria

234. Lateral funiculus of spinal cord has all except : **Delhi 1994**

A. Fasciculus gracilis and cuneate
B. Lateral spinothalamic tract
C. Rubrospinal tract
D. Vestibulospinal tract

235. True about nerve impulse is : **AIIMS 1994**

A. Travels in one direction at synapse
B. Travels in one direction along axon
C. Travels with the speed of electric current
D. If current is increased too slowly, the nerve responds very fast

236. In complete transection of the spinal cord, the muscle supplied by the lower segment display : **AMU 1990**

A. Increase in tone
B. Loss of tone
C. No change in the tone
D. Alternate high and low tone

237. Which of the following parts of the cerebral hemispheres contains the auditory area : **AMU 1990**

A. Precentral gyrus
B. Postcentral gyrus
C. Superior temporal gyrus
D. Cingulate gyrus

238. Striated muscle contains alternating : **AMU 1990**

A. A and Z bands B. I and Z bands
C. A and I bands D. I and II bands

239. The inherent rhythmicity of respiration comes from: **AMU 1991**

A. Vagus nerve B. Pons
C. Cerebral cortex D. Medulla

240. Long term consequence of transection of cord at C_3 : **Punjab 1994**

A. Loss of tendon jerks
B. Lack of reflex micturition
C. Reflex fall in BP as bladder fills
D. Loss of shivering reflex of legs

241. Commonest feature of frontal lobe lesion is : **AI 1994**

A. Psychic blindness B. Aphasia
C. Distractibility D. Amnesia

242. Most sensitive part of axon is : **AI 1994**

A. Dendrite B. Soma
C. Axon tip D. Axon hillock

Ans.									
225. A	226. A	227. C	228. D	229. A	230. D	231. D	232. NONE	233. D
234. D	235. A	236. A	237. C	238. C	239. B	240. D	241. C	242. D

243. In Frontal lobe lesion following are true except : AIIMS 1997
A. Right-Left dissociation
B. Urinary incontinence
C. Personality change
D. Monoporesis

244. Nerve signals are transmitted by : Kerala 1994
A. Miniature end plate potential
B. Action potential
C. Resting membrance potential
D. Post tetanic potential

245. Flocculonodular lobe of cerebellum is concerned with : Kerala 1994
A. Equilibrium B. Hearing
C. Impulse control D. Fine movements

246. Vestibular fibres relay in : Kerala 1994
A. Vermis
B. Lateral geniculate body
C. Flocculonodular lobe of cerebellum
D. Auditory cortex

247. Phagocytosis is done by : AIIMS 1996
A. Microglia B. Oligodendroglia
C. Astrocytes D. All of the above

248. Difference in normal resting cerebral blood flow in gray and white matter is —— ml per 100g/min : AIIMS 1986, 93
A. 20 B. 35
C. 55 D. 75

249. In children, cerebral flow blow is approximately ——that of adult : DNB 1994
A. Half B. Same
C. 2 times D. 3 times

250. Autonomic ganglia are : Delhi 1997
A. Cholinergic B. Adrenergic
C. Noradrenergic D. Dopaminergic

251. Best method to increase the muscle strength is : Kerala 1996
A. Isometric exercises
B. Isotonic exercises
C. Aerobic isotonic exercises
D. Electrical stimulation

252. To generate the swallowing reflex integrity of chain should be upto : Rajasthan 1995
A. Pyramid
B. Trigeminal nerve
C. IX & X Cranial nerve
D. Afferent central fibres to hypothalamus

253. Muscle is stimulated by following except : AIIMS 1997
A. α-motor neurone B. γ-motor neurone
C. Iα fibers D Type-IV afferent

254. The sarcotubular system is mainly concerned with: TNPSC 1997
A. Transmission of action potential
B. Muscle metabolism
C. Muscle degeneration
D. Movement of the muscle

255. Blood brain barrier is not present is : AIIMS 1997
A. Area postrema B. Corpus striatum
C. Corpus callosum D. Cerebral cortex

256. Loss of Acetyl choline receptors in the slow channel syndrome is due to accumulation of which ion in the neuromuscular junction : JIPMER 1998
A. Sodium B. Potassium
C. Calcium D. Magnesium

257. Slow relaxation of muscle is known as : JIPMER 1998
A. Myokymia B. Myotonia
C. Myocalcimia D. Muscle spasm

258. Pre central sulcus & corticospinal tracts are required for : JIPMER 1998
A. Voluntary movement
B. Position sense appreciation
C. Orientation in time & place
D. Stereognosis & spatial skills

259. Endolymph drains into : JIPMER 1998
A. Extradural space
B. Subdural space
C. Sub-arachnoid space
D. Virchow Robin space

260. Thalamus is a relay centre for all of the following sensations except : JIPMER 1998
A. Smell B. Proprioception
C. Pain D. Temperature

261. Regarding the Blood Brain Barrier which of the following is true : JIPMER 1998
A. Presents entry of lipid soluble substances
B. Disrupted by tumors & infection
C. Present throughout the CNS
D. All of the above

262. True about nuclear bag fibre : UP 1998
A. Detects dynamic change
B. Supplied by Ia sensory fibre
C. One of the type of extrafusal fibre
D. One of the type of intrafusal fibre

263. A positive feedback is used to our advantage in the regulation of : Manipal 1992
A. Body temperature
B. Carbon dioxide concentration
C. Mean arterial pressure
D. Uterine contractions during parturition

Ans.									
243. D	244. B	245. A	246. C	247. A	248. C	249. C	250. A	251. A	252. D
253. D	254. B	255. A	256. C	257. B	258. A	259. B	260. A	261. B	262. D
263. D									

264. Which of the following is mismatch? **Manipal 1992**

A. Area 6 : primary gustatory cortex
B. Area 8 : conjugate movement of eyes
C. Area 24 : autonomic responses
D. Area 44 : motor area of speech

265. True statement regarding CSF is : **Manipal 1998**

A. Daily production less than 100 ml.
B. CSF analysis rules out active secretion as a mechanism of CSF formation.
C. It flows from III ventricle to IV ventricle.
D. Produced only by choroid plexus.

266. The correct sequence of parts of body represented on the motor area of cerebral cortex from above downwards is : **CSE 1996**

A. Trunk, arm, thumb, face
B. Trunk, arm, face, thumb
C. Arm, trunk, face, thumb
D. Arm, trunk, thumb, face

267. An efferent from muscle spindles arise from : **CSE 1996**

A. The equatorial region
B. The polar region
C. Both equatorial and polar regions
D. Golgi tendon organs

268. All are synthetic senses except : **TN 1999**

A. 2 point discrimination
B. Stereognosis
C. Vibratory sense
D. Cold sensation

269. Middle cerebellar peduncle transmits———fibres : **TN 1999**

A. Ponto cerebellar B. Tectospinal
C. Spino cerebellar D. Olivocerebellar

270. Receptor which itself is a dendrite of a Nerve : **TN 1999**

A. Olfactory B. Gustatory
C. Visual D. Hearing

271. The cortical representation for control of micturition is : **Kerala 1999**

A. Cingulate gyrus B. Paracentral lobule
C. Frontal lobe D. Occipital lobe

272. If one of your nerves is compressed and this leads to paresthesia for some time, the type of nerve fiber affected is probably : **PGI 1999**

A. A α B. Aαδ
C. C D. B

273. Renshaw cell inhibition is an example of : **AIIMS 1999**

A. Feed-forward inhibition
B. Oscillating motor activity
C. Circuitry forward
D. All of the above

274. Afferent for segmental stretch reflex is: **AIIMS 1999**

A. Secondary muscle spindle
B. Golgi tendon organ
C. Iα
D. Iβ

275. Repeated painful stimuli at the same site showed increase in pain.This is caused by: **AIIMS 1999**

A. Decreases in the receptive area
B. Depletion of neurotransmitter
C. Increase in threshold
D. Decrease in reflex time

276. The distance by which two touch stimuli must be separated to be perceived as two different stimuli is greater on the : **CSE 1999**

A. Lips B. Orsum of hand
C. Finger-tips D. Nape of neck

277. Reticular formation contains areas concerned with the regulation of : **CSE 1999**

A. Hunger and thirst
B. Heart rate and hunger
C. Thirst and respiration
D. Heart rate and respiration

278. Which of the following in cerebellum is excitatory: **Orissa 1998**

A. Purkinje cell B. Granule cell
C. Basket cell D. Golgi cell

279. Match List-I with List-II and select the correct answer using the codes given below the lists : **CSE 1999**

List-I (Functional Division)	List-II (Phylogenetic division)
A. Spinocerebellum	1. Archicerebellum
B. Pontocerebellum	2. Vernal neocerebellum
C. Vestibulocerebellum	3. Paleocerebellum
D. Tectocerebellum	4. Neocerebellum

Codes :

	A	B	C	D
A.	3	4	2	1
B.	4	3	1	2
C.	4	3	2	1
D.	3	4	1	2

280. The symptoms of Parkinson's disease are caused by the lesion of connection of basal ganglia at the site between : **CSE 1999; Delhi 2001**

A. Cerebral cortex and caudate nucleus
B. Putamen and substantia nigra
C. Thalamus and cerebral cortex
D. Caudate nucleus and globus pallidus

Ans. 264. A 265. C 266. A 267. D 268. D 269. A 270. A 271. B 272. B 273. A
274. A 275. D 276. C 277. D 278. C 279. D 280. D

281. **Sympathetic stimulation causes : MAHE 1999**
A. Arteriolar constriction.
B. Ciliary muscle contraction.
C. Decreased gut motility.
D. Decreased salivary secretion.

282. **Consider the following statements : CSE 1999**
Voluntary control of respiration is :
1. Under control of cerebral cortex
2. Mediated by hypothalamus
3. The cause of exercise hyperventilation
4. Not influenced by medullary rhythmicity area
Which of the following statements are correct
A. 1 and 4 B. 1 and 2
C. 1, 2 and 3 D. 2, 3 and 4

283. **Which of the following sensations does not relay through hypothalamus? JIPMER 2000**
A. Smell B. Taste
C. Touch D. Hearing

284. **Distal limb muscle tract relay through: JIPMER 2000**
A. Ventral corticospinal tract
B. Lateral corticospinal tract
C. Tectospinal tract
D. Rubrothalamic tract

285. **Sweating as a result of exertion is mediated through: JIPMER 2000**
A. Adrenal hormones
B. Sympathetic cholinergic
C. Sympathetic adrenergic
D. Parasympathetic cholinergic

286. **A dog was fed always while ringing a bell. Then whenever the bell was rung it salivated here the bell acts as a : AI-2000**
A. Reinforcer B. Conditioner
C. Non-conditioner D. Facilitator

287 **True about alpha block is all except : UP 1999**
A. Low irregular voltage
B. Mental alertness
C. Desynchronisation
D. Synchronisation

288. **Lesion in Inferior frontal gyri shows : UP 2000**
A. Difficulty in articulation
B. Compromised language output
C. Inability to comprehenced written language
D. Inability to comprehenced hearing

289. **Climbing fibers are : UP 2000**
A. Output fibre
B. Excitatory fibre
C. Comes from superior olivary nucleus
D. Comes from multiple source

290. **Which type of cell in the visual cortex responds best to a moving bar of light ? TNPSC 2000**
A. Simple B. Complex
C. Hypercomplex D. Bipolar

291. **The cells of cochlea are called as : TNPSC 2000**
A. Epitheliocytipilon
B. Outer & inner hair cells
C. Transitional apical hair cells
D. None of these

292. **Pyrogens raise body temperature by : TNPSC 2000**
A. Setting the thermostat to higher level
B. Releasing interleukins
C. Decreasing peripheral heat liberating mechanism
D. Causing rigors

293. **Auditory pathways pass through all of the following structures except : Kerala 2000**
A. Cochlear nuclei B. Superior olives
C. Trapezoid body D. Superior colliculus

294. **Which of the following postural reflexes is integrated in the midbrain ? Kerala 2000**
A. Optical righting reflex
B. Placing reaction
C. Labyrinthine righting reflex
D. Hopping reaction

295. **Complete sectioning just above the spinal cord causes : MAHE 2000**
A. Total cessation of respiration
B. Apneustic respiration
C. Cheyne Stokes respiration
D. None of the above

296. **In brain : MAHE 2000**
A. Mesenchephalic nucleus of Cr. V has multipolar neurons.
B. Proprioceptive fibers of Cr. V relay in the mesenchephalic nucleus.
C. Fibers of the external capsule arise in frontoparietal opperculum of insula.
D. Fasciculus retroflexus arises from the interpeduncular nucleus.

297. **All are controlled by autonomic nervous system except : PGI 2000**
A. Aldosterone B. Insulin
C. GH D. Somatostatin

298. **Effectiveness of blood brain barrier is by : AIIMS 2000**
A. Tight endothelial junction
B. Microglial cell
C. Thick basement membrane
D. Tight arrangement of astrocytes

299. **Which of the following is not associated with increase in intracranial pressure : AIIMS 2000**
A. Increase in blood pressure
B. Respiratory depression
C. Tachycardia
D. Deterioration of consciousness

Ans.	281. C	282. C	283. C	284. B	285. B	286. B	287. D	288. B	289. B	290. B
	291. B	292. B	293. D	294. C	295. A	296. B	297. A	298. A	299. C	

300. Initiation of nerve impulse occurs at the axon hillock because : AI 2001
A. It has a lower threshold than the rest of the axon
B. It is unmyelinated
C. Neurotransmitters are release at this place
D. Most excitable and threshold high

301. When a person looks to the right side, the reflex of the impulse comes from : AI 2001
A. Right motor area B. Left motor area
C. Midbrain D. Occiput

302. Which of the following is not true about action potential in skeletal muscle : Delhi 2001
A. Duration of action potential and muscle twitch is same.
B. Action potential spreads along T-tubules which releases Ca^{++}.
C. Is shorter than the action potential of cardiac muscle.
D. Ca^{++} in response to action potential is released from terminal cisterns.

303. Smooth muscle contraction due to release of calcium occurs because of : Delhi 2001
A. ↑cAMP
B. Troponin-C
C. ↑cIMP
D. Calmodulin dependent MLCK

304. During skeletal muscle contraction : Delhi 2001
A. A-band shortens
B. Both H and I-band shorten
C. Both A and I-band shorten
D. Both A and H-band shorten

305. How will you assess the function of nerve after injury : DNB 2001
A. Nerve induction study
B. Open dissection
C. EMG
D. None of the above

306. Following are true about Leptin except : JIPMER 2001
A. Produced by adipose tissue
B. Increased level in obesity
C. Acts on hypothalamus
D. Increases appetite

307. Which ion is more in CSF ? Kerala 2001
A. Cl B. HCO_3
C. Na^+ D. K+

308. NREM sleep neurotransmitter: Rohtak 2001
A. Serotonin B. Substance-P
C. Nor adrenaline D. Adrenaline

309. Regarding presynaptic inhibition, which of the following combinations is true : AIIMS 2001
A. Affected by axo-axonic transmission
B. Prolonged by IPSP
C. Prolonged or shortened by IPSP
D. Not affected by pharmacologic agents
E. Prolonged by anaesthetic agents
F. Prolonged by strychnine
G. Inhibited by picrotoxin
a. a, d and f are true
b. a, e and g are true
c. b, f and d are true
d. a, c and g are true

310. The length of a muscle at which tension is maximum is called : JIPMER 2002
A. Optimal length B. Maximal length
C. Resting length D. Active length

311. A person with eyes closed and mind wondering will have the following wave in EEG : JIPMER 2002
A. Beta waves B. Alpha waves
C. Delta waves D. Theta waves

312. Which of the following is/are true about Miniature end plate potential : SGPGI 2002
A. It forms in neuromuscular end plate of the resting muscle.
B. It disappears on giving Acetylcholine.
C. It follows different laws as compared to end plate potentials.
D. All of the above.

313. True regarding Refractory period is all the following except : SGPGI 2002
A. It is equal to duration of APD
B. Membranes are in a depolarized state
C. The duration is equal to 1 second
D. It is refractory to all stimuli

314. 80% of serotonin is present in : SGPGI 2002
A. Brain B. Spleen
C. Small intestine D. Muscle

315. True about Tropomyosin is : AI 2002
A. Helps in the fusion of actin and myosin.
B. Covers myosin and prevents attachment of actin and myosin.
C. Slides over myosin.
D. Causes Ca^{++} release.

316. Sudden decrease in serum calcium is associated with: AI 2002
A. Increased thyroxine and PTH
B. Increased phosphate
C. Increased sensitivity of muscle and nerve
D. Cardiac conduction abnormality

317. Tapping on foot pad of decerebrate animal result in extension of limbs. This is example of : UP-2002
A. Altitudinal reflex B. Tonic neck reflex
C. Step forward D. Step backward

Ans.									
300. A	301. B	302. A	303. D	304. B	305. A	306. D	307. A	308. A	309. B
310. C	311. B	312. D	313. C	314. C	315. B	316. C	317. A		

318. True about EEG is : **BHU-2002**
A. Bilaterally symmetrical
B. Denotes the intelligence
C. Deep sleep is characterized by slow amplitude waves
D. Contrast medium is used

319. A 10°C decrease in temperature causes decrease in cerebral metabolic rate by : **AIIMS 2002**
A. 10% B. 30%
C. 50% D. 70%

320. The neurons may get irreversibly damaged if exposed to significant hypoxia for : **AIIMS 2002**
A. 8 min B. 2 min.
C. 30 sec. D. 15 sec.

321. A lesion of ventrolateral part of the spinal cord will lead to loss (below the level of lesion) of : **AI 2003**
A. Pain sensation on the ipsilateral side
B. Proprioception on the contralateral side
C. Pain sensation on the contralateral side
D. Proprioception on the ipsilateral side

322. Synaptic conduction is mostly orthodromic because : **AI 2003**
A. Dendrites cannot be repolarised.
B. Once repolarised, an area cannot be depolarised.
C. The strength of antidromic impulse is less.
D. Chemical mediator is located only in the presynaptic terminal.

323. Which of the following is true about the autonomic nervous system : **AI 2003**
A. The sympathetic outflow from the CNS is through both the cranial nerves and the sympathetic chain.
B. The parasympathetic outflow from the CNS is through the cranial nerves only.
C. The superior hypogastric plexus is located at the anterior aspect of the aortic bifurcation and fifth lumbar vertebrae.
D. The superior hypogastric plexus contains sympathetic fibres only.

324. The main excitatory neurotransmitter in the CNS is: **AI 2004**
A. Glycine B. Acetylcholine
C. Aspartate D. Glutamate

325. The force of muscle contraction can be increased by all of the following except : **AI 2004**
A. Increasing the frequency of activation of motor units.
B. Increasing the number of motor units activated.
C. Increasing the amplitude of action potentials in the motor neurons.
D. Recruiting larger motor units.

326. The parvocellular pathway from lateral geniculate nucleus to visual cortex is most sensitive for the stimulus of : **AIIMS 2004; AI 2004**
A. Color contrast
B. Luminance contrast
C. Temporal frequency
D. Saccadic eye movements

327. Which one of the following molecules is used for cell signalling? **AI 2005**
A. CO_2 B. O_2
C. NO D. N_2

328. A child demonstrates irregular spasmodic, involuntary movements of the limbs and facial muscles. He is most likely to have a lesion in the : **DNB 1990**
A. Caudate nucleus
B. Precentral gyrus of cortex
C. Post-central gyrus of cortex
D. Rubrospinal tract

329. The alpha rhythm of EEG : **UPSC 1988**
A. Has amplitude about 50 microvolts, frequency 8-12 HZ
B. Best seen when subject's eyes are closed
C. Indicates that the subject is awake
D. All of the above

330. Dreaming is usually associated with : **NIMHANS 1986; Delhi 1987**
A. Slow waves in EEG
B. Rapid eye movements
C. Increased muscle tone
D. Decreased muscle tone

331. Dorsal root fibres of spinal cord : **DNB 1990**
A. Mainly motor
B. Involved in flare phenomenon of triple response
C. Produces cutaneous vasoconstriction on stimulation
D. Involved in central control of vascular tone

332. Normal swallowing is dependent on the : **Orissa 1990**
A. Trigeminal nerve
B. Ninth and tenth cranial nerves
C. Spinal cord
D. Pyramidal tract

333. Efferent error signals from cerebellum are transmitted to the cerebral cortex via the : **AIIMS 1986**
A. Dentate nucleus B. Fastigial nucleus
C. Globose nucleus D. Emboliform nucleus

334. Symptoms of cerebellar lesion include the following except : **AI 1990**
A. Atonia B. Ataxia
C. Agnosia D. Asynergia

Ans. 318. C 319. D 320. B 321. C 322. D 323. C 324. D 325. C 326. A 327. C
328. A 329. D 330. B 331. B 332. B 333. A 334. C

335. **EEG rhythm recorded from the surface of the scalp during REM sleep : AIIMS 1986**
A. Alpha B. Beta
C. Delta D. Theta

336. **The EEG rhythm having lowest frequency is : Delhi 1987**
A. Alpha B. Beta
C. Delta D. Theta

337. **Cerebral cortex is generally considered to be a functional and anatomical outgrowth of : Orissa 1991**
A. Hypothalamus B. Thalamus
C. Cerebellum D. Midbrain

338. **Least speed of conduction is seen in : WB 2007**
A. Bundle of Files B. SA node
C. AV bundle D. Purkinje system

339. **Axoplasmic flow in neuron by all except : AIIMS 2007**
A. Dynein B. Kinesin
C. Microfilament D. Neurofilament

340. **Cerebral blood flow is regulated by all except : AIIMS 2007**
A. Blood pressure B. Arterial PCO2
C. Potassium ions D. Cerebral metabolic rate

341. **Broca's area is concerned with : AI 2007, 2008**
A. Word formation B. Comprehension
C. Repetition D. Reading

342. **The nucleus involved in Papez circuit is : AI 2007**
A. Pulvinar
B. Intralaminar
C. VLP nucleus
D. Anterior nucleus of Thalamus

343. **The mechanism of hearing and memory, including all except : AI 2007**
A. Changes in level of neurot. ansmitter at synapse
B. Increasing protein synthesis
C. Recruitment by multiplication of neurons
D. Spatial Reorganization of synapse

344. **Which of the following is true regarding physiological changes in the brain during exercise? AI 2008**
A. Blood flow is decreased
B. Blood flow is increased
C. Blood flow remains unaltered
D. Blood flow initially is increased and then decreases

345. **Which of the following is not a Sarcolemma protein? AI 2008**
A. Perlecan B. Dystrophin
C. Dystroglycan D. Sarcoglycan

346. **The most important physiological factor which maintains CSF pressure is ; AIIMS 2008**
A. Rate of CSF formation
B. Rate of CSF absorption
C. Blood flow to the brain
D. Venous pressure

347. **Which of the following factors does not affect the cerebral blood flow ? AIIMS 2008**
A. Cerebral metabolic rate
B. Arterial CO2
C. K+ ions
D. Blood pressure

348. **The increase in threshold of a receptor when a series of stimuli of subthreshold intensity are applied in succession is called : AIIMS 2008**
A. Adaptation B. Accommodation
C. Initiation D. Resistance

349. **The correct order of susceptibility of the different types of nerve fibers to local anaesthetics is : AIIMS 2008**
A. B > C > A B. A > B > C
C. C > A > B D. C > B > A

350. **True for vasomotor center is : AI 2009**
A. Not influenced by cortical centers
B. Stimulated by baroreceptors from arterial organs
C. In sleep medulla stops sending signals which explains decrease in BP
D. Functional interaction with cardio-vagal center

351. **Action potential generated in axon hillock is due to : AI 2009**
A. It has least threshold
B. Neurotransmitters produced
C. Unmyelinated
D. Has more ion channels

Ans.	335. A	336. C	337. B	338. D	339. D	340. C	341. A	342. D	343. C	344. C
345. A	346. B	347. D	348. B	349. D	350. D	351. D				

EXPLANATIONS OF CNS

1. Ans.— B. Accommodation

"All-or-None" Law

Slowly rising currents fail to fire the nerve because the nerve adapts to the applied stimulus, a process called Accommodation.

Once threshold intensity is reached, a full-fledged action potential is produced. Further increases in the intensity of a stimulus produce no increment or other change in the action potential as long as the other experimental conditions remain constant. The action potential fails to occur if the stimulus is subthreshold in magnitude, and it occurs with a constant amplitude and form regardless of the strength of the stimulus if the stimulus is at or above threshold intensity. The action potential is therefore "all-or-none" in character and is said to obey the all-or-none law.

2. Ans. — C Seven pass gated

These receptors are also known as seven transmembrane receptors or 7 TM receptors.

* "Muscarinic" Acetylcholine receptors (Acetyl-choline and Muscarine)
* Adenosine receptors (Adenosine)
* Adrenoceptors (also known as Adrenergic receptors, for adrenaline, and other structurally related hormones and drugs).
* "GABA receptors, Type-B (γ-Aminobutyric acid or GABA)
* Angiotensin receptors (Angiotensin)
* Cannabinoid receptors (Cannabinoids)
* Cholecystokinin receptors (Cholecystokinin)
* Dopamine receptors (Dopamine)
* Glucagon receptors (Glucagon)
* Metabotropic glutamate receptors (Glutamate)
* Histamine receptors (Histamine)
* Olfactory receptors (for the sense of smell)
* Opioid receptors (Opioids)
* Rhodopsin (a photoreceptor)
* Secretin receptors (Secretin)
* Serotonin receptors, except Type-3 (Serotonin, also known as 5-Hydroxytryptamine or 5-HT)
* Somatostatin receptors (Somatostatin)
* Calcium-sensing receptor (Calcium).

3. Ans. — C Decreased muscle tone

* There are two kinds of sleep patterns - *NREM* (non- rapid eye movement) & *REM* (Rapid eye movement), NREM is further divided into 4 phases.
* Before going to sleep patterns know some of the common EEG waves.
* EEG or electronecephalography involves recording the electrical activity of the brain with the help of surface electrodes placed on the scalp.

a. *Alpha Waves*

- It is the wave form seen in adult humans who are awake but at rest with eyes closed. He is mentally relaxed.
- There is a fairly regular pattern of waves at frequency of 8-12 Hz and an amplitude of 50-100 mv.

b. *Beta Waves*

- These are seen when a person is awake and alert. He is *mentally busy* or tense.
- Beta waves have *lower amplitude* (i.e. 20mv) an *higher frequency* (13-30) than alpha waves.
- The alpha rhythm of an individual is promptly replaced by beta rhythm by asking the person to open the eyes or by exposing the person to a sensory stimulus such as a clap, a bang, or a touch. (This is k/a *alpha block*. Also k/a *desynchronization,* because it breaks up the synchronized neural activity producing regular alpha waves).

c. *Theta Waves*

- These are of large amplitude, regular low frequency (4-7 Hz) waves.
- These are seen when a person is in *light sleep.*

d. *Delta Waves*

- These are seen when the person is in *deep sleep.*
- They are *high amplitude, slow waves* with a frequency less than 4 Hz (they have amplitudes two or four times greater than most other types of brain waves).

* Thus, the frequency decreases in the following order :

Beta > Alpha > Theta > Delta *[Mnemonic : BAT - Dance]*

Sleep

* As a person starts falling asleep, his alpha rhythm is gradually replaced by a slower EEG waves of higher amplitude till he has a well defined *delta rhythm.* This gradual transition has been divided into 4 phases 1, 2, 3 & 4. Stage 4 is the phase of typical delta rhythm.

* After about every 90 min., the slow wave (NREM) sleep pattern changes to an altogether different form of sleep waves, altered the *REM sleep.*

- In REM sleep the person continues to sleep *(in fact he threshold for arousal by sensory stimuli is elevated)* but his EEG suddenly becomes *desynchronized* into a low amplitude high frequency waveform, quite indistinguishable from the *beta rhythm* of awake state.
- The similarity of the EEG to that of an awake individual and the difficulty in awaking the person have suggested the term *paradoxical sleep* for REM sleep.
- In REM sleep, the muscle tone is completely lost, but phasic contractions occur in a number of muscles, most notably the eye muscles. The resulting rapid eye movements are basis of the name of this type of sleep.
- *Penile erections* may occur during this type of sleep.
- Most *dreams* occur during REM sleep (dream may also occur during NREM sleep but they are not registered in the memory).

Phases of NREM sleep :

* *Stage 1* - is characterized by low amplitude, high frequency activity, with interspersed *theta waves.*

* *Stage 2* - In stage 2, the EEG slows down but the slow wave activity is interrupted by *sleep spindles,* which are bursts of activity at 10 to 14 Hz (resembling alpha waves) and by *large K-complexes* (large slow potentials).

* *Stage 3* - Shows high amplitude, low frequency waves.

* *Stage 4* - In stage 4, the amplitude becomes still higher and the frequency still lower.

- Stage 3 & 4 are also k/a delta sleep because the EEG waves fall in the range of delta waves.
- Thus, the characteristic of deep sleep is a pattern of rhythmic slow waves indicating marked synchronization.

Brain death is defined by a maintained flat EEG.

4. Ans. — B Small short-duration polyphasic action potential

Small short-duration polyphasic action potentials are seen in myopathy & myaesthemia gravis.

In denervation :

- early in the course, the number of MUPs, (motor unit potential) appearing during contraction is reduced and the configuration of the remaining ones are quite normal.
- In time, the remaining MUPs often increase in size and in amplitude and become longer in duration and sometimes polyphasic.
- After about 2 weeks of denervation, fibrillation potentials can be recorded from the resting muscle. (Fibrillation is the spontaneous contraction of a single muscle fibre. It is ordinarily not visible through the skin).

- Another type of spontaneous activity sometimes recorded from restin denervated muscle is that of positive sharp waves also called as 'saw tooth' potentials.
- In chronic denervation, spontaneous and repetitive fasciculation potentials may be seen (Fasciculation represents the spontaneous firing of an entire motor unit, causing contraction of a group of muscles and in contrast most often the result of reinnervations following nerve or motor neuron damage).
- In chronic denervation sometimes, 'giant potential' can be seen. This is because surviving axons often produce collateral sprouts which re-innervate denervated muscles, thus some motor units become much larger than normal in both amplitude and duration.

Just to recapitulate basic physiology of a Motor unit :

- A motor unit consists of a motor neuron together with all the muscle fibre which it innervates.
- The muscle fibres belonging to a motor unit are scattered throughout a portion of the muscle.
- In any given portion of a muscle, muscle fibres belonging to 20-50 different motor units intermingle with each other.
- The unit of activation of a muscle is a motor unit, and the unit of activation within a motor unit is a muscle fibre.

5. Ans.— C Hypothermia

* Cushing's triad consists of :
  - Bradycardia
  - Hypertension
  - Irregular respiration
* Cushing's reflex of triad is a special type of CNS ischemic response that results from increased pressure of the cerebrospinal fluid around the brain in the cranial vault.
* For instance, when intracranial pressure increases the cerebrospinal pressure.
* This compresses the whole brain as well as the arteries in the brain and cuts off the blood supply to the brain.
* This initiates a CNS ischemic response that causes the arterial pressure to rise, when the arterial pressure has risen to a level higher than the cerebrospinal fluid pressure, blood flows once again into the vessel of the brain to relieve the ischemia (Cushing's reflex).
* Ordinarily, the blood pressure comes to a new equilibrium level slightly higher than the cerebrospinal fluid pressure, thus allowing blood to continue flowing to the brain.
* The Cushing's reaction helps to protect the vital centres of the brain from loss of nutrition if ever the CSF pressure rises high enough to compress the cerebral arteries.
* The rise in the arterial pressure causes a reflex decrease in heart rate via arterial baroreceptors and this is why bradycardia rather than tachycardia is characteristically seen in patients with increased intracranial pressure.

6. Ans.— C Left lateral Spinothalamic tract

* Anterolateral cordotomy of the left lateral Spinothalamic tract will relieve pain in the right leg.
* Spinothalamic tract is the tract carrying pain and temperature.
* It carries pain and temperature sensations from its respective dermatome to the cortex.
* On its entry into the spinal cord it crosses over to the opposite half of the cord almost immediately (actually within one or two spinal cord vertebral segments).
* After the crossing over is complete, it enters the thalamus on the opposite side and then moves on to the cerebral cortex.
* Therefore, any lesion in the spino-thalamic tract will result in loss of pain and temperature sensation contra-laterally below the level of lesion.

7. Ans.— D Awake/alert state

8 Ans.— A Pressure

* Mammalian nerve fibers are divided into 3 groups (by Erlanger and Gasser)—A,B and C
* Group-A fibers are the thickest and the C fibers the thinnest.
* The relative susceptibility of mammalian A, B & C nerve fibers to conduction block produced by various agents :

Susceptibility to	*Most Susceptible*	*Intermediate*	*Least Susceptible*
Pressure	A	B	C
Local Anaesthetics	C	B	A
Hypoxia	B	A	C

- The greater the diameter of a given nerve fiber, the greater its speed of conduction.

9. Ans.— C Microelectrode

"Nerve cells have a low threshold for excitation. The stimulus may be electrical chemical, or mechanical. Two types of physiochemical disturbances are produced local, non-propagated potentials - synaptic, generator or electrotonic potentials and propagated disturbances - the action potential (or nerve impulse).

The electrical events in neurons are rapid being measured in milleseconds (ms); and the potential changes are small, being measured in millivolts (mV). In addition to development of microelectrodes with a tip diameter of less than 1 micron, the principal advances that make detailed study of the electrical activity in nerve possible were the development of electronic amplifiers and cathode ray ascilloscope". —Ganong.

10. Ans.— D ^{125}I-albumin for blood volume

*** Methods for measuring body fluid volumes.**

a. Plasma volume.
- **Evans blue (T-1824)**
- **Serum albumin labelled with radio-active iodine**

b. ECF
- **Insulin**
- **Mannitol**
- **Sucrose**

c. Total body water
- **Deuterium oxide (D2O, heavy water).**
- **Tritium oxide (3H2O).**
- **Aminopyrine**

d. Red cell volume (volume occupied by all the circulating red cells in the body).
- **tagged red blood cells.**

*** Other body fluid volumes can be calculated from these above measured volumes, like :**

*** Interstitial fluid volume = ECF volume — Plasma volume.**

*** Total blood volume = Plasma volume x 100/100- hematocrit**

*** Red cell volume = Total body water — ECF volume.**

*** Intracellular fluid volume = Total body water - ECF volume.**

{Note : Both Antipyrine & Aminopyrine are pyrazolane derivatives & used for measurement of Total body water}

Also Remember :

TBW

(60% of body weight)

Extracellular fluid—Intracellular Fluid

(20%) (40%)

Interstitial fluid Plasma

(Plasma + RBCS)

Total blood volume (8%)

11. Ans.— A. Membrane of effector structures innervated by post-ganglionic parasympathetic nerve endings

12. Ans.— D. All of the above

13. Ans.— A. Decorticate rigidity is greater than decerebrate rigidity

14. Ans.— C. The direction of nystagmus is in the same direction of rotation

15. Ans.— B. Dopamine

Dopamine deficiency leads to Parkinsonism

16. Ans.— B. Intention tremor

17. Ans.— D. Subthalamic nucleus

18. Ans.— E. The cerebellum

The receptor for inverse sketch reflex is in the Golgi tendon organ. There are 3-25 muscle fibres per tendon organ.

19. Ans.— C. The motor cortex

20. Ans.— D. The left posterior-superior temporal gyrus

21. Ans.— C. Inter-collicular transection

22. Ans.— B. Hypothalamus

23. Ans.— C. Layer 4

24. Ans.— B. Beta waves

25. Ans.— B. Thalamus

26. Ans.— D. 40%

27. Ans.— C. A-beta

28. Ans.— D. Rapid shallow breathing

29. Ans.— D. There is involuntary tremor

30. Ans.— C. Recall of events occurring a few weeks previously

31. Ans.— D. Medulla oblongata

32. Ans.— D. Pass in part through reticular formation and in part bypass it

33. Ans.— C. Vasodilator metabolites

Lactic acid is one of them.

34. Ans.— D. Not decreased by curare

35. Ans.— B. Lead to a increased probability of response

36. Ans.— C. 150 cc

Normal CSF pressure is about 130 mm range 60-150 mm H2. Composition of CSF versus plasma is :

	CSF	Plasma
Na (meq/L)	140	140
K ((meq/L)	2.9	4.6
Ca (meq/L)	2.3	4.7
HCO3 (meq/L)	25	25
Cl- (meq/L)	113	99
pH 7.33	7.4	
Protein (mg/dl)	20.0	7500
Glucose (mg/dl)	64	100

37. Ans.— D. It interferes with the action of acetylcholine esterase

38. Ans.— A. Diminished use of contralateral appendages below the lesion

Upper motor neuron lesion	Lower motor neuron lesion
* Paralysis and spasticity	Paralysis and flaccidity
* Hyperactive deep tendon jerks	Absent deep tendon jerks
* A base of wasting	Muscular atrophy
* Corticospinal tract involved	Ventral horn cells or their cranial equivalents involved

39. Ans.— A. Has a totally inhibitory output from its cortex

40. Ans.— D. Basal ganglia complex

41. Ans.— D. Contains a higher concentration of ascorbic acid

42. Ans.— A. Essential part of withdrawal reflex

Interneurons are present in the grey matter of the brain as well as the spinal cord. In the spinal cord, they are present in the dorsal horn as well as the ventral horn and in the intermediate areas between the two. In the ventral horn, their number is 30 times the number of motor neurons. Interneurons are small and highly excitable cells neurons as well as with the motor neurons. These cells phenomena of convergence, divergence, repetitive discharge etc.

43. Ans.— B. Lack nodes of Ranvier

44. Ans.— D. All of the above

Pain and temperature sensations are carried by lateral spinothalamic tract and touch is carried by anterior spinothalamic tract. Dorsal columns carry fine touch, tactile localization, two point discrimination, sense of vibration and pressure with intensity discrimination and sense of position.

45. Ans.— A. Swallowing reflex

The number of swallows per day is about 600 : 200 while eating and drinking, 350 while awake without food and 50 while sleeping.

46. Ans.— B. Some loss of pain sensation

47. Ans.— B. The diameter of axon

48. Ans.— D. Conducts from one node of Ranvier to the next

49. Ans. — A. Spinal cord

50. Ans.— E. All of the above

51. Ans.— C. Cl-

A slight decrease in resting membrane potential, (RNP) leads to increased K^+ effux and Cl^- influx, restoring RMP. However, when depolarization exceeds 7mV, the voltage gated Na+ channels start to open at an increased rate. The number of Na+ channels per sq. micro meter of membrane in myelinated mammalian neurons has been estimated to be 50-75 in cell body, 350-500 in initial segment, less than

25 on surface of myelin, 2000-12000 on the nodes of Ranvier and 20-75 at axon terminals. Along axons of unmyelinated neurons, the number is about 110.

52. Ans.— D. Discriminatory sensation

53. Ans.— A. Cerebral

54. Ans.— B. Lower chloride

Chloride in CSF is 113 meq/Kg H_2O whereas in plasma, it is 99. Bicarbonate, PCO_2 and creatinine are also higher in CSF.

55. Ans.— B. 4

Histologically, the fifth layer of cerebral cortex in this part contains giant cells Betz (mean diameter 16μ) which give rise to thick myelinated corticospinal fiber, supplementary motor area is located on medial superior bank of cingulate gyrus and extending upto upper region of lateral surface infront of area 4. Premotor cortex is Brodmann's areas 6, 8 and 44.

56. Ans.— A. Linear

57. Ans.— A. 65 mm of Hg

58. Ans.— B. Blood glucose levels

59. Ans.— B. Deep sleep

The frequency of waves in EEG are remembered by d-Tab', delta (0-3), Theta (4-7), alpha (8-13) and beta (above 13).

60. Ans.— B. Initiation of muscular movements

61. Ans.— A. Motor cortex

62. Ans.— A. Excessive stimulation of alpha motor neurons of all the muscles

63. Ans.— C. III

64. Ans.— D. All are correct

65. Ans.— C. 3-4 years

66. Ans.— D. Posterior columns

67. Ans.— A. Sensory fibres from thalamus to brain

68. Ans.— D. Tactile discrimination and two point discrimination

69. Ans.— C. Pre-programming of voluntary activity

70. Ans.— B. Present with action

By the age of 3-4 years, nerve conduction velocity in a child is same as that in an adult.

71. Ans.— A. 6 hours

Changes in nerve cell bodies are characterized by disintegration of Nisselgranules into fine dust chromatolysis) and swelling of the same. Usually recovery follows and cell appears normal after about 80 days.

72. Ans.— C. Posterior horn cells

73. Ans.— D. 7%

In brain, autoregulation maintains a normal cerebral blood flow at arterial pressures of 65-140 mmHg.

74. Ans.— C. 8-13

See ques. 42

75. Ans.— B. Inferior border of frontal lobe

76. Ans.— D. 13-30

77. Ans.— D. Acetylcholine

78. Ans. C. Distension

79. Ans. D. Proprioception

Classification of nerve fibres is

	Nerve fibre type	Function diameter (mm)	Fibre velocity (m/s)	Conduction
A	(myelinated)			
	Alpha	Propriception, somatic motor	12-20	70-120
	Beta	Touch, pressure	5-122	30-70
	Gamma	Motor in muscle spindles	3-6	15-30
	Delta	Pain, cold, touch	2-5	12-30
B.	(myelinated)	Pre-ganglionic autonomic	<3	3-15
	Post-ganglionic autonomic			
C.	(unmyelinated)	Pain, temperature	0.301	<2-5

80. Ans.— C. Aδ, C
81. Ans.— B. Optic chiasma
82. Ans.— C. Apneustic respiration
83. Ans.— B. 0.08
84. Ans.— C. 14-16/sec
85. Ans.— C. Recurrent inhibition
86. Ans.— B. 400 mm/day
87. Ans.— D. None of the above
88. Ans.— A. Anorexia
89. Ans.— B. Spike potential
90. Ans.— B. Injection of histamine
91. Ans. — B. 10
92. Ans.— D. Spinal cord
93. Ans.— C. Intensity discrimination
94. Ans.— D. The cartilaginous plates and the lens
95. Ans.— A. Law of projection
96. Ans.— B. Stretch
97. Ans.— B. Serotonin
98. Ans.— C. Antigravity
99. Ans.— C. a + b
100. Ans.— D. A delta and C fibres
101. Ans.— A. Rate of cerebral carbon dioxide formation.
102. Ans.— A. SA node, AV node
103. Ans.— B. Motor area
104. Ans.— A. Astrocytes
105. Ans.— A. Stimulation vagus
106. Ans.— A. Stimulation vagus
107. Ans.— A. Less excitable tissue
108. Ans.— A. Increasing the permeability of a neuron to K+
109. Ans.— A. Serotonin
110. Ans.— C. Dopamine
111. Ans.— B. IX
112. Ans.— A. Energy stored
113. Ans.— C. Low High
114. Ans.— B. IX
115. Ans.— C. L2, 3, 4
116. Ans.— B. Midbrain
117. Ans.— A. A-alpha
118. Ans.— D. C
119. Ans.— B. Axons
120. Ans.— D. All of the above
121. Ans.— D. Loss of inhibition delivered to gamma efferent neurons.
122. Ans.— C. Variable
123. Ans.— A. Activation of stretch receptors in Golgi tendon organ.
124. Ans.— C. Causes a reflex inhibition of homonymous alpha, efferent neurons.
125. Ans.— D. a+b
126. Ans.— C. 3.5 ml/100g brain/min
127. Ans.— C. 49
128. Ans.— B. Cushing reflex
129. Ans.— B. R, W, F
130. Ans.— D. Hypothalamus
131. Ans.— D. Postganglionic parasympathetic neuron
132. Ans.— D. Memory
133. Ans.— B. Basal ganglia lesions
134. Ans.— B. H
135. Ans. D. Na+
136. Ans.— C. 44
137. Ans.— C. CO_2
138. Ans.— C. Cl-
139. Ans.— C. Polysynaptic involving spinal cord
140. Ans.— B. Spinocerebeller tract
141. Ans.— B. Have conduction velocity of about five times that seen in heart muscle.
142. Ans.— C. Motor neuron and its muscle fibres.
143. Ans.— A. 1 4 2 3
144. Ans.— A. Superior
145. Ans.— D. It disappears when the subject closes his eyes
146. Ans.— D. Extrapyramidal system

Its disturbance leads to extrapyramidal syndrome or Parkinsonism.

147. Ans.— A. Cerebral cortex
148. Ans.— D. Spinal cord
149. Ans.— D. 4

The best known motor cortex is in precentral gyrus. However, there is a supplementary motor area on and above the superior bank of cingulate sulcus on the medial side of hemisphere that reaches the premotor cortex on lateral surface of brain.

150. Ans.— D. Both a and c
151. Ans.— D. Result in stimulation of auditory area in occipital cortex

152. Ans.— A. Suprachiasmatic nuclei

153. Ans.— D. A mild collicular section

154. Ans.— D. CO_2

See ques. 104

155. Ans.— A. Reticulocortica

156. Ans.— C. Positive Babinski's sign

157. Ans.— D. EPSPs and IPSPs of cortical cells which behave like dipoles

158. Ans.— C. Capillarie

159. Ans.— C. Changes in arterial PO2

160. Ans.— A. Homonymus upper quadrantinopia

161. Ans.— C. Depolarisation

162. Ans.— B. Loss of tactile and two point discrimination

163. Ans.— D. Sodium

164. Ans.— D. Serotonin

165. Ans.— A. Diverging circuit

Interneurones are important for connection.

166. Ans.— C. Reverbrating circuit

167. Ans.— D. Thrust downward

168. Ans.— C. Exterioceptive system

169. Ans.— A. Gamma-aminobutyric acid (GABA)

GABA is the major inhibitory mediator in the brain where it is trnasmitter at 20% of CNS synapses. It is also present in retina and is the mediator responsible for presynaptic inhibition.

170. Ans.— D. 3 2 1 4

171. Ans.— D. Ca

172. Ans.— D. Type-C

173. Ans.— D. Autonomic ↓ Somatic ↑

174. Ans.— C. Static tremor and rigidity

175. Ans.— D. Heart rate

176. Ans.— B. Parasympathetic system

177. Ans.— C. 10^{12}

178. Ans.— D. Layer-V

It is in the Brodmann Motor Cortex (Area 4)

179. Ans.— B. Hearing

180. Ans.— D. The hippocampus

181. Ans.— B. In the posterior part of the temporal cortex

182. Ans.— C. Glycine

183. Ans.— C. 150-200 mm

184. Ans.— D. Acetylcholine

An average human endplate contains 15-40 million acetylcholine receptors. Each nerve impulse releases about 60 acetylcholine vesicles, and each vesicle contains about 1000 molecules of the neurotransmitter. The amount is enough to activate about 10 times the number of acetylcholine receptors needed to produce a full endplate potential.

185. Ans.— D. Compensated respiratory— ↑ bicarbonate, ↑ pCO2 alkalosis

186. Ans.— A. Anterior hypothalamus

187. Ans.— C. Constriction of bronchial musculture

188. Ans.— D. All the cortex is removed from the brain

189. Ans.— D. Cerebral palsy

190. Ans.— B. The theory that there is change in RNA inside some of the neuron

191. Ans.— C. Flexor reflex

It is flexor withdrawl reflex

192. Ans.— C. 300-400; 40-60

193. Ans.— D. 110

194. Ans.— C. Beta waves (High frequency low voltage waves)

195. Ans.— B. Median eminence of hypothalamus

196. Ans.— C. Depolarization

197. Ans.— C. Replacement of rhythmic EEG pattern with low voltage, irregular waves

198. Ans.— B. Delta waves

199. Ans.— A. Difficulty in interpretation of sound

200. Ans.— C. It can conduct impulses both orthodromically and antidromically

201. Ans.— B. Eccrine sweat glands

202. Ans.— C. Petitmal

Frequency is 3/sec.

203. Ans.— A. Posterior column

204. Ans.— B. Decreased ST interval

205. Ans.— B. Decrease the arterial pressure

206. Ans.— D. Schwann cell

207. Ans.— B. 30

208. Ans.— A. Free nerve ending

209. Ans.— B. More than 20,000/sec

210. Ans.— D. Olfaction

Olfaction is in Frontal lobe

211. Ans.— A. Hyperphagia

212. Ans.— D. 12th

213. Ans.— B. 12 hours

214. Ans.— A. GABA

Amine neurotransmitters are dopamine, norepinephrine, epinephrine, 5HT, histamine. Excitatory are glutamate and aspartate whereas inhibitory are glycine and GABA.

215. Ans.— A. 4 gm

216. Ans.— B. Cerebellar lesions

217. Ans.— B. Nernst

218. Ans.— C. 10-15

219. Ans.— C. Acetylcholine

It was the first neurotransmitter discovered

220. Ans.— D. Cardiac muscle fibres

221. Ans.— D. Osmolality

See explanation of Ques. 36

222. Ans.— B. Cholesterol

See explanation of Ques. 36

223. Ans.— D. Mg++

See explanation of Ques. 36

224. Ans.— C. 7.33

225. Ans.— A. $\frac{1}{100,000}$ to $\frac{1}{500,000}$

226. Ans.— A. Acetylcholine

Choline esterase inhibitors are useful in Alzheimer's disease. Drugs used are Rivastigmine, Tacrine etc.

227. Ans.— C. Retention of urine and faeces

228. Ans.— D. All sensations

229. Ans.— A. Loss of Na+ from the interstitial compartment

230. Ans.— D. Elevation of plasma from free fatty acids

231. Ans.— D. Proprioception

232. Ans.— NONE

233. Ans.— D. ↑ Mitochondria

234. Ans.— D. Vestibulospinal tract

Slow muscle fibres are type-I or red oxidative muscle fibres. Myosin isoenzyme ATPase rate is slow and Ca++ pumping capacity of sarcoplasmic reticulum is with moderate diameter and moderate glycolytic activity but oxidative capacity is high.

235. Ans.— A. Travels in one direction at synapse

236. Ans.— A. Increase in tone

237. Ans.— C. Superior temporal gyrus

238. Ans.— C. A and I bands

239. Ans.— B. Pons

240. Ans.— D. Loss of shivering reflex of legs

241. Ans.— C. Distractibility

The other symptoms like emotional dyscontrol, personality deterioration, incontinence of urine, etc are also seen.

242. Ans.— D. Axon hillock

243. Ans.— D. Monoporesis

244. Ans.— B. Action potential

245. Ans.— A. Equilibrium

246. Ans.— C. Flocculonodular lobe of cerebellum

247. Ans.— A. Microglia

248. Ans.— C. 55

249. Ans.— C. 2 times

250. Ans.— A. Cholinergic

251. Ans.— A. Isometric exercises

252. Ans.— D. Afferent central fibres to hypothalamus

253. Ans.— D. Type-IV afferent

254. Ans.— B. Muscle metabolism

255. Ans.— A. Area postrema

The circumventricular organs or organ like tissue outside the brain are (i) posterior pituitary and median eminence (ii) area postrema (iii) organovasculosum of lamina terminalis (OVLT, supraoptic crest) (iv) Subfornical organ (SFO).

256. Ans.— C. Calcium

257. Ans.— B. Myotonia

258. Ans.— A. Voluntary movement

259. Ans.— B. Subdural space

260. Ans.— A. Smell

261. Ans.— B. Disrupted by tumors & infection

Many drugs may also influence it.

262. Ans.— D. One of the type of intrafusal fibre

263. Ans.— D. Uterine contractions during parturition

264. Ans.— A. Area 6 : primary gustatory cortex

265. Ans.— C. It flows from III ventricle to IV ventricle

266. Ans.— A. Trunk, arm, thumb, face

267. Ans.— D. Golgi tendon organs

268. Ans.— D. Cold sensation

Cold sensation is not synthetic

269. Ans.— A. Ponto cerebellar
270. Ans.— A. Olfactory
271. Ans.— B. Paracentral lobule
272. Ans.— B. A $\alpha\delta$
273. Ans.— A. Feed-forward inhibition
274. Ans.— A. Secondary muscle spindle
275. Ans.— D. Decrease in reflex time
276. Ans.— C. Finger-tips
277. Ans.— D. Heart rate and respiration

The reticular formation : The phylogenetically old reticular core of brain, occupies the midventricular portion of medulla and midbrain. It contains areas regulating HR, BP and respiration.

278. Ans.— C. Basket cell
279. Ans.— D.

A	B	C	D
3	4	1	2

280. Ans.— D. Caudate nucleus and globus pallidus
281. Ans.— C. Decreased gut motility
282. Ans.— C. 1, 2 and 3
283. Ans.— C. Touch

Touch is not relayed through it.

284. Ans.— B. Lateral corticospinal tract
285. Ans.— B. Sympathetic cholinergic
286. Ans.— B. Conditioner
287. Ans.— D. Synchronisation
288. Ans.— B. Compromised language output

Language output is disrupted.

289. Ans.— B. Excitatory fibre
290. Ans.— B. Complex
291. Ans.— B. Outer & inner hair cells
292. Ans.— B. Releasing interleukins
293. Ans.— D. Superior colliculus
294. Ans.— C. Labyrinthine righting reflex

Righting reflexes operate to maintain the normal standing position and keep an animal's head upright. These reflexes are a series of responses integrated for the most part of nuclei of midbrain.

295. Ans.— A. Total cessation of respiration
296. Ans.— B. Proprioceptive fibers of Cr. V relay in the mesenchephalic nucleus
297. Ans.— A. Aldosterone

Aldosterone secretion is increased by :- (i) Glucocorticoid secretion is also increased by surgery, anxiety, physical trauma, haemorrhage (ii) Glucocorticoid secretion unaffected — high K+ intake, low Na+ intake, constriction of IVC in thorax, standing, secondary hyperaldosteronism.

298. Ans.— A. Tight endothelial junction
299. Ans.— C. Tachycardia
300. Ans.— A. It has a lower threshold than the rest of the axon
301 Ans.— B. Left motor area
302. Ans.— A. Duration of action potential and muscle twitch is same
303. Ans.— D. Calmodulin dependent MLCK
304. Ans.— B. Both H and I-band shorten
305. Ans.— A. Nerve induction study
306. Ans.— D. Increases appetite
307. Ans.— A. Cl

See Ques. 2

308. Ans.— A. Serotonin
309. Ans.— B. Prolonged by IPSP
310. Ans.— C. Resting length
311. Ans.— B. Alpha waves
312. Ans.— D. All of the above
313. Ans.— C. The duration is equal to 1 second
314. Ans.— C. Small intestine

Small intestine is a rich site (Carcinoid may produce serotonin excessively.

315. Ans.— B. Covers myosin and prevents attachment of actin and myosin

Tropomyosin has molecular weight of 70,000; they are long filaments located in the groove between 2 chains in actin.

316. Ans.— C. Increased sensitivity of muscle and nerve

Hypocalcemic tetany may produce neuromuscular rigidity, muscle cramps (Chvostek's sign and Trousseau's sign), laryngospasm,.

317. Ans.— A. Altitudinal reflex
318. Ans.— C. Deep sleep is characterized by slow amplitude waves
319. Ans.— D. 70%
320. Ans.— B. 2 minute

321. Ans.— C. Pain sensation on the contralateral side

"Anterior spino thalamic tract (ventro-lateral) is a sensory tract which carry sensations of pain & temperature. It is the tract of crossed variety so that when it is cut at spinal cord level it will lead to loss of pain & temperature on contralateral side of body paresthesias and even convulsions.

322. Ans.— D. Chemical mediator is located only in the presynaptic terminal

One way conduction :

"Chemical mediators at synaptic junctions explains one way conduction. The mediator is located in the synaptic knobs of the presynaptic fibres but not in the post synaptic membranes."

323. Ans.— C. The superior hypogastric plexus is located at the anterior aspect of the aortic bifurcation and fifth lumbar vertebra

Synpathetic outflow also known as "Thoraco-lumber outflow". Hence the name indicates it comes through ventral renal of Thorasic & lumber region.

Parasympethetic outflow known as craniosacral so it comes out bia cranial nerves & sacral nerves (2 & 4).

Superior hypogastric pluxes is located at the anterior aspect of the Aortic Bifurcation. It contains both sympathetic & parasympathetic fibres.

324. Ans.— D. Glutamate

Glutamate is the main excitatory transmitter in the brain and spinal cord and it is the transmitter responsible for 75% of the excitatory transmission in brain.

Inhibitory amino acid:

- **Glycine in brain stem and spinal cord.**
- **GABA in brain (cerebellum, cerebral cortex, etc.)**

Excitatory amino acid :

- **Glutamate in cerebral cortex and brain stem**
- **Asparate in spinal cord**

325. Ans.— C. Increasing the amplitude of action potentials in the motor neurons

Force of muscle contraction depends upon

- Resting length of muscle
- Isometrical contraction
- Recruitment
- Repetition of stimuli
- Fast muscle fibers

326. Ans.— A. Color contrast

"The colour sensitive LGN cells project to the primary visual cortex (area 17) forming peg shaped regions".

From Lateral Geniculate Nucleus

Magnocellular pathway	Parvocellular pathway
- From layer 1 and 2	- From layer 3- 6
- Carries signal for detection of movement, depth and flicker	- Carries signal for color vision, texture, shape and fine details

327. Ans.— C. NO.

- **The nervous system is a special case of cell-to-cell signalling. Here the signalling molecule (Neurotransmitter) travel from the signalling cell (a neuron) to the target cell (another neuron/muscle/gland cell) across a junction (synapse).**

Gases which acts like a neurotransmitter in CNS :

1. **NO**
2. **CO**

328. Ans.— A. Caudate nucleus

329. Ans.— D. All of the above

330. Ans — B. Rapid eye movements

331. Ans.— B. Involved in flare phenomenon of triple response

332. Ans.— B. Ninth and tenth cranial nerves

333. Ans.— A. Dentate nucleus

334. Ans.— C. Agnosia

335. Ans.— A. Alpha

336. Ans.— C. Delta

337. Ans.— B. Thalamus

338. Ans.— D. Purkinje system

The conduction speeds in cardiac tissue SA are :

	Conduction rate (m/s)
SA Node	0.05
Atrial pathways	1.0
AV node	0.05
Bundle of His	1.0
Purkinje system	4.0
Ventricular muscle	1.0

339. Ans.— D Neurofilament

Axoplasmic flow can be fast or slow :

Fast axoplasmic flow	Slow axoplasmic flow
Can be anterograde or retrograde	Only anterograde
Rate of anterograde transport—400 mms/day Rate of retrograde transport—200 mms/day	Rate —0.5-10 mm s/day
Occurs along microtubules	Occurs along microtubules
Molecular motor involved in anterograde transport is kinesin Molecular motor involved in retrograde transport is Dynein	

340. Ans. — C Potassium ions

Factors affecting cerebral blood flow

a. Cerebral metabolism b. Cerebral perfusion pressure
c. Arterial PCO2 d. Arterial PO2
e. Temperature f. Blood viscosity
g. Autonomic system

341. Ans.— A Word formation

Broca'a area (Area 44) is located in the inferior frontal gyrus. Immediately anterior to the primary motor cortex and above the sylvian fissure and is associated with 'word formation'.

Repetition is impaired with lesions in Broca's area, Wernicke's area and the arcuate fasciculus. This is not a characteristic function of Broca's area.

342. Ans.— D Anterior Nucleus of Thalamus

'The Anterior Thalamic Nucleus project the cingulate cortex and from there connections to the hippocampus complete a complex closed described as the Papez Circuit'.

343. Ans. — C Recruitment by multiplication of neurons

Neurons are 'permanent cells' that do not undergo mitotic division in post natal life. Thus recruitment by multiplication of neurons is the single best answer of exclusion.

- **Changes in the level of neurotransmitter of synapse**
- **Increasing Protein Synthesis**
- **Structural changes (Spatial reorganization) in Synapses**
- **Recruitment by multiplication of neurons**

However, relation of new cells to memory processing needs further research before it can be established.

Recruitment by multiplication of neurons is therefore the single best answer of exclusion.

344. Ans.— C Blood flow remains unaltered

- **Brain autoregulates between 60 mm Hg and 140 mm Hg, which maintains blood flow at a constant rate despite fluxes in the blood pressure.**
- **The factors that affect cerebral blood flow are :**

a. O2 or the lack of it
b. H+ ions
c. CO2 levels.

- **Cardiac output and regional blood flow in a sedentary man.**

	Quiet standing	**Exercise**
Cardiac output	5900	24,000
Blood flow to :		
Heart	250	1000
Brain	**750**	**750**
Active skeletal muscle	650	20,850
Inactive skeletal muscle	650	300
Skin	500	500
Kidney, liver, gastrointestinal tract, etc.	3100	600

345. Ans.— A Perlecan

- ***Perlecan* is a large multi-domain proteoglycan that binds to and cross-links many extracellular matrix (ECM) components and cell-surface molecules.**
- **Perlecan is synthesized by both vascular endothelial and smooth muscle cells and deposited in the extracellular matrix.**
- **Perlecan is a key component of the vascular extracellular matrix, here it interacts with a variety of other matrix components and helps to maintain the endothelial barrier function.**
- **Perlecan is a potent inhibitor of smooth muscle cell proliferation and is thus thought to help to maintain vascular homeostasis.**
- **Perlecan can also promotes growth factor (e.g. FGF2) activity and thus stimulate endothelial growth and re-generation.**

346. Ans.— B. Rate of CSF absorption

* **"Regulation of Cerebrospinal Fluid Pressure by the Arachnoidal Villi-The normal rate of cerebrospinal fluid formation remains very nearly constant.**

347. Ans.— D Blood pressure

* **"As in most other vascular areas of the body, cerebral blood flow is highly related to metabolism of the tissue."**

* **Brain Blood Flow is Virtually Constant Despite Changes in Arterial Blood Pressure.**

348. Ans.— B Accommodation

* ***"The relation between the strength and the duration of a threshold stimulus is called the strength-duration curve. Slowly rising currents* fail to fire the nerve because the nerve adapts to the applied stimulus, a process called accommodation."**

349. Ans. — D C > B > A

Relative Susceptibility of Mammalian A, B, and C Nerve Fibers to Conduction Block Produced by Various Agents.

Susceptibility to:	*Most Susceptible*	*Intermediate*	*Least Susceptible*
Hypoxia	B	A	C
Pressure	A	B	C
Local anaesthetics	C	B	A

350. Ans. D. Functional interaction with cardiovagal center

Factors affecting the activity of the vasomotor area in the medulla

Direct stimulation

- **CO_2**
- **Hypoxia**

Excitatory inputs

- **From cortex via hypothalamus**
- **From pain pathways and muscles**
- **From carotid and aortic chemoreceptors**

Inhibitory inputs

- **From cortex via hypothalamus**
- **From lungs**
- **From carotid, aortic, and cardiopulmonary baroreceptors**

351. Ans. D. Has more ion channels

It contains the highest no. of voltage gated sodium channels.

2.

IMPORTANT TEXT OF CVS

CORRELATION OF PLASMA K+ LEVEL AND THE ECG, ASSUMING PLASMA CA++ IS NORMAL.

Normal tracing (plasma K^+4-5.5 mEq/liter). PR interval = 0.16 sec; QRS interval = 0.06 sec; QT interval = 0.4 sec (normal for an assumed heart rate of 60).

Hypokalemia (plasma K^+ ± 3.5 mEq/liter). PR = 0.2 sec; QRS interval = 0.06 sec; ST segment depression. A prominent U wave is now present immediately following the T. The actual QT interval remains 0.4 sec. If the U wave is erroneously considered a part of the T, a falsely prolonged QT interval of 0.6 sec will be measured.

Hypokalemia (plasma K^+ ± 2.5 mEq/liter). The PR is lengthened to 0.32 sec; the ST segment is depressed; the T wave is inverted; a prominent U wave is seen. The true QT interval remains normal.

Hyperkalemia (plasma K^+ ± 7.0 mEq/liter). The PR and QRS intervals are within normal limits. Very tall, slender, peaked T waves are now present.

Hyperkalemia (plasma K^+ ±8.5 mEq/liter). There is no evidence of atrial activity; the QRS complex is broad and slurred and the QRS interval has widened to 0.2 sec. The T waves remains tall and slender. Further elevation of the plasma K^+ may result in ventricular tachycardia and ventricular fibrillation.

MCQ's OF CVS

What is important in CVS

Rhythmic excitation of heart, Normal ECG (Values of different components), Cardiac output, Venous return and their regulation, Coronary circulation.

1. Which one of the following is the correct statement regarding coronary blood flow ? AIIMS 2006, 2008

A. Coronary blood flow is directly related to perfusion pressure and inversely related to resistance.
B. Coronary blood flow is inversely related to perfusion pressure and directly related to resistance.
C. Coronary blood flow is directly related to perfusion pressure and also to resistance.
D. Coronary blood flos is inversely related to both pressure and resistance.

2. Which bacteria acts by mechanism of cyclic AMP activaion ? AIIMS 2006

A. V. cholera B. Clostridium difficile
C. B. cereus D. B. fragilis

3. Which of the following statements is true regarding Golgi tendon? AIIMS 2006

A. Measures dynamic length
B. Measures static length
C. Sends signal to α motor neuron of the same muscle
D. Measures total tension

4. The sodium-potassium pump is an example of : AIIMS 2006

A. Active transport
B. Passive transport
C. Facilitated diffusion
D. Osmosis

5. Which one of the following acts as second messengar ? AIIMS 2006

A. Mg++ B. Cl-
C. Ca++ D. PO4+3

6. The ECG of a 40-year old male was recorded using standard bipolar limb leads. The sum of voltages of the three standard leads was found to be 5 millivolts. This indicates : AIIMS 2005

A. A normal heart
B. Right ventricular hypertrophy
C. Left ventricular hypertrophy
D. Increased cardiac muscle mass

7. When the aviator is subjected to negative G : AIIMS 2004

A. The hydrostatic pressure in veins of lower limb increases
B. The cardiac output decreases
C. Black out occurs
D. The cerebral arterial pressure rises

8. All of the following factors normally increase the length of the ventricular cardiac muscle fibers except : AI 2005

A. Increased venous tone
B. Increased total blood volume
C. Increased negative intrathoracic pressure
D. Lying to standing change in posture

9. S.A. node acts as a pacemaker of the heart because of the fact that it : AI 2005

A. Is capable of generating impulses spontaneously
B. Has rich sympathetic innervations
C. Has poor cholinergic innervations
D. Generates impulses at the highest rate

10. Patients having acute cardiac failure do not show oedema, because : AI 2004, 2006

A. The plasma oncotic pressure is high
B. There is renal compensation
C. There is an increase in cardiac output
D. There is a fall in the systemic capillary hydrostatic pressure.

11. During the cardiac cycle the opening of the aortic valve takes place at the : AI 2004

A. Beginning of systole
B. End of isovolumetric contraction
C. End of diastole
D. End of diastasis

Ans. 1. A 2. A 3. D 4. A 5. C 6. D 7. D 8. D 9. D 10. D 11. B

12. **As a part of space research program, a physiologist was asked to investigate the effect of flight-induced stress on blood pressure. Accordingly, the blood pressure of the cosmonauts were to be measured twice: once before the take-off and once after the spacecraft entered the designated orbit around the earth. Fora proper comparison, the preflight blood pressure should be recorded in : AI 2003**
A. The lying down position
B. The sitting position
C. The standing position
D. Any position, as long as the post-flight recording is made in the same position.

13. **Two students, Vineet and Kamlesh were asked to demonstrate in dogs the role of sinus nerve in hypovolemic shock. Vineet severed the sinus nerves when the mean blood pressure (MBP) was 85 mm Hg and Kamlesh cut the sinus nerve when the mean blood pressure was 60 mm Hg. On cutting the sinus nerve : AI 2003**
A. Vineet recored the increase in MBP but Kamlesh recorded an decrease in MBP.
B. Vineet recorded a decrease in MBP but Kamlesh recorded an increase in MBP.
C. Both recorded an increase in MBP.
D. Both recorded a decrease in MBP.

14. **Which of the following factors probably affects myocardial blood flow to the greatest extent under normal conditions? PGI 1991**
A. Degree of parasympathetic stimulation
B. Rate of release of adenosine from the myocardium
C. Degree of sympathetic stimulation of coronary vessels.
D. Myocardial carbon dioxide concentration

15. **The main inhibitory center of heart is : AIIMS 1996**
A. Nucleus tractus solitarius
B. Nucleus ambiguous
C. Nucleus parabrachialis
D. Dorsal nucleus of vagus

16. **Which of the following area has more coronary blood flow : AMC 1992**
A. Right B. Left
C. Apical D. Both a or b have equal

In Question 17 to 21, match the following : AIIMS 1984, 94
A. Ist heart sound B. 2nd heart sound
C. 3rd heart sound D. Beginning of T-waves
E. P-wave on ECG

17. **S-wave on ECG**
18. **Onset of 'a' wave in atrial pressure curve**
19. **Maximum aortic pressure**
20. **Period of maximal ventricular flow**
21. **A-V valve opens**

22. **All of the following ions cause vasodilation except: AIIMS 1983, 93**
A. Mg++ B. K+
C. Ca++ D. Kinins

23. **Normal systolic pressure in pulmonary artery is : AIIMS 1986, 96**
A. 0-10 mm Hg B. 10-20 mm Hg
C. 25-32 mm Hg D. 90-120 mm Hg

24. **O_2 content of saturated arterial blood is : AP 1999**
A. 11.2 ml/100 ml B. 14.5 ml/100 ml
C. 19.4 ml/100 ml D. 21.3 ml/100 ml

25. **Which of the following is responsible for the plateau phase of cardiac action potential : AP 1999**
A. Opening of slow calcium channels
B. Opening of K channels
C. Opening of Na+ channels
D. Closing of Na channels

26. **Cardiac output in L/min divided by heart rate equals : AIIMS 1993**
A. Cardiac efficiency B. Cardiac index
C. Mean stroke volume D. Mean arterial pressure

27. **In an average adult the stroke volume per minute is : AMU 1999**
A. 20-40 cc B. 40-50 cc
C. 60-70 cc D. 80-100 cc

28. **Platue phase of action potential is seen in : AIIMS 1997**
A. SA node B. AV node
C. Atrial fibers D. Ventricular fibers

29. **Linear velocity of blood at normal cardiac output in the aorta is : Rohtak 1998**
A. 32 cms/sec. B. 64 cms/sec.
C. 8 cms/sec. D. 50 cms/sec.

30. **The portion of the electrocardiogram related to the propagation of the cardiac impulse between the SA node and the AV node is the : UP 1992**
A. QT interval B. PR interval
C. ST interval D. RR interval

31. **Electrocardiographic leads designated V1, V2 etc. refer to : TN 1989, 93**
A. Unipolar limb leads B. Unipolar chest leads
C. Bipolar limb leads D. Bipolar chest leads

32. **Parasympathetic stimulation would decrease the following except : Kerala 1988, 91**
A. SA node rhythmicity
B. Heart rate
C. A.V. conduction time
D. Atrial contractility

33. **Work performed by the left ventricle is greater than that performed by the right ventricle due to differences in : AMU 1996**
A. Blood velocity B. Stroke volume
C. Arterial pressures D. Atrial pressures

Ans.									
12. A	13. C	14. B	15. B	16. A	17. A	18. E	19. D	20. C	21. B
22. C	23. C	24. C	25. A	26. C	27. C	28. D	29. A	30. B	31. B
32. C	33. C								

34. What is not true for extrasystole in ventricle? **NIMHANS 1987, 97**

A. Fails to produce radial pulse
B. Hints at serious heart ailment
C. Associated with abnormal QRS complex
D. Tendency to be followed by a compensatory pause

35. What is not true for jugular venous pulse? **Kerala 1989, 91**

A. Pressure typically raised in right ventricular failure.
B. Pressure typically raised in partial obstruction of superior vena cava.
C. Commonly pulse not visible with normal heart.
D. Pulse exaggerated in tricuspid incompetence.

36. Murmur may be found using a stethoscope over all, except : **Rohtak 1986, 93**

A. Dilatation in arteries
B. Vessels in which turbulance
C. In early diastole in healthy adults
D. Larger arteries in healthy adults

37. During B.P. measurement if the muffled sound does not disappear with return of mercury to 'O', the conclusion is : **Rohtak 1986, 92**

A. Aortic stenosis
B. Low haematocrit
C. Zero diastolic pressure
D. Patent ductus arteriosus

38. Which is going to best declare the case as that of interatrial septal defect with other cardiac abnormalities? **DNB 1991**

A. Elevated pressure in left atrium
B. Elevated pressure in right atrium
C. Elevated PO2 in pulmonary artery
D. Systolic murmur

39. Pulmonary embolism is a complication of all, except : **AIIMS 1983, 94**

A. Vit. K deficiency B. Oral contraception
C Prolonged bed rest D. Surgical procedure

40. The component of cardiac tissue having the highest propagation velocity is : **Delhi 1988, 92**

A. Purkinje fibres B. AV node
C. Atrial muscle D. Ventricular muscle

41. Auscultation of heart provides evidence of all, except : **AP 1991**

A. Ventricular septal defect, if a loud diastolic murmur is heard.
B. Mitral regurgitation if a systolic murmur is heard which is propagating into axilla and back of left side.
C. Mitral stenosis if an early diastolic murmur is heard.
D. Aortic stenosis if a systolic murmur is mainly propagated into neck vessels is heard.

42. First component of first heart sound is usually clearly heard on ventral surface of chest at : **Rohtak 1991**

A. 2nd intercostal space to right of sternum
B. 2nd intercostal space to left of sternum
C. 5th intercostal space to left of sternum
D. 5th intercostal space over sternum

43. Second component of first heart sound is associated with what phenomenon during cardiac cycle : **DNB 1992**

A. Closure of pulmonary valves
B. Closure of aortic valves
C. Closure of mitral valves
D. Closure of tricuspid valves

44. The natural rate of rhythmic contraction is greatest in which part of the heart? **AIIMS 1997**

A. Ventricular myocardium
B. Atria
C. Sinoartrial node
D. Purkinje fibers

45. The velocity of impulse transmission is slowest in the : **AIIMS 1984, 87; Delhi 1995**

A. A-V node
B. Ventricular myocardium
C. Atria
D. Purkinje system

46. Circus movements in the heart can be caused by all of the following except : **Delhi 1982, 94**

A. Increased myocardial conduction velocity
B. Decreased myocardial refractory period
C. Damage to the Purkinje system
D. Atrial or ventricular dilatation

47. A decrease in the velocity of impulse conduction through the A-V node will usually cause : **AMC 1983, 91**

A. The PQ interval to increase
B. The PQ interval to decrease
C. Disappearance of the T-wave
D. Increased heart rate

48. The rate of conduction of action potentials in Purkinje fibers is about : **PGI 1986, 87, 90**

A. 0.02 meters/sec B. 2.0 meters/sec
C. 6.0 meters/sec D. 0.6 meters/sec

49. The T-wave of the normal electrocardiogram corresponds to : **AIIMS 1982, 92**

A. Ventricular depolarization
B. Ventricular repolarization
C. Isovolumetric contraction
D. Atrial systole

Ans.	34. B	35. C	36. D	37. B	38. C	39. A	40. A	41. A	42. C	43. D
	44. C	45. A	46. A	47. A	48. B	49. B				

50. Isometric ventricular contraction is characterized by : Delhi 1984, 90
A. ↑ Pressure in both atria
B. ↑ Coronary blood flow
C. ↓ Pressure in both atria
D. None of the above

51. Which of the following about cardiac output is correct : Delhi 1985; DNB 1998
A. Not necessarily increases with heart rate
B. Increases to 50L/mt in exercise
C. Proportional to B.P.
D. Proportionally falls with increase in heart rate

52. The first heart sound (S1) occurs due to closure of AV valves during : UPSC 1983; Delhi 1995
A. Isotonic relaxation
B. Isotonic contraction
C. Isovolumetric contraction
D. Isovolumetric relaxation

53. 'a' wave of venous pulse is caused by : PGI 1990
A. Auricular contraction
B. Ventricular contraction
C. Auricular relaxation
D. Ventricular relaxation

54. Cardiac index is the ratio of : PGI 1982, 93
A. Cardiac output and body weight
B. Cardiac output and surface area
C. Cardiac output and work of heart
D. Stroke volume and surface area

55. QRS complex indicates : AI 1996
A. Atrial depolarization
B. Ventricular depolarization
C. Artrial repolarization
D. Ventricular repolarization

56. The basis for Koratkoff's sounds is stated to be : Delhi 1983, 95
A. AV valve closure B. Aortic valve closure
C. Arterial expansion D. Arterial turbulance

57. Opening of aortic valves is initiated when : AP 1989, 91
A. Ventricular pressure exceeds aortic pressure
B. Ventricles contract
C. Ventricles relax
D. Aortic contracts

58. Essential hypertension is generally associated with an early increase in : Bihar 1989, 94
A. Oxygen use B. Coronary flow
C. Cardiac work D. Cardiac output

59. A hypertrophied ventricle will depolarize : Bihar 1989, 97
A. More rapidly than other ventricle
B. Shift the electrical axis to involved side
C. Before the other ventricle
D. None of the above

60. Changes in mean electrical axis of the ventricles may be caused by : Bihar 1991
A. Muscular necrosis
B. Bundle branch block
C. Change in body position
D. Hypertrophy of one ventricle
E. All of the above

61. Pulse pressure in a particular vessel is determined chiefly by : Bihar 1991
A. Distance from heart
B. Frictional characteristics of lumen
C. Distensibility
D. Cross-sectional area

62. Sympathetic stimulation of heart causes : AIIMS 1983, 99
A. Increased coronary flow
B. Increased excitability of heart
C. Increased force of myocardial contraction
D. All of the above

63. Parasympathetic stimulation of heart causes : AIIMS 1983, 92
A. Decreased rate of S.A. node
B. Increased excitability of A-V junctional fibres
C. Prevents ventricular contraction
D. None of the above

64. Increased pressure within carotid sinus produces : AIIMS 1985, 93
A. Reflex increase in venous pressure
B. Reflex hyperpnoea
C. Reflex bradycardia
D. Increase in heart rate

65. What is not true of 'a' wave of venous pulsations in neck ? DNB 1989, 95
A. Exaggerated in tricuspid stenosis
B. Abolished in atrial fibrillation
C. Occurs just after in carotid artery
D. Exaggerated in complete heart block when P-wave falls between QRS and T-waves

66. First heart sound occurs during the period of : DNB 1992
A. Isotonic relaxation
B. Isovolumetric relaxation
C. Isovolumetric contraction
D. Isotonic contraction

67. Fibres of A-V junction : AMU 1991
A. Modified muscle fibres
B. Modified nerve fibres
C. Highly contractile
D. Conduct impulse rapidly

Ans.	50. A	51. A	52. C	53. A	54. B	55. B	56. D	57. A	58. C	59. B
	60. E	61. C	62. D	63. A	64. C	65. C	66. C	67. A		

68. **When bundle of His compietely interrupted the : AMU 1992**
A. Atria beat irregularly
B. QRS complex varies in shape
C. P-R interval longer than normal but constant from heat to beat
D. Ventricles typically contract at about 30-40 beats/min

69. **Sympathetic activity in heart increases in all, except : AMU 1991**
A. During excitement
B. During exercise
C. When decrease in parasympathetic nerve activity
D. When arterial pressure falls

70. **The first heart sound occurs synchronously with : NIMHANS 1991**
A. Rise in atrial pressure and rise in ventricular pressure
B. P-wave of ECG
C. Closure of aortic and pulmonary valves
D. B and C

71. **The second heart sound differs from first heart sound is that : TN 1992**
A. Is occasionally split
B. Has higher frequency
C. Duration greater than first sound
D. Due partly to turbulence set up by valve closure

72. **Conduction velocity is least in : JIPMER 1990, 93**
A. SA node B. AV node
C. His bundle D. Purkinje fibres

73. **Absolute refractory period of heart is the gap of time in which : AIIMS 1998**
A. Heart is in diastole
B. Unresponsive to neural stimuli
C. No action potential from another part of heart will reexcite the heart muscle
D. None of the above

74. **Dicrotic notch in aortic pressure curve is : AIIMS 1996**
A. Magnified by aortic regurgitation
B. Absent in arteriosclerosis
C. Of no diagnostic value
D. Coincident with 2nd heart sound

75. **When pacemaker is another area of heart, it denotes : AIIMS 1986, 92**
A. Wrong with conducting tissue
B. Wrong with S-A node
C. Wrong with neural controlling system
D. None of the above

76. **Sympathetic vasoconstrictor tone is diminished in response to increased activity of : PGI 1985, 91**
A. Carotid body chemoreceptors
B. Carotid sinus pressoreceptors
C. Pain receptors
D. Medullary chemoreceptors

77. **Ventricular filling : Rohtak 1986, 96**
A. Produces 3rd heart sound in some healthy persons.
B. Depends mainly on contraction of atria.
C. Begins during isometric ventricular relaxation.
D. Will not occur unless atrial pressure is higher than atmospheric pressure.

78. **All are true for veins, except : Rohtak 1986, 97**
A. Innervated by sympathetic constrictor fibres.
B. Contain major part of blood volume.
C. Respond to an increase in intraluminal pressure by constriction.
D. Receive nutrition through vasa vasorum which arises from veins.

79. **Blood flow through left coronary artery : AIIMS 1985, 91**
A. Regulated by sympathetic vasodilator nerves
B. Increases when myocardial hypoxia
C. Greatest during early systole
D. Decrease in reflex response to fall in blood pressure

80. **In man, cardiac cycle duration (sec.) is : DNB 1992**
A. 0.4 B. 0.8
C. 1. D. 1.6

81. **In systole, coronary blood flow falls by ———% : Rajasthan 1998**
A. 80 B. 60
C. 40 D. 10

82. **Repolarization of ventricles must : PGI 1980, 91**
A. Begin in septum
B. Begin in apical epicardium
C. Begin at AV node
D. Occurs last at apex

83. **Q-wave in healthy individual denotes a dipole in : PGI 1982, 96**
A. Apex with axis of 180°
B. Base with axis of 180°
C. Base with axis of 180°
D. Apex with axis of 180°

84. **Carotid sinus on pressure causes : PGI 1997**
A. Reflex bradycardia B. ↑ RR
C. ↑ HR D. ↓ RR

85. **Heart sound indicating condition of myocardium is : PGI 1993; WB 1998**
A. S1 B. S2
C. S3 D. S4

86. **Stimulation of stretch receptors present in the left ventricle causes hypotension and bradycardia. This phenomenon is known as : Delhi 1997**
A. Brainbridge reflex
B. Bezold-Jarisch reflex
C. Cushing's reflex
D. Herring Breuer reflex

Ans.										
	68. D	69. C	70. A	71. B	72. B	73. C	74. D	75. B	76. B	77. A
	78. D	79. B	80. B	81. C	82. C	83. A	84. A	85. C	86. B	

87. Splitting in S2 is due to : AIIMS 1996
A. Atrial systole
B. Delay in closure of aortic valves
C. Delay in closure of mitral valves
D. Delay in closure of pulmonary valves

88. SA node is the pace maker because of its : PGI 1982
A. Neural control
B. Location in atrium
C. Strength of impulse formation
D. Rate of impulse formation

89. R-wave in healthy subjects denote a dipole with an electrical axis of : AIIMS 1994
A. 0° B. -60°
C. 60° D. 120°

90. Under resting conditions, the cardiac output is ----------- L/min : PGI 1992
A. 2 B. 4
C. 5.25 D. 7.5

91. Blood flow through left coronary artery is : AIIMS 1996
A. Greatest during early systole
B. Increased when myocardial hypoxia
C. Regulated by sympathetic vasodilator nerves
D. Decreased in reflex response to fall in blood pressure

92. Mary's law denotes relationship between heart : PGI 1994
A. Contraction and conductivity
B. Rate and contraction
C. Contraction and volume
D. Rate and blood pressure

93. The coronary blood flow (ml per minute) is : Delhi 1980, 91
A. 250 B. 500
C. 750 D. 840

94. Heart rate is maximum in a normal : AIIMS 1994
A. Foetus B. Newborn
C. Adults D. Oldage

95. The average coronary blood flow in human being at rest is —— of cardiac output : PGI 1993
A. 4-5% B. 5-10%
C. 10-15% D. 15-20%

96. 'Vulnerable period' of heart is a time occurring during— wave and represents a period when premature beats may lead to fibrillation : AIIMS 1999
A. P B. Q
C. R D. T

97. Normal QRS interval is approximately : AIIMS 1994
A. 0.2 sec B. 0.4-0.6 sec
C. 0.08-0.1 sec D. 1.0-1.5 sec

98. The last part of ventricle to activate after atrial activation is : AMC 1986, 91
A. Epicardium of apex
B. Endocardium of apex
C. Base of right ventricle
D. Base of left ventricle

99. The first part of ventricle to contract after atrial systole is : AMC 1982; DNB 1988, 93
A. Base of left ventricle B. Base of right ventricle
C. Apex of heart D. Right ventricle

100. If in an ECG, PRT waves are normal but S wave is absent, it indicates : AIIMS 1983, 93
A. Myocardial depression
B. Left bundle branch block
C. No cardiac abnormality
D. Activation of part of base terminal

101. A sign of nodal rhythm is : AIIMS 1981, 93
A. Prolonged PR interval
B. Prolonged QRS complex
C. Increased sympathetic tone to SA node
D. Increased parasympathetic tone to SA node

102. Prolonged P R interval indicates increased : AIIMS 1980, 92
A. Sympathetic tone to SA node
B. Parasympathetic tone to SA node
C. Parasympathetic tone to AV node
D. Sympathetic tone to AV node

103. Repolarization wave of ECG is : PGI 1980; AIIMS 1982, 94
A. T-wave B. S-wave
C. R-wave D. a+b

104. The jumping of depolarization from node-to-node is called : AIIMS 1982, 92
A. Absolute refractory period
B. Relative refractory period
C. Saltatory conduction
D. Orthodromic conduction

105. U-waves may seen with : AMU 1987, 95
A. Hyperkalemia
B. Hyponatremia
C. Quinidine administration
D. Angina

106. Which of the following is wrongly matched about ECG waves and their duration : UPSC 1982, 91
A. P wave—0.10 sec
B. S wave —0.04 sec.
C. QRS complex— max 0.10 sec.
D. Q wave— 0.10 sec.

Ans.										
	87. D	88. D	89. C	90. C	91. B	92. D	93. A	94. A	95. A	96. D
	97. C	98. D	99. C	100. C	101. D	102. C	103. D	104. C	105. C	106. D

107. Systolic and diastolic murmurs over body of sternum is mostly on account of : AIIMS 1993
A. Aortic insufficiency and stenosis
B. Aortic and pulmonary insufficiency
C. Aortic and pulmonary stenosis
D. Decreased hematocrit

108. Principal source of energy to heart in healthy individual is : PGI 1991
A. Glucose B. Amino acids
C. Free fatty acids D. Lactate and pyruvate

109. 'P' wave of ECG occurs at : AMC 1993
A. Beginning of ventricular contraction
B. End of ventricular contraction
C. Beginning of atrial contraction
D. End of atrial contraction

110. Under basal conditions, calorie provided by various components of diet are (%) : DNB 1991

	Carbohydrate	Ketone	Fat
A.	45	15	40
B.	50	5	45
C.	35	5	60
D.	25	15	60

111. Repolarization of ventricular muscle : DNB 1998
A. Occurs last at apex
B. Begins in septum
C. Begins in apical epicardium
D. Begins at AV node

112. Stimulation of baroreceptors leads to : PGI 1984; AI 1990
A. ↑ BP ↑ HR B. ↓ BP ↓ HR
C. ↑ ICT D. ↓ ICT

113. Venous return is increased in : Delhi 1996
A. Inspiration B. Expiration
C. Peak of a or b D. Extremes of a or b

114. In pacemaker of heart, after the impulse, action potential comes back to firing level due to : Delhi 1995
A. ↑ Na^+ permeability B. ↓ K^+ permeability
C. Ca^{++} channels D. Opening of K^+ channels

115. Independent P-wave and QRS complex indicates : PGI 1981, 93
A. Failure of conduction in AV node
B. Depression of SA node
C. Slowing of conduction of AV node
D. Early repolarisation of ventricle

W.116. Increased venous return leads to increased contraction by way of the Frank Starling mechanism, which one of the following would not happen : Rajasthan 1992
A. ↑ end diastolic sarcomere length
B. ↑ myocardial tension during systole
C. ↑ stroke volume
D. ↑ end diastolic volume

117. According to Starling's law, cardiac output can be increased by : Delhi 1998
A. Heart rate
B. BP
C. End diastolic volume
D. End systolic volume

118. Coronary blood flow at rest in man is : Delhi 1992
A. 100 ml/min B. 200 ml/min
C. 250 ml/min D. 500 ml/min

119. The cause of post extrasystolic potentiation is : PGI 1983, 98
A. Ca^+ B. K^+
C. Na^+ D. Mg^{++}

120. Pressure (mmHg) in right ventricle during systole is : Rohtak 1996
A. 0 B. 25
C. 80 D. 121

121. Blood flow is more in a majority in : AMU 1995
A. Right coronary artery
B. Left coronary artery
C. Equal
D. Not fixed

122. In arteriolar constriction, capillaries are supplied by : Delhi 1997
A. Pulsatile flow
B. Non-pulsatile flow
C. Newtonian flow
D. Any of the above

123. Right ventricular pressure is high in all of the following except : AP 1996
A. Tetralogy of fallot
B. Eisenmenger's syndrome
C. Pulmonary stenosis
D. None of the above

124. The ECG waves produced by ventricular repolarization is : AP 1996
A. P B. Q
C. R D. T

125. U-waves are produced in ECG : TN 1996
A. Just after Q-waves B. Just before R-waves
C. Just before S-waves D. Just after T-waves

126. Intrinsic autoregulation of heart is by : Delhi 1996
A. Mean arterial pressure
B. Cardiac output work
C. Sympathetic system
D. Right atrial pressure

127. The duration (sec.) and frequency of S1 is : DNB 1990
A. 0.15, 30 B. 0.12, 50
C. 0.20, 50 D. 0.20, 70

Ans.								
107. A	108. C	109. C	110. C	111. C	112. B	113. A	114. B	115. A
116. NONE	117. C	118. C	119. A	120. B	121. A	122. C	123. D	124. D
125. D	126. B	127. A						

128. **Cardiac output is maximally increased in : AMU 1982, 92**
A. Anxiety B. Eating
C. Exercise D. Pregnancy

129. **Cardiac index in a normal person is : TN 1996**
A. 2.1 B. 3.2
C. 4.6 D. 5.9

130. **Heart sound heard immediately before the first heart sound when atrial pressure is high : AP 1996**
A. First B. Second
C. Third D. Fourth

131. **Heart rate is accelerated by the following, except : DNB 1999**
A. Inspiration B. Grief
C. Exercise D. Anger

132. **Heart rate is slowed by the following, except : Delhi 1990**
A. Expiration
B. Fear
C. Increased intra-cranial pressure
D. Hypoxia

133. **The duration (sec) and frequency (Hz) of S2 is : AIIMS 1982, 92**
A. 0.12, 50 B. 0.15, 60
C. 0.15, 75 D. 0.15, 80

134. **Bainbridge reflex : AIIMS 1982, 95**
A. Increases the heart rate
B. Decreases the heart rate
C. a or b
D. Does not alter the heart rate

135. **The duration of S3 is : PGI 1980, 92**
A. 0.1 sec. B. 0.2 sec.
C. 0.3 sec. D. 0.4 sec.

136. **An irregular, rapid heart rate with normal QRS complexes and no P-waves suggests : AMC 1996**
A. Sinus arrhythmia
B. Second degree heart block
C. Paroxysmal tachycardia with a ventricular pacemaker
D. Atrial fibrillation

137. **The delay between the P-wave and the Q-wave in the normal electrocardiogram is primarily caused by : PGI 1986, 93**
A. A slow transmission through the A-V node and junctional fibres
B. Delay at the internodal pathways
C. Circus movement
D. The slow rate of conduction in atrial heart muscle

138. **A stronger than normal heart may be observed during : AIIMS 1993**
A. Sympathetic stimulation
B. Myocardial ischemia
C. Stokes-Adams syndrome
D. Atrial fibrillation

139. **The heart is predisposed to ventricular fibrillation: AIIMS 1997**
A. When action potentials follow a short but circular pathway
B. During sinus bradycardia
C. If conduction velocity through the myocardium is decreased
D. All of the above

140. **In an electrocardiogram recorded from the standard limb leads, the QRS complex was smallest in lead-II. Also, it was prodominantly positive (R taller than S-wave) in lead-I and predominantly negative (R shorter than S-wave) in lead-III. The mean electrical axis of the heart in this case must be closed to : CSE 1998**
A. + 60 degrees B. + 90 degrees
C. +120 degrees D. -30 degrees

141. **Fourth heart sound is heard in : AIIMS 1986; UPSC 1994**
A. Early diastol B. Late diastole
C. Early systole D. Late systole

142. **PR interval is : Kerala 1998**
A. From the beginning of P to the end of R.
B. Time taken for the conduction of impulse through the atria & SV node.
C. Time taken for the impulse of travel across the AV node.
D. None

143. **Which one of the following effects in the heart would not be a result of increased vagal nerve activity : Delhi 1996**
A. Acetylcholine release at the nerve endings
B. Decreased S-T interval
C. Bradycardia
D. Hyperpolarization of the S-A node

144. **Increased venous return leads to increased cardiac output by way of the Frank-Starling mechanism. Which one of the following would not happen : DNB 1988, 96**
A. Increased end diastolic sarcomere length
B. Increased myocardial tension during systole
C. Increased stroke volume
D. Decreased end diastolic volume

145. **Just before atrial depolarization and contraction : PGI 1987, 92**
A. The heart is completely polarized
B. A period of diastasis occurs
C. The pulmonic valve is closed
D. All of the above

Ans.	128. C	129. B	130. D	131. B	132. D	133. A	134. A	135. A	136. D	137. A
	138. A	139. A	140. D	141. B	142. C	143. B	144. D	145. D		

146. A possible cause of sinus bradycardia is : Rohtak 1995

A. Complete heart block
B. Decreased sympathetic outflow
C. Atropine
D. Decreased vagal outflow
E. All of the above

147. All of the following factors increase cardiac output except : AMC 1993

A. Pregnancy in late stages
B. Histamine
C. Eating
D. Sitting from lying position

148. Sodium enters the cardiac cycle in : PGI 1983; Delhi 1987, 92

A. Repolarization B. Depolarization
C. Phase of relaxation D. End of cardiac cycle

149. With normal cardiac function, a 10mm. Hg change in which of the following pressures would have the greatest effect on cardiac output : PGI 1980, 95

A. Pressure in the carotid arteries
B. Pressure in the renal artery
C. Aortic pressure
D. Right atrial pressure

150. Pre-load include all, except : Rajasthan 1992

A. Muscle contractility B. Stroke volume
C. Peripheral resistance D. Force of contraction

151. Isovolumetric relaxation preceeds : PGI 1996

A. Ventricular ejection B. Ventricular relaxation
C. Atrial contraction D. Atrial relaxation

152. Isovolumetric contraction does not coincide with : PGI 1996

A. AV valves closure
B. Rise of volume
C. Ventricles contract
D. Little muscle shortening

153. Pulse pressure is : AIIMS 1993

A. 1/2 diastolic + 1/3 systolic
B. Diastolic + 1/2 systolic
C. 1/3 diastolic + 1/2 systolic
D. Systolic - diastolic BP

154. Left atrial filling pressure closely approximates : AIIMS 1993

A. CVP
B. Intra-cranial pressure
C. PCWP
D. Intra-pleural pressure

155. A prominent 'V' wave may suggest : PGI 1993

A. Atrial flutter with changing block
B. Ventricular septal defect
C. Tricuspid incontinence
D. Pulmonary hypertension

156. 1 Torr is approximately equal to ------- mm Hg : DNB 1992

A. 0. B. 1.0
C. 2.0 D. 7.2

157. Normal pH of arterial plasma is : DNB 1991

A. 7.10 B. 7.20
C. 7.33 D. 7.40

158. Which of the following statements is not true about right ventricular infarction : Karnataka 1994

A. Generally associated with inferior wall myocardial infarction.
B. JVP is raised.
C. Management includes fluid restriction.
D. Diagnosis is confirmed by right sided chest leads on ECG.

159. The P-wave of the ECG occurs : Karnataka 1994

A. At the beginning of Atrial contraction
B. After the Atrial contraction
C. At the beginning of the ventricular contraction
D. At the end of the ventricular contraction

160. Blood supply to splanchnic area is ↓ in exercise due to : AIIMS 1993

A. Venoconstriction with ↑ blood flow
B. Venodilatation with ↓ blood flow
C. Venodilatation with ↑ blood flow
D. Venodilatation with normal blood flow

161. Sympathetic stimulation causes all except : AIIMS 1993

A. ↑ HR B. ↑ contraction
C. ↑ refractory period D. ↑ conduction

162. A cardiac left to right shunt congenital defect becomes significant when pulmonary blood flow reaches a volume -------- times as great as systemic flow : AMU 1999

A. Same B. 1.5
C. 2 D. 2.5

163. Heart pumps out blood : AMU 1991

A. To provide nutrition to cells
B. To remove waste product from the body
C. To maintain temperature of the body
D. All of the above

164. In haemorrhagic shock, one would expect a decrease in all the following except : AMU 1989

A. Cardiac work B. Oxygen usage
C. Coronary flow D. Plasma PCO_2

165. Loss of blood volume by about 10% of total over the period of 20 minutes causes : Punjab 1994

A. ↓ BP, normal venous pressure (VP)
B. ↓ BP, ↓ VP
C. Normal BP, normal VP
D. Normal BP, ↓ VP

Ans.	146. B	147. D	148. B	149. D	150. C	151. B	152. B	153. D	154. C	155. C
	156. B	157. D	158. A	159. A	160. A	161. C	162. C	163. D	164. D	165. C

166. Baroreceptors signal at which B.P. (mm Hg) range: **AI 1994**

A. 0-150 B. 50-150
C. 0-250 D. 150-250

167. Regarding capillaries all are true except : **AI 1994**

A. Largest cross section area
B. Incapable of constricting in response to vitamins
C. Contain more blood than veins
D. Sustain tangential pressures

168. Slow blood transfusion over 3 hours, most blood will be pooled in : **AI 1994**

A. Veins B. Arteries
C. Capillaries D. Heart

169. Plateau phase of action potential is due to: **Assam 1995**

A. Na+ influx
B. K+ effux
C. Na+Ca2+slow channel
D. All of the above

170. True statement regarding diastasis is : **Rajasthan 1994**

A. It occurs during the emptying phase of ventricles.
B. Blood flow in this period is rapid.
C. Third heart sound coincides with this period.
D. A-V valve opens at the beginning of this period.

171. Inter-ventricular pressure is less than intra-atrial pressure in : **Rajasthan 1995**

A. Isometric contraction
B. Isometric relaxation
C. Maximum ejection phase
D. First rapid filling

172. Consider the statements : **TNPSC 1997**

I. Nodal Rhythm is the rhythmicity exhibited by Sinoatrial Node.
II. The velocity of conduction of cardiac impulse is maximum in Purkinje Tissue.
III. Conduction is delayed in ventricular hypertrophy.
IV. Determination of cardiac output is the useful test to study the conducting tissues of heart.

A. II, III correct B. I, II correct
C. I, II, III correct D. II, III, IV correct

173. Pacemaker potential : **CSE 1995**

A. Is in the form of plateau potential
B. Is due to a slow diastolic depolarization
C. Is a graded potential
D. Develops in the right atrial fibres

174. Cardiac muscle action potential is shown in the given diagram and its phases have been marked. Consider the following statements in this regard : **CSE 1995**

1. Phase-I is due to closure of Na+ channels and CI influence.
2. Phase-II is due to opening of Ca2+ channels and closure of K+ channels.
3. Phase-III is due to closure of Ca2+ channels and prolonged opening of K+ channels.
4. Phase-IV is due to opening of Na2+ channels and effux.

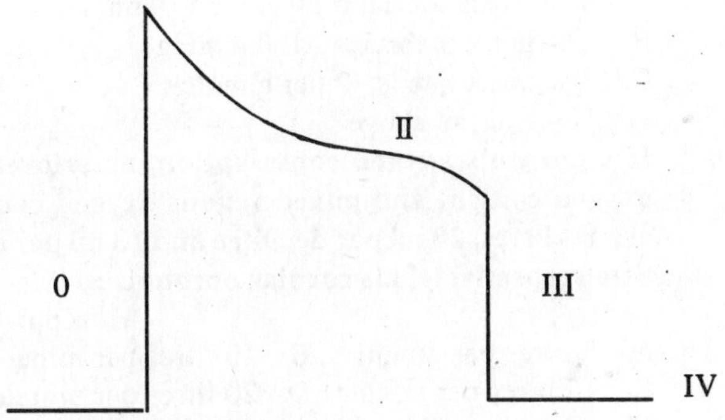

Of these statement :

A. 1 and 2 are correct B. 2 and 4 are correct
C. 1 and 3 are correct D. 2 and 3 are correct

175. Consider the following statement : **CSE 1995**

I Experimental hypertension can be produced to stimulating sinoaortic nerve.
II: Sino-aortic nerve normally stimulates vasomotor centre.

Of these statements :

A. I is true but II is false
B. Both I and II are true
C. I is false but II is true
D. Both I and II are false

176. Consider the following statements : **CSE 1996**

The mean electrical axis of the heart

1. Is about 60°
2. Is directed in ventricular hypertrophy
3. Deviates inventricular hypertrophy

A. 1 and 3 are correct
B. 2 and 3 are correct
C. 1 and 2 are correct
D. 1,2 and 3 are correct

177. Consider the following statements : **CSE 1996**

Cardiac output is increased by sympathetic stimulation due to :

1. Increased in the force of contraction
2. Increased in the heart rate
3. Starling's effect
4. Brainbridge reflex

Of these statements

A. 1 and 4 are correct
B. 1 and 2 are correct
C. 1,2 and 3 are correct
D. 2,3 and 4 are correct

Ans. **166. B** **167. C** **168. C** **169. C** **170. C** **171. D** **172. C** **173. A** **174. D** **175. B** **176. B** **177. D**

178. If the cardiac output, stroke volume, systolic arterial pressure, diastolic arterial pressure and right artrial pressure are 5 litres per minute, 50 ml, 140 mmHg, 80 mmHg and 0 mmHg respectively, which of the following statements is likely to be correct ? Manipal 1992

A. The mean arterial pressure is 110 mmHg
B. The pulse pressure is 100 mmHg
C. The heart rate is 72 per minute
D. None of the above

179. If a person's oxygen consumption, arteriovenous oxygen content and mixed venous oxygen content are 1.4 litres, 20 ml per decilitre and 13 ml per decilitre respectively, his cardiac output is : Manipal 1992

A. 5 litres per minute B. 10 litres per minute
C. 15 litres per minute D. 20 litres per minute

180. The absolute refractory period in the heart : Manipal 1995

A. Is that phase of the cardiac cycle when the heart does not respond to a stimulus, however strong.
B. Corresponds in time with the duration of the action potential.
C. Is longer than the refractory period in the skeletal muscle.
D. All of the above.

181. During cardiac cycle, the rate of increase in intraventricular pressure is the maximum in : CSE 1997

A. Rapid ejection
B. Rapid filling of ventricule
C. Isometric contraction
D. Reduced ejection

182. Consider the following statements : CSE 1997
The ECG record does not show the repolarization of auricle because it is hidden by the :

1. Repolarization of ventricles
2. Depolarization of auricles
3. Depolarization of ventricles
4. Inter-atrial septal depolarization

Of these statements

A. 1,2 and 4 are correct B. 1 and 4 are correct
C. 2 and 3 are correct D. 3 alone is correct

183. The correct sequence of the given electromechanical events as they occur during the cardiac cycle is: CSE 1998

A. 1st heart sound, QRS complex of EKG, c-wave of jugular pulse.
B. QRS complex of EKG, c-wave of jugular pulse, 1st heart sound.
C. C-wave of jugular pulse, 1st heart sound, QRS complex of EKG.
D. QRS complex of EKG, 1st heart sound, c-wave of jugular pulse.

184. Consider the following statements : CSE 1998
Major portion of ventricular filling

1. Is during rapid filling phase of ventricle
2. Occurs during atrial systole
3. Is possible even if atria fail as a pump

Of these statements :

A. 1,2 and 3 are correct B. 1 and 2 are correct
C. 2 and 3 are correct D. 1 and 3 are correct

185. In WPWS, there is an aberrant spread of impulses from : Kerala 1999

A. AV node to ventricle
B. Atria to ventricle
C. SA node to Bundle of His
D. Atrium to Bundle of His

186. Bradycardia in athletes is due to : Kerala 1999

A. Increased sympathetic action
B. Increased vagal tone
C. Decreased vagal tone
D. Decreased sympathetic tone

187. The feature of JVP in cardiac tamponade is : PGI 1999

A. Prominent x descent with prominent 'y' descent
B. Prominent x descent with absent 'y' descent
C. Absent x descent with prominent 'y' descent
D. Absent x descent with absent 'y' descent

188. Which of the following event is represented by the 'P' wave of the E.C.G. : Orissa 1998

A. S.A. node depolarisation
B. A.V. node depolarisation
C. Atrial muscle depolarisation
D. Bundle of His depolarisation

189. Which of the following are associated with papillary muscles of the heart ? CSE 1999

1. Helping the a-v valves to close
2. Preventing excessive bulging of a-v valves into atria
3. U wave of the ECG
4. Helping the a-v valves to open

Select the correct answer using the codes given below:
Codes :

A. 2 and 4 B. 3 and 4
C. 1 and 3 D. 1 and 2

190. Sudden drop in systemic B.P. occurs at : MAHE 1999

A. Arteries B. Arterioles
C. Capillaries D. Veins

191. When BP increased in carotid sinus it causes : MAHE 1999

A. Decreased vagal tone
B. Decreased sympathetic discharge to heart
C. Increased vagal tone
D. None of the above

Ans.	178. D	179. D	180. D	181. A	182. D	183. D	184. D	185. B	186. B	187. B
	188. C	189. A	190. B	191. C						

192. The natural anticoagulant in the animal body is : TNPSC 1998

A. Heparin B. Hyaluronidase
C. Vitamin-K D. Dicumarol

193. Loss of blood more than 500 ml is sensed by : TNPSC 1998

A. Carotid baroreceptors
B. Atrial receptors
C. Juxtaglomerular apparatis
D. All of the above

194. Proto-diastole : TNPSC 1998

A. Precedes isovolumic contraction
B. Follows isovolumic contraction
C. Precedes isovolumic relaxation
D. Follows isovolumic relaxation

195. Lowest myocardial O2 consumption is required for: TNPSC 1998

A. Pressure work B. Volume work
C. Electrical activity D. Basal needs

196. Consider the statements : TNPSC 1998

The normal blood pressure response to standing is :

I. Slight decrease in systolic pressure
II. Slight increase in diastolic pressure
III. Slight increase in mean pressure
IV. No change

Of the statements choose the correct answer :

A. I alone is correct
B. I and II are correct
C. I, II and III are correct
D. All are correct

197. False statement regarding blood pressure is : TNPSC 1998

A. Pulse pressure is the difference between systolic and diastolic pressures.
B. Mean pressure is the average of systolic and diastolic pressures.
C. Cuff method underestimates true systolic pressure.
D. Cuff method underestimates true diastolic pressure when phase-V is taken as the end point.

198. Palpable pulsus alternans indicates a systolic pressure difference of at least : TNPSC 1998

A. 10 mm Hg B. 16 mm Hg
C. 21 mm Hg D. 25 mm Hg

199. One of the following is true about A-V node blood supply : TNPSC 1998, 2000

A. Right coronary artery—60%
B. Left coronary artery—40%
C. Both coronaries
D. None is true

200. Which of the following is properly matched : TNPSC 1998

A. Pacemaker of heart - Venous Return
B. Vasomotor centre - Vagus nerve
C. Stokes Adam Syndrome - Tachycardia
D. Peripheral Resistance - Arterioles

201. Ventricular mechanoreceptor is stimulated by: UP 1999

A. Hypervolumia B. Valsalva manoeuver
C. Hypovolumia D. Acidosis

202. In lying position : TNPSC 2000

A. Heart rate is decreases
B. Venous return increases
C. Cerebral blood flow is unchanged
D. All of these

203. Myocardial blood flow to the left ventricle increase in all of the following except : TNPSC 2000

A. Early systole
B. Myocardial hypoxia
C. Adenosine infusions
D. Stimulation of sympathetic nerves to the heart

204. Which of the following inhibits vasomotor center? Kerala 2000

A. Hypercapnia
B. Stimulation of baroreceptors
C. Stimulation of chemoreceptors
D. Anger and excitement
E. Hypoxia

205. Single most important factor in control of automatic contractility : AI 2001

A. End diastolic volume
B. Right atrial volume
C. SA node pacemaker potential
D. Sympathetic stimulation

206. Which is true about measurement of BP with sphygnomonmeter : AI 2001

A. Less than intravascular pressure
B. More than intravascular pressure
C. Equal to IVP
D. Depend upon blood flow

207. All of the following is correct regarding capillaries except : AI 2001

A. Greatest surface area
B. Least diameter
C. Contains more blood than veins
D. Least responsive to epinephrine

208. Which of the following regulates the fine control of blood pressure : Delhi 2001

A. Medulla B. Hypothalamus
C. Midbrain D. Median eminence

Ans. 192. A 193. D 194. B 195. B 196. C 197. B 198. A 199. C 200. D 201. B 202. D 203. D 204. B 205. C 206. A 207. C 208. A

209. Cardiac output is increased by receptors : **DNB 2001**

A. Chronotropic B. Inotropic
C. Both D. None

210. Correct about first heart sound is : **Kerala 2001**

A. S1 shorter than S2
B. S1 frequency lower than S2
C. Due to closure of semilunar valves
D. Due to start of systole

211. The work done by left ventricle is greater than of right ventricle because : **JIPMER 2002**

A. LV has thick wall
B. ↑ preload
C. Increased afterload
D. Increased stroke volume

212. Beta-II receptors are found in : **SGPGI 2002**

A. Arterioles B. Veins
C. SA node D. Myocardium

213. Increased blood pressure mediates reflex bradycardia through impulses in all the following nerves except : **SGPGI 2002**

A. Accessory cervical B. Nerve of Herrings
C. Glossopharyngeal D. Vagus

214. EPSP in cardiac muscle is maintained by : **A.P.-2002; AI 2003**

A. Mg2+ B. K+
C. Ca2- D. Na+

215. False about ECG in hyperkalemia is : **BHU-2002**

A. Peaked P-wave
B. Peaked T-wave
C. QRS
D. Decreased QT

216. Cardiac output measured by thermodilution technique is unreliable in all of the following situations except : **AI 2003**

A. Ventricular septal defect
B. Tricuspid regurgitation
C. Low cardiac output
D. Pulmonary regurgitation

217. During the cardiac cycle the opening of the aortic valve takes place at the : **AI 2004**

A. Beginning of systole
B. End of isovolumetric contraction
C. End of diastole
D. End of systole

218. All of the following factors normally increase the length of the ventricular cardiac muscle fibres except : **AI 2005**

A. Increased venous tone
B. Increased total blood volume
C. Increased negative intrathoracic pressure
D. Lying-to-standing change in posture

219. S.A. node acts as a pacemaker of the heart because of the fact that it : **AI 2005**

A. Is capable in generating impulses spontaneously
B. Has rich sympathetic innervations
C. Has poor cholinergic innervations
D. Generates impulses at the highest rate

220. Spike is seen in electric discharge from : **PGI 1994**

A. SA node B. Atria
C. Ventricle D. All of the above

221. The pressure (mm Hg) in left ventricle diastole is : **PGI 1986; Delhi 1990**

A. 0 B. 25
C. 80 D. 120

222. Wenckebach phenomenon is : **Delhi 1996**

A. PR interval prolongation followed by dropped QRS interval
B. Sharp QRS complex
C. ST interval prolongation
D. Multiple extra systoles

223. A continuous murmur over manubrium is likely due to : **PGI 1984; Delhi 1985, 97**

A. AS B. MS
C. AR D. PDA

224. Major part of total peripheral resistance is provided by : **AIIMS 1996**

A. Venules B. Capillaries
C. Arterioles D. Small arteries

225. Velocity of blood flow is inversely proportional to: **AIIMS 1996**

A. Viscosity B. Flow
C. Cross-sectional area D. Length

226. Diastolic pressure is mainly determined by: **AIIMS 1996**

A. Capillary permeability
B. Venous capacitance
C. Venous elasticity
D. Peripheral resistance

227. The resistance of a blood vessel is 16 PRU. Doubling the vessel diameters would change the resistance to : **AIIMS 1999**

A. 1 PRU B. 2 PRU
C. 8 PRU D. 12 PRU

228. For cardiac muscle, Vmax can be used as a measure of : **AIIMS 1996**

A. Excitability B. Contractility
C. Rhythmicity D. Conductivity

229. Sympathetic stimulation of which vessels causes the greatest increase in total peripheral resistance? **PGI 1996**

A. Veins B. Venules
C. Capillaries D. Arterioles

Ans.									
209. A	210. B	211. C	212. A	213. A	214. C	215. A	216. C	217. B	218. D
219. D	220. D	221. A	222. A	223. D	224. C	225. C	226. D	227. A	228. C
229. D									

230. **Major blood reservoirs of the body include all of the following except : AIIMS 1997**
A. Thoracic vena cava
B. Liver sinuses
C. Major abdominal veins
D. Venous plexus of the skin

231. **Which of the following is probably most important mediating angiotensin induced long-term elevation of arterial blood pressure? PGI 1990**
A. Simulation of aldosterone secretion
B. Constriction of non-renal peripheral artherioles
C. Increased sympathetic stimulation
D. Renal effect to decrease sodium and water excretion

232. **Cardiac output is normally controlled primarily by the : PGI 1991**
A. Need of the tissues for blood
B. Right atrial pressure
C. Mean systemic pressure
D. Venous resistance

233. **In gross -osteum secundum ASD, increased work is done by : WB 2007**
A. Left atrium B. Left ventricle
C. Right atrium D. Right ventricle

234. **True about blood pressure measurement is all/except : AIIMS 2007**
A. Cuff width should be 40% of arm circumference.
B. Diastolic blood pressure is indicated by fourth Korotkoff sound.
C. Small cuff measures spuriously elevated Diastolic blood pressure.
D. Monkenberg sclerosis causes pseudohypertension.

235. **Heart muscle, true are all except : AI 2007**
A. Act as syncitium
B. Has multiple nuclei
C. Has ap junctions
D. Has branching

236. **Which of the following adaptations will be apt to increase the work capacity at high altitude : AI 2007**
A. Increasing workload, decreasing duration of exercise
B. Increasing workload, increasing duration of exercise
C. Decreasing workload, increasing duration of exercise
D. Decreasing workload, decreasing duration of exercise

Ans. 230. A 231. D 232. C 233. D 234. B 235. B 236. C

EXPLANATIONS OF CVS

1. Ans.— A **Coronary blood flow is directly related to perfusion pressure and inversely related to resistance.**

Coronary blood flow, like blood flow in any other organ is directly related to the perfusion pressure and inversely related to resistance.

2. Ans.— A **V. cholera**

Cholera is the best known bacterial secretory diarrhea. Its enterotoxin stimulates cyclic adenosine monophosphate in the enterocyte, which promotes salt and water secretion.

3. Ans.— D **Measures total tension**

* When muscles contract (possibly due to the stretch reflex), they produce tension at the point where the muscle is connected to the tendon, where the golgi tendon organ is located.
* The golgi tendon organ records the change in tension, and the rate of change of the tension, and sends signals to the spine to convey this information.
* When this tension exceeds a certain threshold, it triggers the lengthening reaction which inhibits the muscles from contracting and causes them to relax. Other names for this reflex are the inverse myotatic reflex, autogenic inhibition, and the clasped-knife reflex.
* This basic function of the golgi tendon organ helps to protect the muscles, tendons, and ligaments from injury.
* The lengthening reaction is possible only because the signalling of golgi tendon organ to the spinal cord is powerful enough to overcome the signalling of the muscle spindles telling the muscle to contract.

4. Ans. — A **Active transport**

Transport of substances through the cell membrane

* Cell membrane is a lipid bilayer that allows the diffusion of only water and lipid soluble substances (O_2, N_2 & CO_2) through it.
* Lipid bilayer is impermeable to most essential molecules and ions. These are transported inside the cell with the help of transport proteins.
* These transport proteins are of two types:

1. Ion channels—Some transport proteins provide watery spaces all the way through the molecule. This allows free movement of water as well as selected ions or molecules through them.
2. Carrier proteins—These carrier proteins bind with molecules or ions that are to be transported and then changes its configuration. This confirmational change in the carrier protein transports the substance across the membrane.

Transport by carrier proteins are of 2 types :

a. Faciliated diffusion - When carrier protein moves substances in the direction of their chemical or electrical gradient. Here no energy input is required e.g. glucose transport by glucose transporter, which moves glucose down its conc. gradient from the ECF to cytoplasm of cell.

b. Active transport - When carrier protein trnasports substance against their electrical and chemical gradients. This form of transport requires energy.

In man this energy is provided by hydrolysis of ATP therefore active transport proteins are ATPases, the most important of which is Na^+, K^+ ATPase also k/a Na^+ - K^+ pump.

5. Ans.— C **Ca^{++}**

* Second messengers are molecules that relay signals received at receptors on the cell surface (such as the arrival of protein hormones, growth factors, etc.) to target molecules in the cytosol and/or nucleus.
* Not only they relay the signals, they greatly amplify the strength of the signal.

* There are three major classes of second messengers.
  1. Cyclic nucleotides (e.g. cAMP & cGMP)
  2. Products of membrane phospholipid breakdown-inasitol trisphosphate (IP3) and diacylglycerol (DAG)
  3. Calcium ions

* Calcium ions are probably the most widely used second messengers.

6. Ans.— D Increased cardiac muscle mass

* Guyton writes :
  "Normally, the voltages in the three standard bipolar limb leads, as measured form the peak of the R-wave to the bottom of the S-wave, vary between 0.5 to 2.0 millivolts, with lead III usually recording the lowest voltage and lead II the highest.
  - In general when the sum of the voltages of all the QRS complexes of the three standard leads is greater than 4 millivolts the patient is considered to have a high voltage electrocardiogram.
  - The cause of high-voltage QRS complexes most often is increased muscle mass of the heart which is ordinary than 4 millivolts the patient is considered to have a high voltage electrocardiogram.
  - The cause of high-voltage QRS complexes most often is increased muscle mass of the heart, which ordinary results from hypertrophy of the muscle is response to excessive load on one part of the heart or the other . The increased quantity of muscle causes generation of increased quantities of electricity around the heart. As a result, the electrical potentials recorded in the electrocardiographic leads are considerably greater than normal"

* It is not able to differentiate whether it is right or left heart hypertrophy.

7. Ans.— D The cerebral arterial pressure rises.

Because of rapid changes in velocity and direction of motion in aeroplanes several types of acceleratory forces often effect the body during flight.

When a man is simply sitting in his seat, the force with which he is pressing against the seat results from the pull of gravity and is equal to his weight.

The intensity of this force is said to be + 1G.

If this force increases, it becomes more positive.

If the airoplane goes through an outside loop so that the man is held down by his seat belt, negative G is applied to his body

Effects of Negative and Positive-G

	Positive-G		Negative-G
1.	Blood is centrifuged loward the lower limbs, veins increases	1.	Blood is centrifuged towards the head, so that the cerebral blood pressure can rise.
2.	Cardiac out put decreases	2.	Cardiac out put increases
3.	Black out of vision occurs	3.	Red out occurs

8. Ans.— D Lying to standing change in posture :

When a person moves from a supine position to standing position a significant volume of blood pools in the lowe extremity because of high compliance of veins and venous return decreases. As a result of decreased venous return the length of ventricular cardiac muscle fibres is decreased and in accordance with 'Frank-Sterling relationship' the stroke volume and cardiac output decreaes.

9. Ans.— D Generates impulses at the highest rate :

"The sinus node controls the beat of the heart because its rate of discharge is greater than that of any other part of the heart. Therefore, the sinus node is the pacemaker of the heart" - Guyton

Although, the AV node and Purkinje fibres are also capable of generating impulses spontaneously, it is the sinus node which controls the hearts rhythmicity and acts as the pacemaker of the heart.

This is attributed to the fact that the discharge rate of the SA node is considerable faster than the natural self-excitatory discharge of either the AV node or the Purkinje fibres. Each time the sinus node discharges its impulse is conducted into both, the AV node and Purkinje fibres and discharges their excitable membranes. Then these tissues as well as the sinus node recover and start almost at the same time, but the sinus node discharges again much more rapidly and discharges the AV node & Purkinje fibres again before they can reach their own threshold for self-excitation.

10. Ans.— D There is fall in systemic capillary hydrostatic pressure :

Edema normally occurs due to increased hydrostatic pressure that pushes fluid out or due to reduced oncotic pressure that fails to pull the fluid.

'Acute heart failure is usually predominantly systolic and sudden reduction in cardiac output often results in systemic hypotensin without peripheral edema' — *Harrison 15th /321*

Acute heart failure is thus associated with a fall in hydrostatic pressure and not an increase, and therefore explains lack of peripheral edema.

Peripheral edema appears later consequent to fluid retention by the kidney a renal compensation'.

11. Ans.— B End of isovolumetric contraction :

Beginning of systole	AV valves close
End of isovolumetric contraction	Semiulnar valves open
End of diastole	AV valves close
End of diastasis	AV valves are open and semiulnar valves are closed

12. Ans.— A The lying down position

The confounding variable in this question is 'gravity'. Gravity is present on earth but is not present in space.

So, we have to take the B.P. in a position which sort of nulifies the effect of gravity on earth.

The best position is the lying down position because then the whole body is at the same height with respect to the heart.

13. Ans.— C Both recorded as increase in MBP

Carotid sinus contain baro-receptors which fire at increasing frequency when the B.P. rises.

The baro-receptor discharge inhibits the tonic discharge of vasoconstrictor nerves and excites the vagal innervation of heart, both producing a drop in blood pressure.

Thus, if the nerve from these baro-receptors is severed, the inhibitory effect on vasoconstrictor nerves in removed. This will lead to an increase in mean blood pressure.

Note : However, that the baroreceptors do not fire when mean B.P. is below 30 mm Hg. (Fire maximally at mean B.P. of 150 mm Hg.)

Thus, if the nerve is severed when the mean B.P. is below 30 mm Hg. There would not be any effect seen since technically these baroreceptors are already shut off.

However, in our question, both Vineet and Kamlesh severed the nerve when the mean B.P. was above 30 mm Hg.

Therefore, in both cases, the baroreceptors were already firing and by severing the nerve, this inhibitory impulse was stopped. Thus, mean blood pressure will rise in both cases.

Note : Severing only the carotid sinus nerve will not lead to drastic increases in B.P. because the Aortic arch baroreceptors are still functional & will prevent excessive rise in B.P. However, if both carotid body & Aortic arch receptors are disconnected, the B.P. rises to more than 200-300 mm Hg.

14. Ans.— B. Rate of release of adenosine from the myocardium

15. Ans.— B. Nucleus ambiguous

16. Ans.— A. Right

17. Ans.— A. Ist heart sound

18. Ans.— E. P-wave on ECG

19. Ans.— D. Beginning of T-waves

20. Ans.— C. 3rd Heart sound

21. Ans.— B. 2nd Heart sound

22. Ans.— C. Ca++

23. Ans.— C. 25-32 mm Hg

24. Ans.— C. 19.4 ml/100 ml

Gas content of blood is

ml/dL of blood containing 15 gm of Hemoglobin

Arterial blood	**Venous blood**
(PO2 95 mm Hg	(PO2-40 mm Hg)
PCO2 40 mm HG	PCO2 - 46 mmHg
Hb-97% saturate)	Hb - 75% saturated

Gas	Dissolved	Combined	Dissolved	Combined
O2	0.29	19.5	0.12	15.1
CO2	2.62	46.4	2.98	49.7
N2	0.98	0	0.98	0

25. Ans. — A. Opening of slow calcium channels

26. Ans. — C. Mean stroke volume

Cardiac output in a resting supine man is 5L/min (stroke vol (70mL) X Heart rate (72/min) and stroke volume is 70 mL. The output per sqm of body surface is cardiac index (which is 3.2L).

27. Ans. — C. 60-70 cc

28. Ans. — D. Ventricular fibers

29. Ans. — A. 32 cms/sec.

Normal arm to tongue circulation is 15 sec.

30. Ans. — B. PR interval

31. Ans. — B. Unipolar chest leads

32. Ans. — C. A.V. conduction time

33. Ans. — C. Arterial pressures

34. Ans. — B. Hints at serious heart ailment

35. Ans. — C. Commonly pulse not visible with normal heart

36. Ans. — D. Larger arteries in healthy adults

Murmurs are not seen in healthy adults.

37. Ans. — B. Low haematocrit

38. Ans. — C. Elevated PO2 in pulmonary artery

39. Ans. — A. Vit.-K deficiency

Vit-K deficiency causes bleeding.

40. Ans. — A. Purkinje fibres

41. Ans. — A. Ventricular septal defect, if a loud diastolic murmur is heard

42. Ans. — C. 5th intercostal space to left of sternum

43. Ans. — D. Closure of tricuspid valves

44. Ans. — C. Sinoartrial node

45. Ans. — A. A-V node

46. Ans. — A. Increased myocardial conduction velocity

47. Ans. — A. The PQ interval to increase

48. Ans. — B. 2.0 meters/sec

49. Ans. — B. Ventricular repolarization

50. Ans. — A. ↑ Pressure in both atria

51. Ans. — A. Not necessarily increases with heart rate

If stroke volume falls, the rise in heart rate can not increase cardiac output.

52. Ans. C. Isovolumetric contraction

53. Ans. A. Auricular contraction

54. Ans. B. Cardiac output and surface area

55. Ans. B. Ventricular depolarization

Normal QRS interval is 0.08 sec. (range upto 0.10 sec). It reflects ventricular depolarization and atrial repolarization.

56. Ans. — D. Arterial turbulance

The cuff pressure at which the sounds are first heard is the systolic pressure. As the cuff pressure is lowered further, the sounds become louder, then dull and muffled, finally, in most individuals, they disappear. These are sounds of Korotkoff. However, in adults after exercise and in children, the diastolic pressure correlates best with the pressure at which the sounds becomes muffled. This is also true in diseases such as hyper-thyroidism and aortic insufficiency.

57. Ans. — A. Ventricular pressure exceeds aortic pressure

58. Ans. — C. Cardiac work

In over 90% of patients, the cause is unknown. When the resistance against the left ventricle must pump (after load) is elevated for a prolonged period, the cardiac muscle hypertrophies (which carry a poor prognosis.

59. Ans. — B. Shift the electrical axis to involved side

There is shift in electrical axis to the involved side.

60. Ans. — E. All of the above

61. Ans. — C. Distensibility

Pulse pressure is difference between the systolic and diastolic pressure, which is normally about 50 mm Hg.

Mean pressure is the average pressure throughout the cardiac cycle. Pulse pressure falls slightly in medium and large sized vessels but rapidly in small arteries and arterioles. The magnitude of fall of pressure depends on whether the arterioles or vessels are constricted or dilated.

62. Ans. — D. All of the above

63. Ans. — A. Decreased rate of S.A. node

This is due to baro-receptors.

64. Ans. — C. Reflex bradycardia

65. Ans. — C. Occurs just after in carotid artery

'a' wave seen in jugular pulse and is due to atrial systole.

66. Ans. — C. Isovolumetric contraction

First heart sound is a low, lightly prolonged 'lub' caused by vibrations set up by sudden closure of mitral or tricuspid, valves at the start or ventricular systole.

67. Ans.— A. Modified muscle fibres

68. Ans.— D. Ventricles typically contract at about 30-40 beats/min

69. Ans.— C. When decrease in parasympathetic nerve activity

70. Ans.— A. Rise in atrial pressure and rise in ventricular pressure

71. Ans.— B. Has higher frequency

72. Ans.— B. AV node

Conduction speed (m/s) of various cardiac tissues are SA node (0.05), AV node (0.05), atrial pathways (1.0), Bundle of His (1.0), Purkinje system (1.0) and ventricular muscle (1.0)

73. Ans.— C. No action potential from another part of heart will reexcite the heart muscle

74. Ans.— D. Coincident with 2nd heart sound

75. Ans.— B. Wrong with S-A node

SA node is pacemaker of the heart.

76. Ans.— B. Carotid sinus pressoreceptors

77. Ans.— A. Produces 3rd heart sound in some healthy persons

78. Ans.— D. Receive nutrition through vasa vasorum which arises from veins

79. Ans.— B. Increases when myocardial hypoxia

80. Ans.— B. 0.8

Duration of cardiac cycle (at heart rate of 75/min) is 0.80 sec (and at heart rate of 200/min, it is 0.30) out of which duration of systole is 0.27 sec and diastole is 0.53 sec.

81. Ans.— C. 40

82. Ans.— C. Begin at AV node

83. Ans.— C. Apex with axis of 180°

It is due to baroreceptors.

84. Ans.— C. Reflex bradycardia

85. Ans.— C. S3

86. Ans.— D. Bezold-Jarisch reflex

87. Ans.— D. Delay in closure of pulmonary valves

88. Ans.— D. Rate of impulse formation

89. Ans.— C. 60°

90. Ans.— C. 5.25

Under normal conditions (rest), cardiac output is 4.7 L and in exercise, it may rise upto 22L approximately.

91. Ans.— B. Increased when myocardial hypoxia

92. Ans.— D. Rate and blood pressure

93. Ans.— A. 250

94. Ans.— A. Foetus

Heart rate falls in sleep and rises by emotion, exercise, fever and other stimuli.

95. Ans.— A. 4-5%

96. Ans.— D. T

97. Ans.— C. 0.08-0.1 sec.

98. Ans.— D. Base of left ventricle

99. Ans.— C. Apex of heart

100. Ans.— C. No cardiac abnormality

101. Ans.— D. Increased parasympathetic tone to SA node

102. Ans.— C. Parasympathetic tone to AV node

103. Ans.— D. a+b

Ventricular depolarisation and atrial repolarization are seen in QRS complex (average 0.08 sec) whereas ventricular depolarization plus ventricular repolarization are indicated by QT interval (average 0.40 sec). ST interval (average 0.40 sec.) (QT minus QRS) indicates ventricular repolarisation (average 0.32 sec).

104. Ans.— C. Saltatory conduction

105. Ans.— C. Quinidine administration

106. Ans.— D. Q wave - 0.10 sec.

107. Ans.— A. Aortic insufficiency and stenosis

108. Ans.— C. Free fatty acids

The supply of free fatty acis (FFA) is regulated by two bipasses-lipoprotein lipase (which hydrolyses triglycerides in chylomirons and VLDL, providing FFA and glycerol) and intracellular hormone sensitive lipase of adipose tissue.

109. Ans.— C. Beginning of atrial contraction

110. Ans.— C. 35 5 60

111. Ans.— C. Begins in apical epicardium

112. Ans.— B. ↓ BP ↓ HR

113. Ans.— A. Inspiration

114. Ans.— B. ↓ K^+ permeability

115. Ans.— A. Failure of conduction in AV node

116. Ans.— NONE

Question is wrongly framed

117. Ans.— C. End diastolic volume

Starling's law of the heart or Frank Starling law is that energy of contraction is proportional to the initial length of the cardiac muscle fiber"., (i.e. the extent of the preload) is proportionate to the end of diastolic volume. The relation between ventricular stroke volume and end-diastolic volume is called Frank Starling curve.

118. Ans. — C. 250 ml/min
119. Ans. — A. Ca^+
120. Ans. — B. 25
121. Ans. — A. Right coronary artery
122. Ans. — C. Newtonian flow
123. Ans. — D. None of the above
124. Ans. — D. T
125. Ans. — D. Just after T-waves
They are seen in hypokalemia
126. Ans. — B. Cardiac output work
127. Ans. — A. 0.15, 30
128. Ans. — C. Exercise
129. Ans. — B. 3.2
130. Ans. — D. Fourth
131. Ans. — B. Grief
132. Ans. — D. Hypoxia
133. Ans. — A. 0.12, 50
134. Ans. — A. Increases the heart rate
Rapid infusion of blood or saline in anaesthesized initial animals sometimes produces a rise in heart rate. If heart rate is low. The effect was decribed by Bainbridge in 1915 is called Bainbridge reflex.
135. Ans. — A. 0.1 sec.
136. Ans. — D. Atrial fibrillation
137. Ans. — A. A slow transmission through the A-V node and junctional fibres
138. Ans. — A. Sympathetic stimulation
139. Ans. — A. When action potentials follow a short but circular pathway
140. Ans. — D. -30 degrees
141. Ans. — B. Late diastole
142. Ans. — C. Time taken for the impulse of travel across the AV node
Normal PR interval is 0.18 sec (range 0.12 to 0.20 sec.) and reflect atrial depolarization and conduction through AV-node.
143. Ans. — B. Decreased S-T interval
144. Ans. — D. Decreased end diastolic volume
145. Ans. — D. All of the above
146 Ans. — B. Decreased sympathetic outflow
147. Ans. — D. Sitting from lying position
148. Ans. — B. Depolarization
149. Ans. — D. Right atrial pressure
150. Ans. — C. Peripheral resistance
151. Ans. — B. Ventricular relaxation
152. Ans. — B. Rise of volume
153. Ans. — D. Systolic - diastolic BP
Normal pulse pressure is 50 mm Hg.
154. Ans. — C. PCWP
155. Ans. — C. Tricuspid incontinence
156. Ans. — B. 1.0
157. Ans. — D. 7.40
158. Ans. — A. Generally associated with inferior wall myocardial infarction
159. Ans. — A. At the beginning of Atrial contraction
160. Ans. — A. Venoconstriction with ↑ blood flow
161. Ans. — C. ↑ refractory period
Refractory period does not increase with sympathetic stimulation (but may rather fall).
162. Ans. — C. 2
163. Ans. — D. All of the above
164. Ans. — D. Plasma PCO_2
165. Ans. — C. Normal BP, normal VP
166. Ans. — B. 50-150
167. Ans. — C. Contain more blood than veins
168. Ans. — C. Capillaries

Characteristics of various types of blood vessels in humans

Vessel	Lumen diameter	Wall thickness	Approx. Total cross-sectional area	% of blood volume contain
Aorta	2.5 cm	2 mm	4.5	2
Artery	0.4 cm	1 mm	20	8
Arteriole	40 µm	20µm	400	1
Capillary	5 µm	1µm	4500	5
Venule	20 µm	2 µm	4000	54
Vein	0.5 cm	0.5 µm	40	
Vena cava	3 cm	1.5 mm	18	

In systemic vessels, there is an additional 12% in the heart and 18% in pulmonary circular.

169. Ans. — C. Na+Ca2+slow channel
170. Ans. — C. Third heart sound coincides with this period
171. Ans. — D. First rapid filling
172. Ans. — C. I, II, III correct
173. Ans. — A. Is in the form of plateau potential
174. Ans. — D. 2 and 3 are correct
175. Ans. — B. Both I and II are true
176. Ans. — B. 2 and 3 are correct
The normal direction of mean QRS vector is generally - 30 to 110 degrees. Mean QRS vector is called electrical axis of heart.

177. Ans. — D. 2,3 and 4 are correct

178. Ans. — D. None of the above

179. Ans. — D. 20 litres per minute

180. Ans. — D. All of the above

During phases 0-2 and about half of phase 3 (until the membrane potential reaches approximately -50 mV during repolarization), cardiac muscle cannot be excited again which is called absolute refractory period. It remains relatively refractory until phase 4.

181. Ans. — A. Rapid ejection

182. Ans. — D. 3 alone is correct

183. Ans. — D. QRS complex of EKG, 1st heart sound, c-wave of jugular pulse

184. Ans. — D. 1 and 3 are correct

185. Ans. — B. Atria to ventricle

In WPWS, there is accelerated AV-conduction. There is additional aberrant muscular or nodal tissue connection (bundle of knet) between atrial and ventricals. There is short PR interval, prolonged. QRS deflection slow on the uptake with normal PJ interval (short of P-wave to end of QRS complex)

186. Ans. — B. Increased vagal tone

187. Ans. — B. Prominent x descent with absent 'y' descent

188. Ans. — C. Atrial muscle depolarisation

189. Ans. — A. 2 and 4

190. Ans. — B. Arterioles

191. Ans. — C. Increased vagal tone

192. Ans. — A. Heparin

193. Ans. — D. All of the above

194. Ans. — B. Follows isovolumic contraction

195. Ans. — B. Volume work

196. Ans. — C. I, II and III are correct

197. Ans. — B. Mean pressure is the average of systolic and diastolic pressures

198. Ans. — A. 10 mm Hg

199. Ans. — C. Both coronaries

200. Ans. — D. Peripheral Resistance- Arterioles

201. Ans. — B. Valsalva manoeuver

Valsalva maneuver is initial treatment for PAT (Paroxysmal atrial tachycardia) and now electrical ablation is also used.

202. Ans. — D. All of these

203. Ans. — D. Stimulation of sympathetic nerves to the heart

204. Ans. — B. Stimulation of baroreceptors

Baroreceptors are stretch receptors in the walls of heart and blood vessels. The carotid sinus and aortic arch receptors monitor the arterial circulation.

205. Ans. — C. SA node pacemaker potential

206. Ans. — A. Less than intravascular pressure

207. Ans. — C. Contains more blood than veins

208. Ans. — A. Medulla

209. Ans. — A. Chronotropic

210. Ans. — B. S1 frequency lower than S2

211. Ans. — C. Increased afterload

212. Ans. — A. Arterioles

213. Ans. — A. Accessory cervical

214. Ans. — C. Ca2-

Calcium is importent for EPSP

215. Ans. — A. Peaked P-wave

In hyperkalemia, there is no evidence of atrial activity. QRS complex is broad and slurred and QRS complex is about 0.2s. Slender peaked T-waves are also seen.

216. Ans. — C. Low cardiac output

In contrast to the Flick method, the indicator dilution method is least reliable when the cardiac output is low.

217. Ans. — B. End of isovolumetric contraction

At the end of isovolumetric contraction, aortic and pulmonary valves open

Mitral and Tricuspid valve close

↓

Isovolumic or Isometric contraction

↓

Aortic and pulmonary valve open

Aortic and pulmonary valve close

↓

Isovolumic or isometric relaxation

↓

Mitral and Tricuspid valve open

↓

Events of the cardiac cycle at a heart rate of 75 beats/min. The phases of the cardiac cycle identified by the numbers at the bottom are as follows: 1. atrial systole; 2. isovolumetric ventricular contraction; 3. ventricular ejection; 4. isovolumetric ventricular relaxation; 5. ventricular filling.

218. Ans. — D. Lying-to-standing change in posture

Factors Affecting the Length of Ventricular Cardiac Muscle Fibers

	Increase		Decrease
1.	↑ Stronger atrial contraction	1.	Standing*
2.	↑ Total blood volume	2.	↓ intracardiac pressure
3.	↑ Venous tone	3.	↓ Ventricular compliance
4.	↑ Pumping action of skeletal muscle		
5.	↑ Negative intrathoracic pressure		

* Sitting or standing from lying position causes 20-30% Decrease in cardiac output.

219. Ans. — D. Generates impulses at the highest rate

"The SA node normally discharges most rapidly, depolarisation spreading from it to the other regions before they discharge spontaneously. The SA node is therefore the normal cardiac pacemaker, its rate of discharge determining the rate at which heart beats."

220. Ans.— D. All of the above

221. Ans.— A. 0

222. Ans.— A. PR interval prolongation followed by dropped QRS interval

223. Ans.— D. PDA

224. Ans.— C. Arterioles

225. Ans.— C. Cross-sectional area

Velocity (V) is proportional to flow (Q) divided by the area of the conduct (A)

$$V = \frac{Q}{A}$$

226. Ans.— D. Peripheral resistance

227. Ans. — A. 1 PRU

228. Ans.— C. Rhythmicity

229. Ans.— D. Arterioles

230. Ans.— A. Thoracic vena cava

231. Ans.— D. Renal effect to decrease sodium and water excretion

232. Ans. — C. Mean systemic pressure

Conditions affecting cardiac output are— *Increase*- anxiety and excitement (50-100%), eating (30%), exercise (upto 700%), high environmental temperature, pregnancy, epinephrine]; *Decrease* [sitting or standing from lying position (20-30%), rapid arrythmias, heart disease]; no change (sleep, moderate changes in environmental temperature).

233. Ans.— D Right ventricle

It is the most common type. It occurs in 10% of patients with congenital heart disease. It common in females.

234. Ans.— B Diastolic blood pressure is indicated by fourth Korotkoff sound.

* Spuriously high blood pressure is noted in :

1. Small cuff
2. Obesity
3. Thick calcified arteries e.g. Monkenberg's arteriosclerosis, atherosclerosis

235. Ans. — B Has multiple nuclei

The myocardium consists of discrete individual cells, each cell having a single nucleus.

236. Ans.— C Decreasing workload, increasing duration of exercise

The limiting factor at high altitude is the 'rate of oxygen uptake' which is a function of the workload (Resistance). Increasing the workload (resistance) will increase required rate of oxygen uptake which is not available.

Hence a higher working capacity cannot be obtained by increasing the workload.

To increase the work capacity therefore we should increase the duration of exercise.

3.

IMPORTANT TEXT OF LUNGS

RENAL HANDLING OF VARIOUS PLASMA CONSTITUENTS IN A NORMAL ADULT HUMAN ON AN AVERAGE DIET. P, PROXIMAL TUBULES; L LOOPS OF HENLE; D, DISTAL TUBULES; C, COLLECTING DUCTS.

		Per 24 hours			*Percentage*	
Substance	*Filatered*	*Reabsorbed*	*Secreted*	*Excreted*	*Reabsorbed*	*Location*
Na+ (mEq)	26,000	25,850		150	99.4	P, L, D, C
K+ (mEq)	900	900	100	100	100	P, D
Cl^- (mEq)	18,000	17,850		150	99.2	P, L, D, C
HCO_3^- (mEq)	4,900	4,900		0	100	P, D
Urea (mmols)	870	460		410	53	P, L, D, C
Creatinine (mmols)	12	1	1	12	...	...
Uric acid (mmols)	50	49	4	5	98	P
Glucose (mmols)	800	800		0	100	P
Total solute (mOsm)	54,000	53,400	100	700	87	P, L, D, C
Water (ml)	180,000	179,000		1000	99.4	P, L, D, C

CHARACTERISTICS OF A SUBSTANCE SUITABLE FOR MEASURING THE GFR BY DETERMINING ITS CLEARANCE.

Freely filtered

Not reabsorbed or secreted by tubules

Not metabolized

Not stored in kidney

Not protein-bound (substances bound to albumin and globulin not filtered)

Not toxic

Has no effect on filtration rate

Preferably easy to measure in plasma and urine

FACTORS AFFECTING THE GLOMERULAR FILTRATION RATE.

1. Changes in renal blood flow
2. Changes in glomerular capillary hydrostatic pressure
   a. Changes in systemic blood pressure
   b. Afferent or efferent arteriolar constriction
3. Changes in hydrostatic pressure in Bowman's capsule
   a. Ureteral obstruction
   b. Edema of kidney inside tight renal capsule
4. Changes in concentration of plasma proteins: dehydration, hypoproteinemia, etc (minor factors)
5. Increased permeability of glomerular filter; various diseases
6. Decrease in total area of glimerular capillary bed
   a. Diseases which destroy glomeruli with or without destruction of tubules
   b. Partial nephrectomy

RESPIRATORY SYSTEM

LUNG VOLUMES AND SOME MEASUREMENTS RELATED TO THE MECHANICS OF BREATHING.

IRV = Inspiratory reserve volume
ERV = Expiratory reserve volume
TV = Tidal volume
RV = Residual volume

		Volume (liters)		
		Men	Women	
Vital capacity	IRV	3.3	1.9	Inspiratory capacity
	TV	0.5	0.5	
	ERV	1.0	0.7	
	RV	1.2	1.1	Functional residual capacity
Total lung capacity		6.0	4.2	

Respiratory minute volume (rest): 6 liters/min
Alveolar ventilation (rest): 4.2 liters/min
Maximal voluntary ventilation (BTPS): 125-170 liters/min
Timed vital capacity: 83% of total in sec; 97% in 3 sec

MCQ's OF LUNGS

What is important in Lungs

Pulmonary function tests (various capacities) and effect of common diseases on them, Transport of Gases (O_2, CO_2), Regulation of Respiration

1. The intrapleural pressure is negative both during insipiration and expiration because : AIIMS 2005, 2008
A. Intrapulmonary pressure is always negative
B. Thoracic cage and lungs are elastic structure
C. Transpulmonary pressure determines the negativity
D. Surfactant prevents the lungs to collapse

2. Pulmonary function abnormalities in interstitial lung diseases include all of the following except : AI 2005
A. Reduced vital capacity
B. Reduced FEV1/FVC ratio
C. Reduced diffusion capacity
D. Reduced total lung capacity

3. Pulmonary surfactant is secreted by : AI 2005, 2006
A. Type-I pneumocytes
B. Type-II pneumocytes
C. Clara cells
D. Bronchial epithelial cells

4. In which of the following a reduction in arterial oxygen tension occurs ? AI 2005
A. Anaemia
B. CO poisoning
C. Moderate exercise
D. Hypoventilation

5. CO_2 is primarily trasnported in the arterial blood as : AI 2005
A. Dissolved CO_2
B. Carbonic Acid
C. Carbamino-hemoglobin
D. Bicarbonate

6. Maximum mid exp. flow rate indicates flow obstruction in : AIIMS 1996, 98
A. Large airways B. Small airways
C. Trachea D. Trachea & bronchi

7. Respiratory minute volume in a normal person is : UPSC 1985, 95
A. 1.2 L/min B. 2.1 L/min
C. 4.2 L/min D. 6.0 L/min

8. In sternuous exercise, PO_2 (mmHg) falls from : AIIMS 1982, 93
A. 40 to 1 B. 60 to 35
C. 25 to 10 D. 35 to 0

9. During exercise, O_2 entering the blood may increase from 250 ml/min at to rest as high as : Delhi 1986, 96
A. 4 L/mi B. 10 L/min
C. 20 L/min D. 30 L/min

10. The point at which breathing can no longer be voluntarily inhibited is called : AIIMS 1982, 96
A. Herring Breuer reflex B. Breaking point
C. Saturation point D. Any of the above

11. The stimulatory effects of hypoxia on ventilation do not clearly manifest until they become enough to override the counterbalancing inhibitory effects of a decline in : PGI 1982, 92
A. Arterial H^+ B. Arterial H^+ and PCO_2
C. Venous H^+ D. PO_2

12. There is no stimulation of ventilation by hypoxia until the alveolar PO_2 falls below : AMU 1982, 92
A. 60 mm Hg B. 58 mm Hg
C. 50 mm Hg D. 45 mm Hg

13. Stimuli affecting respiratory centre include :
A. CO_2 and O_2 B. Proprioceptors
C. Baroreceptors D. All of the above

14. Carbon dioxide affects respiratory centre via : AIIMS 1984, 94
A. Aortic bodies
B. Carotid bodies
C. Inflation and deflation receptors
D. CSF H^+ concentration

15. The respiratory minute volume is proportionate to the metabolic rate and the link between metabolism and ventilation is : AMU 1987, 97
A. CO_2 B. O_2
C. Proteins D. All of the above

Ans. 1. B 2. B 3. B 4. D 5. D 6. B 7. B 8. A 9. A 10. B
11. B 12. A 13. D 14. D 15. A

16. Of the approximately 49 ml of CO2 in each dl of arterial blood, the quantity of dissolved, carbamino compounds and in HCO3 form is : AIIMS 1984, 95

	Dissolved	Carbamino Compounds	HCO3-
A.	2.6 ml	2.6 ml	43.8 ml
B.	43.8 ml	2.6 ml	2.6 ml
C.	43.8 ml	3.7 ml	0.4 ml
D.	2.6 ml	43.8 ml	3.7 ml

17. Which is untrue about chloride shift : DNB 1989, 94
A. Essentially complete in 1 sec.
B. Chloride, content of arterial blood is more than venous blood.
C. Vice versa of 'b' choice.
D. Diffusion of Cl^- into the red cells.

18. The ambient pressure increases by — atmosphere for every 10 m of depth in sea water and every 10.4 of depth in fresh water : AMC 1980, 93
A. 0.3 B. 0.8
C. 1.0 D. 1.8

19. Cheyne-stokes breathing is seen in : AMU 1983, 96
A. CHF B. Uremia
C. Brain D. Any of the above

20. Hyperbaric oxygenation is useful in all except : AMC 1983, 98
A. Congenital heart disease
B. Gas gangrene
C. Carbon monoxide poisoning
D. Nitrogen toxicity

21. The Alveolar ventilation in an individual with Tidal Volume : 600 ml, Dead space 150 ml & respiratory rate - 15/min is : JIPMER 1993
A. 2 L/min B. 4.5 L/min
C. 6.75 L/min D. 9 L/min

22. When the atmospheric pressure is halved, which of the following is not likely to develop: AIIMS 1985, 95
A. An increase in pulmonary ventilation
B. A fall in arterial pO2
C. A rise in arterial pH
D. A rise in cerebral blood flow

23. Contraction of smooth muscle in respiratory tract occurs in response to all, except : AIIMS 1985, 98
A. Irritation of bronchial mucosa
B. Stimulation of local beta adrenoreceptors
C. A decrease in the pCO2 in the bronchial air
D. A cold stimulus to the bronchial mucosa

24. The surfactant material lining the lung alveoli : AIIMS 1986, 94
A. Decreases the surface tension of alveolar fluid.
B. Increases the compliance of lungs.
C. Has increasingly less effect, the more lungs are inflated.
D. Is decreased when pulmonary blood flow is interrupted.
E. All of the above

25. An increase in ventilation occurs in all except : AIIMS 1984, 98
A. Fall in plasma bicarbonate
B. Sleep
C. Fall in pH of CSF
D. Rise in blood adrenaline level

26. During the initial part of inspiration, which of the following does not occur ? DNB 1990, 95
A. An intrapulmonary pressure falls
B. Intrathoracic pressure rises
C. Intraabdominal pressure rises
D. The partial pressure of O2 in dead space rise

27. What is not true for respiration centre ? AMU 1991, 98
A. Situated in the medulla and pons.
B. Sends out regular bursts of impulses to expiratory muscles during quiet respiration.
C. Sends out regular impulses to expiratory muscles during quiet respiration.
D. Is inhibited during swallowing and vomiting.

28. What factor determines the quantity of gas that will diffuse through a barrier? DNB 1998
A. Surface area available for diffusion and thickness of barrier
B. Molecular weight of diffusing particle
C. Solubility of particle in medium
D. Driving pressure
E. All of the above

29. Apnoea means : DNB 1992, 98
A. Cessation of breathing
B. Shallow breathing
C. Distressed breathing
D. Increased breathing rate

30. Destruction of lung tissue and defective gaseous exchange causes all, except : AP 1989, 90
A. Prominent P-wave
B. Decreased cerebral blood circulation
C. Increased red cell number
D. Pulmonary hypertension

31. The diffusing capacity for carbon dioxide compared to that for oxygen is : Delhi 1984, 94
A. 20 times B. 10 times
C. 5 times D. 2 times

32. At a tidal volume of 500 ml, physiological dead space 150 ml and respiratory rate 12/min. the alveolar ventilation in ml/minute is : AMC 1985, 95
A. 6000 B. 4200
C. 180 D. 900

Ans. 16. A 17. C 18. C 19. D 20. D 21. C 22. D 23. B 24. E 25. B
26. B 27. C 28. E 29. A 30. B 31. A 32. B

33. **Total vital capacity is decreased but timed vital capacity is normal in :** **UPSC 1987, 97**
A. Bronchial Asthma B. Scoliosis
C. Chronic bronchitis D. All the above

34. **The intrapleural pressure (mm Hg) at the end of deep inspiration is :** **Delhi 1993, 98**
A. -4 B. +4
C. -18 D. +18

35. **An increase in ventillation occurs in all situations except :** **AIIMS 1984, 94**
A. Decrease plasma HCO3-
B. Sleep
C. Decreased pH in CSF
D. Increased blood adrenaline

36. **When CO_2 in inspired air increases beyond 10% at atmospheric pressure, it causes :** **PGI 1983, 98**
A. Decreased ventillation
B. Depression of CNS
C. Diminished sensory acquity
D. All of the above

37. **What occurs in acclimatization to a high altitude :** **AMC 1983, 96**
A. Hyperventilation
B. Polycythemia
C. O2 dissociation curve shifts to right
D. Decreased concentration of systemic capillaries

38. **Arterial pO2 is reduced in :** **PGI 1987, 93**
A. Anaemia
B. KCN poisoning
C. Pulmonary hypoventilation
D. CO poisoning

39. **When CO_2 is removed in the lungs, which of the following also occur :** **PGI 1986, 91**
A. Efflux of HCO_3^- from RBC
B. Efflux of Cl- from RBC
C. Efflux of CO_2
D. Efflux of O_2 and influx CO_2

40. **The renal body fluid volume mechanism for regulating arterial pressure is important for :** **AIIMS 1985, 95**
A. Raising the pressure when a person stand suddenly after having been in a lying position.
B. Minimizing a decrease in arterial pressure following severe hemorrhage.
C. Increasing arterial pressure during sternuous physical exercise.
D. Maintaining arterial pressure at a normal level over a period of weeks, months or years.

41. **The most important substance controlling alveolar ventilation is :** **Delhi 1989, 95**
A. O_2 B. CO_2
C. H_2O D. None of the above

42. **Surfactant is decreased or absent in :** **AMC 1988, 98**
A. Emphysema
B. Bronchial asthma
C. Respiratory Distress Syndrome (RDS) in children
D. RDS in adults

43. **CO_2 enters capillaries by :** **AIIMS 1987, 97**
A. Diffusion B. Permeation
C. Osmosis D. Active transport

44. **Carbon monoxide is released in lungs from :** **Delhi 1990, 96**
A. Iron of hema molecule
B. Plasma
C. Transferrin
D. Serum

45. **Effort during normal respiration is done for purpose:** **Delhi 1990, 98**
A. Lung elasticity
B. Respiratory air passages
C. Alveolar air spaces
D. Creating negative pleural pressure

46. **A person ascends to 12,000 feet, develops acute breathlessness; this is due to :** **AI 1990, 98**
A. Decreased pulmonary blood flow
B. Carbon dioxide washout
C. Decreased hypoxic stimulation of respiration
D. Mechanical interference of thorax

47. **A patient is respiring 21/mt (Pulm. ventilation) and has respiratory rate of 20/mt. Which of the following is true :** **Delhi 1985, 95**
A. Doing exercise
B. Has respiratory acidosis
C. Cheyne Stokes breathing
D. Respiring in dead space

48. **An increase in ventillation occurs in all except :** **AIIMS 1987, 97**
A. Decreased Plasma HCO3-
B. Decreased pH of CSF
C. Increased Blood adrenaline
D. None of the above

49. **Maximum voluntary ventillation (L/min) is :** **AMC 1985, 86, 96**
A. 90-120 B. 125-170
C. 170-210 D. 210-250

50. **CO2 influences respiration by acting at :** **AMC 1987, 98**
A. Cerebrum B. Carotid body
C. Whole of Medulla D. Respiratory centre

51. **Alveolar ventillation (L/mt) at rest is :** **AIIMS 1985, 95**
A. 3. B 4.2
C. 6 D. 125

Ans.										
	33. B	**34. A**	**35. B**	**36. D**	**37. C**	**38. C**	**39. B**	**40. D**	**41. B**	**42. C**
	43. A	**44. C**	**45. A**	**46. B**	**47. D**	**48. D**	**49. B**	**50. D**	**51. B**	

Match the following (Questions 52 to 55) : **PGI 1984, 94**

A. 3000 ml B. 4600 ml
C. 500 ml D. 3500 ml

52. **Tidal volume**
53. **Inspiratory reserve volume**
54. **Vital capacity**
55. **Inspiratory capacity**

56. **The substance synthesized or stored in lung tissue and released into blood :** **PGI 1985, 95**
A. Histamine
B. Kallikrein
C. Prostoglandins-E and F
D. All of the above

57. **FRC comprises of :** **AI 1993, AMC 1989, 93**
A. Dead space volume
B. Residual volume
C. Volume of air present after normal expiration.
D. Volume which can be inhaled after normal inspiration.

58. **Surfactant is secreted by :** **Delhi 1993; Kerala 1998**
A. Pneumocyte-I B. Pneumocyte-II
C. Goblet cells D. Pulmonary vessels

59. **Spirometry measures all of the following except :** **Delhi 1992, 99**
A. Tidal volume B. Vital capacity
C. FEV1 D. None of the above

60. **Normal value of FEV1 in an adult male is :** **Rohtak 1987, JIPMER 1992**
A. 95% B. 80%
C. 65% D. 50%

61. **Oxygen toxicity limits exposures to less than —— hours and pressures to — atmospheres or less respectively :** **AIIMS 1982, 92**
A. 3, 5 B. 5, 3
C. 1, D. 2, 1

62. **At 3000 m above sea level, PO2 is about :** **AMC 84, 86, 95**
A. 70 mm Hg B. 60 mm Hg
C. 50 mm Hg D. 45 mm Hg

63. **As one ascends higher than 3000 m sea level, there is :** **AMC 1987, 97**

	PO2	PCO2
A.	Decrease	Increase
B.	Decrease	Decrease
C.	Increase	Increase
D.	Increase	Decrease

64. **Air in the pleural cavity causes all, except :** **UPSC 1981, 94**
A. Reduction in residual volume
B. Abnormal dullness to percussion of the affected side
C. Less obvious rib contours on the affected side
D. Reduced vital capacity

65. **Circulation time through pulmonary capillaries is :** **AIIMS 1980, 95**
A. Less than 1 sec B. 10 sec
C. 20 sec D. 30 sec

66. **Pulmonary venules are constricted by the following except :** **AP 1987, 97**
A. 5 HT B. Histamine
C. E. Coli endotoxin D. Isoproternol

67. **If respiratory rate is 10/min, the alveolar ventillation is 4500 ml, and when respiratory rate becomes 30/min the alveolar ventilation will be :** **AMC 1986, 96**
A. 500 ml B. 1000 ml
C. 1500 ml D. 4500 ml

68. **FEV1/FVC is reduced to :** **AIIMS 1995, 96**
A. Asthma B. Pleural effusion
C. Fibrosis D. All of the above

69. **Total dead space can be calculated from :** **UPSC 1980, 93**
A. PCO2 of expired air
B. PCO2 of alveolar gas
C. Tidal volume
D. All of the above

70. **Diffusion capacity of lungs for O2 at rest in ml/min/mm Hg is :** **AIIMS 1981, 95**
A. 5 B. 10
C. 20 D. 50

71. **In health, physiologic dead space is :** **PGI 1982, 96**
A. Double than that of anatomic dead space
B. Less than that of anatomic dead space
C. Triple than that of anatomic dead space
D. Equal

72. **In cigarette smoking, surfactant is :** **PGI 1982, 92**
A. Increased
B. Decreased
C. Increased followed by decrease
D. Unaltered

73. **Inspiratory capacity is total of :** **UPSC 1984, 95**
A. Residual volume (RV) + Inspiratory reserve volume (IRV)
B. IRV + TV
C. IRV + ERV
D. ERV + RV

74. **Inspiratory capacity is :** **AIIMS 1986, 97**
A. 3.8 litres in women B. 3.3 litres in women
C. 2.4 litres in women D. 1.8 litres in women

75. **Functional residual capacity in a male is :** **UPSC 1985, 95**
A. 3. 8 litres B. 3.3 litres
C. 2.8 litres D. 2. 2 litres

76. **Timed vital capacity in 1 sec is :** **AMU 1987, 98**
A. 73 % B. 83%
C. 87% D. 97%

Ans.									
52. C	**53. A**	**54. B**	**55. D**	**56. D**	**57. C**	**58. B**	**59. D**	**60. B**	**61. B**
62. B	**63. B**	**64. B**	**65. A**	**66. D**	**67. C**	**68. A**	**69. D**	**70. C**	**71. D**
72. B	**73. B**	**74. C**	**75. D**	**76. B**					

77. Work done in quiet breathing is : Rohtak 1986, 96
A. 0.1 Kg-m/min B. 0.2 Kg-m/min
C. 0.5 Kg-m/min D. 2.5 Kg-m/min

78. Maximum work of breathing is : Rohtak 1985, 95
A. 0.5 Kg-m/breath B. 2.0 Kg-m/breath
C. 5.0 Kg-m/breath D. 10 Kg-m/breath

79. Which of the following volume is equal in both men and women: AIIMS 1984, 95
A. Inspiratory reserve volume
B. Tidal volume
C. Residual volume
D. Vital capacity

80. Vital capacity in men is : AMC 1985, 95
A. 4.2 litres B. 4.8 litres
C. 6.0 litres D. 6.8 litres

81. There are about : AMC 1987, 97
A. 50 million alveoli in man
B. 100 million alveoli in man
C. 300 million alveoli in man
D. 500 million alveoli in man

82. The total area of the alveolar walls in contact with capillaries in both lungs is about : AP 1985, 95
A. 10 sq. m B. 30 sq. m
C. 70 sq. m D. 120 sq. m

83. Tidal volume in both men and women is : JIPMER 1985
A. 250 ml B. 500 ml
C. 1000 ml D. 1200 ml

84. Times vital capacity in 3 sec is : TN 1985, 96
A. 83% B. 87%
C. 97% D. 99.9 %

85. The following active substances are metabolized by the lung : AP 1987, 98
A. Kallikrein
B. Serotonin
C. Angiotensin-I —> Angiotensin-II
D. All of the above

86. The blood in the systemic arteries which bypass the pulmonary capillaries is about : NIMHANS 1986
A. 0% B. 2%
C. 10% D. 15%

87. Pulmonary blood volume increases by upto : CMC 1988, 98
A. 50 ml in a normal individual when he lies down.
B. 100 ml in a normal individual when he is lies down.
C. 200 ml in a normal individual when he lies down.
D. 400 ml in a normal individual when he lies down.

88. Pulmonary arterioles are constricted by the following except : DNB 1989, 98
A. Norepinephrine B. Epinephrine
C. Angiotensin-II D. Acetylcholine

89. Respiratory quotient of cerebral tissue is : AMC 1986, 96
A. 0.75-0.95 B. 0.95-0.99
C. 1.0-1.1 D. 1.1-1.2

90. A man breathes about : AMC 1982, 92
A. 100 ml of air per breath
B. 250 ml of air per breath
C. 500 ml of air per breath
D. 1000 ml of air per breath

91. CO_2 which is excreted per minute is : Delhi 1985, 96
A. 50 ml B. 100 ml
C. 200 ml D. 400 ml

92. In a healthy adult, 24 hour production of CO2 is about : AIIMS 1981, 92
A. 120 litres B. 250 litres
C. 330 litres D. 410 litres

93. The percentage of oxygen transported from the lung to the tissues in chemical combination is : PGI 1981,91
A. 28 B. 75
C. 89 D. 97

94. The volume of gas contained in the lung at the end of maximum inspiration is : UPSC 1982, 92
A. Functional residual capacity
B. Inspiratory capacity
C. Inspiratory reserve volume
D. Total lung capacity

95. Diffusion capacity of lungs for carbon monoxide is : AMU 1984, 94
A. 0-5 ml/min/mmHg B. 5-10 ml/min/mmHg
C. 10-30 ml/min/mmHg D. 40-80 ml/min/mmHg

96. Timed vital capacity in 2 sec. is : AIIMS 1982, 92
A. 83% B. 87%
C. 94% D. 97%

97. Anatomical dead space is : AP 1987, 97
A. 50-100 ml B. 100-250 ml
C. 250-400 ml D. 400-500 ml

98. Hering Breuer reflex : AIIMS 1987, Bihar 1991, 99
A. Initiates the rhythmicity of normal breathing
B. Influences only the depth of normal breathing
C. Influences depth and rate of normal breathing
D. All of these
E. Both b+c

99. Cheyne stokes respiration is characterized by : Bihar 1991, 98
A. Continuous hyperpnoea
B. Increased sensitivity of resp. center
C. Fluctuating PO2 and stable PCO2
D. Decreased sensitivity of resp. center
E. Normal circulation time from lung to brain

Ans.										
77. C	78. D	79. B	80. B	81. C	82. C	83. B	84. C	85. D	86. B
87. D	88. D	89. B	90. C	91. C	92. C	93. D	94. D	95. C	96. C
97. B	98. A	99. B							

100. More resistance in expiration is due to : AIIMS 1986, 92

A. Airflow during expiration
B. Compression of airway
C. Change from linear to turbulent flow
D. Saturation with moisture

101. Three week residence at 4000 m altitude may result in : AMC 1984, 94

A. Metabolic acidosi B. Metabolic alkalosis
C. Respiratory acidosis D. Respiratory alkalosis

102. Arterial blood gas analysis in carbon monoxide poisoning is : AIIMS 1994, 96

A. PO_2 normal, O_2 saturation less
B. PO_2 less, O_2 saturation normal
C. PO_2 less, O_2 saturation decreased
D. PO_2 less, O_2 saturation normal

103. Which gas is not responsible for Green House effect : AIIMS 1994, 97

A. Carbon dioxide B. Ozone
C. Nitrogen D. Nitrous oxide

104. Peak expiratory flow rate (PEFR) is : AMC 1984, 86, 87, 98

A. 5 L/mt B. 20 L/mt
C. 50 L/mt D. 400-500 L/mt

105. When vagus nerve is severed, the respiration is : AIIMS 1984, 98

A. Decreased B. Increased
C. Ceased D. No change

106. When dead space is ↑, it affects alveolar : MP 1998, 99

A. PCO2 B. PO2
C. Both PCO2 and PO2 D. Neither PCO2 nor PO2

107. Contraction of which of the following muscles is most important for causing forceful expiration : PGI 1983,90, 95

A. Internal intercostals B. Diaphragm
C. External intercostals D. Abdominals

108. The major cause of the hyperpnea of muscular exercise is : AIIMS 1985, 96

A. Stimulation of the respiratory centre by the cerebral cortex and the joint proprioception.
B. Hypercapnia
C. Hypoxemia
D. Alkalosis
E. Peripheral chemoreceptors

109. If a person has a tidal volume of 411 ml, physiological dead space volume of 100 ml. and a respiratory minute ventilation of 360 ml/min., what is his alveolar ventilation : AIIMS 1982, 92

A. 3600 ml/min B. 3000 ml/min
C. 2700 ml/min D. 1500 ml/min

110. The major factor regulating alveolar ventilation during rest is : Delhi 1986; AMC 1987, 97

A. Arterial PO2
B. Arterial PCO2
C. Arterial pH
D. Nervous output from the joint proprioceptor

111. Which of the following does not occur in high altitude acclimatisation : AMC 1986; PGI 1984, 98

A. Reticulocytosis
B. Increase serum erythropoietin
C. Increased serum cortisol
D. Increased blood glucose

112. Rise of pulmonary arterial pressure is caused by : PGI 1984, 98

A. Hypoxia B. Acidosis
C. Alkalosis D. All of the above

113. A swimmer breathing through a snorkel has a respiration rate of 10/min., a tidal volume of 550 ml and an effective anatomic dead space of 250 ml. What is his alveolar ventilation rate : AIIMS 1984,94

A. 2500 ml/min. B. 3000 ml/min.
C. 3500 ml/min. D. 4000 ml/min.

114. The tidal volume can never become greater than the: PGI 1986 ,96

A. Anatomic dead space
B. Vital capacity
C. Functional residual capacity
D. Residual volume
E. Inspiratory capacity

115. The partial pressure of oxygen in the arterial blood is normally lower than that of the alveolar gas primarily because : PGI 1988, 98

A. Blood move through the lungs too fast.
B. Oxygen requires a pressure gradient to diffuse into blood.
C. Some portions of the lungs are ventilated but not perfused.
D. Some portions of the lungs are perfused but not ventilated.

116. In the tissues, the pCO2 remains normally : CSE 1997, 98

A. Of the order of 50 mmHg
B. Of the order of 40 mmHg
C. Of the order of 100 mmHg
D. Above 100 mmHg

117. In respiratory alkalosis : Manipal 1995, 98

A. The plasma bicarbonate concentration is either low or normal
B. The cerebral blood flow increases
C. The urine is acidic
D. All of the above

Ans.									
100. B	101. D	102. A	103. D	104. D	105. A	106. B	107. D	108. A	109. C
110. B	111. D	112. A	113. B	114. B	115. D	116. C	117. A		

118. **All of the following statements about the residual volume are true except : Manipal 1995, 96**
A. It is the volume of gas that remains in the lung after a maximal expiration.
B. It averages 4-5 litres in a 70-kg adult male.
C. It may be measured by an indicator dilution technique.
D. It increases with age.

W.119. **During inspiration, the : Manipal 1995, 96**
A. Heart rate tends to decrease
B. Jugular venous pressure tends to fall
C. Muscles of the anterior abdominal wall relax
D. Intrapulmonary pressure falls below the intrapleural pressure

120. **Best airway measurement is : Rajasthan 1998, 99**
A. FEV
B. FEV1
C. Vital capacity
D. Inspiratory Reserve volume

Match the values of pressure listed Ques. 121 to 123 below with the appropriate arterial and venous gases: AIIMS 1986, 96
A. 20 mm Hg
B. 40 mm Hg
C. 45 mm Hg
D. 100 mm Hg
E. 569 mm Hg

121. **Arterial pO_2**
122. **Venous pCO_2**
123. **Arterial pCO_2 and venous pO_2**

124. **The partial pressure of water vapor in the lungs : AIIMS 1982, 98**
A. Increases with hyperventilation
B. Is relatively constant with changes in altitude
C. Is proportional to the CO2 concentration
D. Becomes negative wh arometric pressure falls below 47 mm Hg.

125. **Mucociliary action of uppe respiratory tract is : Kerala 1994, 95**
A. Protective function
B. Is of no physiological importance
C. Hinders inspiration
D. Increases the velocity of inspired air

126. **Hyperpnea in exercise is because of : Delhi 1986, 96**
A. Hypercapnia
B. Hypoxaemia
C. Reflex
D. Stimulation of cortex and proprioceptors

127. **At 3000m height, PO_2 is approximately ______ mmHg : DNB 1999**
A. 60
B. 70
C. 80
D. 90

128. **Alveolar hyperventillation causes : Delhi 1986, 96**
A. Respiratory acidosis
B. Respiratory alkalosis
C. Metabolic acidosis
D. Metabolic alkalosis

129. **Normally, insensible water loss through respiratory tract and skin per day is: Delhi 1983, 94**
A. 600-800 ml
B. 100-200 ml
C. 250-300 ml
D. > 1000 ml

130. **Pulmonary wedge pressure corresponds to : AIIMS 1985, 95**
A. Right atrial pressure
B. Right ventricular pressure
C. Left atrial pressure
D. Left ventricular pressure

131. **If the RR is 10/min Tidal vol. - 600 ml and min. volume - 6 L; alveolar ventillation is : Kerala 1997, 98**
A. 4500 ml
B. 6000 ml
C. 3600 ml
D. 9000 ml

132. **True about decrease in respiration is : Delhi 1985, 88, 92**
A. Stops during swallowing
B. Asphyxia
C. Hypoxic hypoxia
D. Paradoxical respiration

133. **Respiratory centre controlled by Pons is : Delhi 1986, 88, 98**
A. Gasping
B. Pneumotoxic
C. Inspiratory
D. Expiratory

134. **FeV2/FeV less than 60% is seen in : UPSC 1986; Delhi 1983, 94**
A. Emphysema
B. Rectus excavatum
C. Interstitial lung disease
D. Pulmonary oedema

135. **In Interstitial lung disease, not seen is : UPSC 1986; Delhi 1988, 94**
A. ↑ pO_2 in blood
B. ↑ pCO_2 in blood
C. Response to O_2 therapy
D. FeV2/FeV are decreased in same ratio

136. **Air taken in and out per breath is : PGI 1993**
A. Tidal volume
B. Vital capacity
C. Alveolar ventilation
D. FEV

137. **Oxygen debt : UPSC 1982, 95**
A. Is impossible to incur when breathing pure oxygen.
B. Can never occur in healthy individual.
C. Is often evidenced by an increase in lactic concentration in the blood.
D. Is caused by lack of anaerobic metabolism.

Ans.	118. B	119. B, C	120. B	121. D	122. C	123. B	124. B	125. A	126. B	127. A
	128. B	129. A	130. C	131. A	132. A	133. B	134. A	135. C	136. A	137. C

138. The most important factor that tends to collapse the lungs (the recoil tendency) is the : AIIMS 1984, 99
A. Elastic fibre in the lungs
B. Intrapleural fluid pressure
C. Total intrapleural pressure
D. Surface tension of the alveolar fluid
E. Tension in the intercostal muscles

139. Oxygen therapy has significant value in all the following types of hypoxia except : Delhi 1996
A. Atmospheric hypoxia
B. Hypoventilation hypoxia
C. Hypoxia due to pulmonary edema
D. Hypoxia due to decreased hemoglobin in the blood
E. Histotoxic hypoxia due to cyanide poisoning

140. Most potent respiratory stimulant is : PGI 1984; Delhi 1986; AI 1999
A. Oxygen B. Carbon dioxide
C. H+ D. K+

141. Which of the following condition is having an elevated arterial pCO2 value : DNB 1991; Rajasthan 1993, 95
A. ARDS B. Fat embolism
C. Pulmonary oedema D. Emphysema

142. The partial pressure of oxygen in the arterial blood is normally lower than that of the alveolar gas primarily because : Rajasthan 1993, 96
A. The lungs use oxygen.
B. Blood moves through the lungs fast.
C. Some portions of the lungs are ventilated but not perfused.
D. Some portions of the lungs are perfused but not ventilated.

143. Compensatory responses to metabolic acidosis include all except : Rajasthan 1993, 98
A. Hyperventilation
B. An increase in titrable acid excretion
C. An increase in NH excretion
D. An increase in glycolysis by H+ activation of phosphofructokinase

144. Respiratory movements are associated with (and partly, cause) fluctuations in blood pressure. The highest rise of systolic pressure occurs at the time of the : Karnataka 1987, 98
A. Late inspiration-early expiration
B. End of expiration
C. Beginning of inspiration
D. Late expiration-early inspiration

145. Structures through which O_2 must diffuse in passing from alveolar lumen to Hb : Karnataka 1989, 90
A. Surfactant containing liquid
B. Alveolar membrane, basement membrane
C. Capillary endothelium, plasma and R.B.C. membrane
D. All of the above

146. A total vital capacity of loss more than 80% of predicted values indicate : Karnataka 1989, 92
A. Respiratory center damage
B. Restrictive pulmonary disease
C. Metabolism is depressed
D. Obstructed air passages

147. The majority of observers can only detect cyanosis when the arterial oxygen saturation falls below : Karnataka 1989, 93
A. 70% B. 80%
C. 85% D. 90%

148. When gases flow through an orifice, the factor least likely to affect the turbulance is the : Karnataka 1999
A. Viscosity of the gas B. Density of the gas
C. Pressure of the gas D. Diameter of the orifice

149. Normal partial pressure of oxygen in arterial blood in health at sea level : Karnataka 1989, 94
A. 60-100 mmHg B. 60-80 mmHg
C. 80-100 mmHg D. 100-200 mmHg

150. Normal arterial oxygen concentration is : Karnataka 1989, 90
A. 100% B. 95-98%
C. 90-95% D. 80-85%

151. Respiratory alkalosis occurs in : AIIMS 1993, 96
A. Diabetic ketoacidosis
B. Pyloric stenosis
C. Primary aldosteronism
D. Excessive ventilation

152. Respiratory acidosis is characterized by : AIIMS 1993, 97
A. $\downarrow$ plasma HCO_3 $\downarrow$ pCO_2
B. $\uparrow$ pCO_2, $\downarrow$ pH
C. $\downarrow$ pH and $\downarrow$ pCO_2
D. $\uparrow$ pCO_2, $\uparrow$ pH

153. Which of the following tends to decrease with age : PGI 1993, 95
A. Vital capacity B. Systolic B.P.
C. Pulse pressure D. Residual volume

154. Decreased FEV_1 and increased Tidal volume is seen in : PGI 1993; Delhi 2001
A. Emphysema B. COAD
C. Br. asthma D. TB

155. Oxygen dissociation curve shifts to right in : PGI 1993, 96
A. Hyperkalemia B. Hypokalemia
C. Metabolic alkalosis D. Anemia

Ans. 138. D 139. E 140. B 141. D 142. D 143. D 144. B 145. D 146. D 147. B 148. C 149. C 150. B 151. D 152. B 153. A 154. A 155. D

156. Commonest cause of Cheyne-stokes breathing is : Karnataka 1994, 97

A. Contusion of the brain
B. Destructive disease of the brain
C. Increased intracranial tension
D. Cardiac failure

157. A case of restrictive lung disease differs from obstructive lung disease in having a lower : Karnataka 1994, 96

A. Residual volume B. Vital capacity
C. Total lung capacity D. All of the above

158. True about respiratory center : AIIMS 1993

A. Continuously sends stimulatory impulses to exp. muscles
B. Has got connection with cardiac center
C. Inhibited by swallowing and vomiting
D. Directly stimulated by ↓ PaO_2

159. Aerobic capacity is increased by : AIIMS 1994, 96

A. Regular 3 months exercise
B. Prolonged exercise routine
C. Spurts of exercise
D. Sternous exercise

160. Following lung volumes are measured in laboratory examination except : Punjab 1994, 95

A. FEV B. Tidal volume
C. Residual volume D. Vital capacity

161. Hyperventilation occurs due to all of the following except : AI 1994

A. Decrease in pH of CSF
B. Increase in circulating catecholamines
C. CO poisoning
D. Aspirin poisoning

162. Anemic hypoxia is characterized by : AI 1994

A. Low arterial pO_2 B. Low arterial O_2 content
C. Cyanosis D. Decreased blood flow

163. Severe hypoxia may produce : AMU 1985

A. BP rise
B. BP fall
C. BP fall followed by BP rise
D. No change

164. Dyspneic index = % breathing reserve (MVV-Maximum Voluntary ventillation, RMV-Resp. minute volume) : AIIMS 1986, 96

A. $\frac{\text{MMV-RMV}}{\text{MVV}} \times 100$
B. $\frac{\text{(MVV-RMV)-2}}{\text{MVV}} \times 100$
C. $\frac{\text{RMV+MVV}}{\text{RMV}} \times 100$
D. $\frac{\text{MVV - RMV}}{\text{RMV}} \times 100$

165. A patient with impaired ability to excrete CO_2 is likely to have all, except : PGI 1981, 92

A. A raised blood bicarbonate level.
B. An acid urine.
C. A lowered arterial blood PO_2 when breathing air at atmospheric pressure.
D. Cool extremities.

166. Patients with restrictive lung diseases differ from those with obstructive airways disease by having : AIIMS 1982, 95

A. Lower ratio of forced expiratory volume in one second/vital capacity.
B. Lower peak flow rate.
C. Lower residual volume and total lung capacity.
D. All of the above.

167. The instrument used for measuring the vital capacity and FEV is : DNB 1990, 95

A. Wright peak flow meter
B. Vitalograph
C. Carlen's catheter
D. None of the above

168. About 90% of the CO_2 entering the blood is carried as : Delhi 1988, 98

A. Dissolved CO_2 B. Carbonic anhydrase
C. Carbamino CO_2 D. Carbonic acid
E. Bicarbonate

169. Normal adult lung weights is : AIIMS 1986, 95

A. 100-200 gms B. 200-300 gms
C. 300-400 gms D. 500-600 gms

170. Angular acceleration while flying may result in a pilot : PGI 1984, 94

A. Hypotension B. Unconsciousness
C. Vertebral fractures D. All of the above

171. Initiation of respiration is done by : JIPMER 1998

A. Dorsal respiratory group
B. Pneumotaxis centre
C. Nucleus parabrachialis
D. Ventral respiratory group

172. Normal PaO_2 (mmHg) is : PGI 1995, 99

A. 40-60 B. 80-108
C. 60-80 D. 110-120

173. At inspiration, the pleural pressure is : WB 1996, 98

A. More positive B. Zero
C. More negative D. Atmospheric

174. The difference between amount of O_2 entering body (ml/per min) and CO_2 excreted (ml/min) is ——— ml/min : AIIMS 1994

A. 20 B. 50
C. 0 D. -10

175. Ventilation/perfusion ratio is maximum in : AIIMS 1996

A. Apical region B. Middle region
C. Base D. Same all over

Ans.									
156. D	157. D	158. C	159. A	160. C	161. C	162. B	163. A	164. A	165. D
166. C	167. B	168. E	169. C	170. C	171. A	172. C	173. C	174. B	175. A

176. Diffusion capacity of O_2 of lungs is —— ml/min/ mmHg at breast : **DNB 1996, 97**

A. 10 B. 20
C. 30 D. 45

177. In physiological shunt,——— % blood bypasses pulm capillaries : **DNB 1996, 98**

A. 0.5 B. 1
C. 2 D. 4

178. Lung diffusion capacity is measured with : **NIMNS 1996**

A. CO2 B. CO
C. O2 D. H2

179. Sympathetic stimulation on the bronchus causes : **TNPSC 1997, 98**

A. Bronchial constriction
B. Increased secretion of glands into Bronchi
C. No effect
D. Bronchial Dilatation

180. Increased alveolo-arteriolar ratio is seen in following except : **AIIMS 1997**

A. Right to Left shunt
B. Alveolar hypoventilation
C. Diffusion decreases
D. None

181. Maximum resistance during expiration is due to : **AIIMS 1997**

A. Collapse of alveoli
B. Expiratory Muscular fatigue
C. Dynamic collapse of air ways
D. Breaking action of inspiratory airways

182. False about focal Bronchoconstriction during expiration : **TN 1999**

A. Local pulmonary Hypertension
B. ↑ respiratory effort
C. ↑ respiratory minute volume
D. None of the above

183. J receptors when stimulated causes : **Kerala 1999**

A. Increased heart rate B. Apnoea
C. Tachypnoea D. Bradypnoea

184. Which of the following is false: **AIIMS 1999**

A. FEV is the fraction of total lung volume in one second.
B. PEFR is maximum expiratory flow of lung capacity.
C. Respiratory minute volume is the amount of the air inspired per minute.
D. MBC is the largest volume of gas can be moved into and out of lungs in one second by effort.

185. Normal PO2 in an 85-years healthy male in his room air breath is: **AIIMS 1999**

A. 80 B. 60
C. 45 D. 110

186. The normal adult Vd/Vt ratio is : **PGI 1999**

A. <20 B. < 35
C. < 40 D. <50

187. In high altitude mountain sickness, feature of pulmonary edema is : **PGI 1999**

A. Decreased pulmonary capillary permeability
B. Increased pulmonary capillary pressure
C. Normal left atrial pressure
D. Increased left ventricular back-pressure

188. During inspiration the intrapleural pressure becomes : **Orissa 1998**

A. Equal to Zero
B. More positive
C. More negative
D. Equal to atmospheric pressure

189. pCO2 affects respiration primarily by stimulating : **Orissa 1998**

A. Carotid and Aortic bodies
B. Pulmonary 'J' receptors
C. Medullary chemoreceptors
D. Baroreceptors

190. About α1 antitrypsin true is : **MAHE 1999**

A. Deficiency in lung causes increased compliance.
B. Deficiency causes decreased elastase enzyme.
C. In smokers with deficiency have increased destruction of lungs.
D. All of the above.

191. Which of the following is most useful test in idiopathic pulmonary fibrosis : **Delhi 2000**

A. FEV1/FVC B. VC
C. MEP D. RV

192. Nitrogen washout method is mainly used to measure : **Delhi 2000**

A. ERV B. FEFR
C. V D. FRC

193. Following lung volume may be normal emphysema except : **Delhi 2000**

A. TLC B. MEP
C. FEV1/FVC D. FEFR

194. CO inhibits respiratory chain by A/E : **UP 1999**

A. Binding with oxygen
B. Binding with haemoglobin
C. Producing hypoxia
D. Producing carboxyhemoglobin

195. Sudden cessation of respiration at terminal stage shows : **UP 2000**

A. Dynamic compression of airway
B. Collapsed alveoli
C. Expiratory muscle fatigue
D. Breaking action of inspiratory muscle

Ans.	176. B	177. C	178. B	179. D	180. C	181. D	182. C	183. C	184. D	185. A
	186. C	187. B	188. C	189. C	190. C	191. B	192. D	193. D	194. A	195. A

196. **In voluntary hyperventilation, muscle sprain is due to : UP 2000**
A. Sympathetic stimulation cause release of acetylcholine at neuromuscular junction
B. Decrease of Ca++ in serum
C. Increase of Ca++ in serum
D. Increase actin and myosin ratio

197. **Which of the following does not affect respiration ? TNPSC 2000**
A. Arterial H+ concentration
B. Arterial Na+ concentration
C. Cerebrospinal fluid CO2 concentration
D. Cerebrospinal fluid H+ concentration

198. **Which occurs after hyperventilation with 6% CO2 ? TNPSC 2000**
A. Apnea
B. Continued hyperventilation
C. Cheyne-Stokes breathing
D. Kussmaul's breathing

199. **When tidal volume is 600 ml. Dead space is 150 ml and rate of respiration is 10/min., alveolar ventilation will be : Kerala 2000**
A. 4.5 litre/min B. 5.0 litre/min
C. 6.0 litre/min D. 4.0 litre/min
E. 5.5. litre/min

200. **A patient is having normal lung compliance and increased airway resistance. What is the most economical way of breathing for him : AIIMS 2000**
A. Slow and deep B. Slow and shallow
C. Rapid and deep D. Rapid and shallow

201. **A low lander goes to the mountains. When he reaches about 5,000 feet high, he develops dyspnea. Which of the following is the correct explanation for his symptom: AIIMS 2000**
A. Carbon dioxide wash out
B. Increased blood flow to the pulmonary tissues
C. CNS depression
D. Increased work of breathing

202. **Alveolar ventillation is (VC-5000 ml, PR-14/min, TV-500 ml dead space—150 ml) : Kerala 2001**
A. 4900 ml B. 3500 ml
C. 2500 ml D. 6000 ml

203. **Activation of which receptor causes pulmonary vasoconstriction : Kerala 2001**
A. Alpha 2 adrenergic B. M3 cholinergic
C. H2 histaminic D. ETA epithelial receptor

204. **In hyperventilation, muscle spasm occurs because of : AIIMS 2001**
A. Increased sympathetic activity
B. Increased parasympathctic activity
C. Decreased Ca++ ions
D. Increased gamma efferent activity

205. **Bellow's spirometry measures : Maharashtra -2000**
A. TLC B. RV
C. Closing volume D. EERV

206. **True about 'dead space' in tracheobronchial tree is: A.P. 2002**
A. Increases in coughing
B. Humidifies air
C. Increases with adrenaline
D. In all respiratory diseases the anatomical dead space coincides with physiological dead space.

207. **Pulmonary surfactant is secreted by : AI 2005**
A. Type-I pneumocytes B. Type-II pneumocytes
C. Clara cells D. Bronchial epithelial cells

208. **From lung to tissues O_2 transported is : Delhi 1982**
A. 70% B. 86%
C. 91% D. 97%

209. **In an normal adult, the ratio of physiological and anatomical dead space is : AMC 1987; PGI 1984, 85**
A. 2 : 1 B. 1 : 3
C. 3 : 1 D. 1 : 1

210. **In a normal adult, 24 hour production of CO_2 is about : UPSC 1980, 90**
A. 150 L B. 280 L
C. 330 D. 410 L

211. **Consider the following statements : CSE 1995, 99**
Periodic (Cheyne-Stokes) breathing is seen
1. After voluntary apnoea
2. After voluntary hyperpnoea
3. At high altitude
4. During wakeful states of adult human being
Of these statements :
A. 1 and 2 are correct B. 2 and 3 are correct
C. 2, 3 and 4 are correct D. 1, 3 and 4 are correct

212. **Muscles of inspiration include which of the following? WB 2007**
A. Diaphragm and internal intercostals
B. Diaphragm and abdominal muscles
C. Abdominal muscles and external intercostals
D. Diaphragm and external intercostals

213. **Cell stability is maintained by : WB 2007**
A. Na+ ions B. K+ ions
C. Ca+ ions D. Mg ions

214. **The mechanism of action of surfactant is : AIIMS 2007**
A. Breaks the structure of water in the alveoli
B. Lubricate the flow of CO2 diffusion
C. Makes the apillary surface hydrophillic
D. All of the above

Ans.									
196. A	197. B	198. C	199. A	200. A	201. A	202. A	203. D	204. C	205. D
206. B	207. B	208. D	209. D	210. B	211. A	212. D	213. B	214. C	215. C

215. Pulmonary circulation is characterized by : AIIMS 2008

A. Vasoconstriction in response to hypoxia
B. Vasodilatation in response to hypoxia
C. Vasoconstriction in response to hypercapnia
D. Resistance is greater than systemic circulation

216. For severe bullous emphysema, total lung volumes are measured by : AIIMS 2008

A. Helium dilution technique
B. Transdiaphragmatic pressure
C. Body plethysmography
D. Diffusion capacity of CO

Ans. **215. C** **216. C**

EXPLANATIONS OF LUNGS

1. **Ans.— B Thoracic cage and the lungs are elastic structures**
   * **Both the thoracic cage and the lungs are elastic structures.**
   * **Being elastic structure they both tend to recoil, but in opposite directions.**
   * **The thoracic cage has inherent tendency to expand, while trying to expand, it draws the parietal pleura with it (because parietal pleura is strongly attached to the inner side of the chest wall).**
   * **The lungs have an inherent tendency to collapse because of their elasticity and surface tension of thin layer of fluid lining of the alveoli.**
   * **As the visceral pleura is strongly attached with the lungs, the pull in the opposite directions of the visceral and parietal pleura, creates a negative intra-pleural pressure.**

2. **Ans.— B. Reduced FEV1/FVC ratio**

3. **Ans.— B Type-II Pneumocytes :**

   Surfactant is produced by type-II alveolar epithelial cells - Ganong 21st/658

   (Alveolar epithelial cells are termed as pneumocytes)

   Surfactant Review

   * **The major constituent of surfactant is : Di-palmitoyl-phosphatidyl cholineQ**
   * **Surfactant reduced the alveolar surface tension and**
     - **prevents alveolar collapseQ**
     - **prevents pulmonary edemaQ**
   * **Respiratory distress syndrome/Hyaline membrane disease is produced due to deficiency of surfactant.**

   Clinical Relevance :

   Thyroid hormone increases activity of Type-II pneumocytesQ RDS is more common with Low Thyroid hormones (Hypothyroidism)

   Glucocorticoids enhance maturation of surfactantQ RDS is more common in premature bodies.

   (There is an increase in maternal & fetal cortisol near term)

   Insulin inhibits activity of type-II pneumocytesQ RDS is common in Diabetic mothers.

   (Fetal hyper-sinsulinemia occurs in diabetic mothers)

   * **Surfactant Deficiency may also occur with:**
     - **Occlusion of Main bronchus Q**
     - **Occlusion of Pulmonary artery Q**
     - **Long term inhalation of 100% O2**
     - **Cigarette smokers Q**

4. **Ans.— D Hypoventilation :**

   Arterial oxygen tension may be reduced either from a defect in oxygenation (e.g. Type-I failure) or ventilation (type-II failure). It is not reduced in anaemia, CO poisoning or moderate exercise.

5. **Ans.— D Bicarbonate :**

   'Transport of carbon dioxide in the form of bicarbonate ions accounts for approximately 70% of the carbon dioxide transported from the tissues to the lungs. Thus, this is by far the most important of all methods of transport.'—*Guyton*

   ***Transport of carbon dioxide :* Carbon dioxide is transported in following three forms :**

Forms	According to Guyton	According to Ganong
As Bicarbonate	70%	43.8% (43.8 ml/100 ml of blood)
As Carbaminocompounds	23%	2.6% (2.6 ml/100 ml of blood)
As dissolved CO2	7%	2.6% (2.6ml/100 of blood)

   Although, there is a significant conflict in the amount by which CO2 is transported in various forms between the text in Guyton and Ganong, the most important of all modes of transport is certainly bicarbonate.

6. Ans.— B. Small airways
7. Ans.— B. 2.1 L/min
8. Ans.— A. 40 to 1
9. Ans.— A. 4 L/min
10. Ans.— B. Breaking point
11. Ans.— B. Arterial H^+ and PCO_2
12. Ans.— A. 60 mm Hg
13. Ans.— D. All of the above

All the mentioned stimuli affect respiratory rate

14. Ans.— D. CSF H^+ concentration
15. Ans.— A. CO_2
16. Ans.— A. 2.6 ml 2.6 ml 43.8 ml
17. Ans.— C. Vice versa of 'b' choice

About 70% of bicarbonate ions formed in RBC's are transferred to plasma in exchange for chloride ions called chloride shift (which is essential for the transport of CO2 as bicarbonate. It occurs very rapidly.

18. Ans.— C. 1.0
19. Ans.— D. Any of the above
20. Ans.— D. Nitrogen toxicity

The problem of nitrogen narcosis can be avoided by breathing mixtures of O_2 and helium.

21. Ans.— C. 6.75 L/min
22. Ans.— D. A rise in cerebral blood flow
23. Ans.— B. Stimulation of local beta adrenoreceptors
24. Ans.— E. All of the above
25. Ans.— B. Sleep
26. Ans.— B. Intrathoracic pressure rises

Intrathoracic pressure decreases during inspiration.

27. Ans.— C. Sends out regular impulses to expiratory muscles during quiet respiration
28. Ans.— E. All of the above
29. Ans.— A. Cessation of breathing
30. Ans.— B. Decreased cerebral blood circulation
31. Ans.— A. 20 times

Carbon monoxide has much higher solubility than CO2 or O2

32. Ans.— B. 4200

Alveolar ventilation is tidal volume minus physiological dead space multiplied by respiratory rate.

33. Ans.— B. Scoliosis
34. Ans.— A. -4
35. Ans.— B. Sleep
36. Ans.— D. All of the above
37. Ans.— C. O2 dissociation curve shifts to right

Ascent to high altitude triggers a substantial rise in 2, 3 - DPG concentration in red cells with a consequent increase in P50 and increase in availability of O_2 to tissues. The rise in 2, 3 DPG which has a half life of 6 hours, is secondary to the rise in blood pH.

38. Ans.— C. Pulmonary hypoventilation
39. Ans.— B. Efflux of Cl- from RBC
40. Ans.— D. Maintaining arterial pressure at a normal level over a period of weeks, months or years
41. Ans.— B. CO_2

Alveolar ventillation is equal to respiratory rate multiplied by the volume of air entering the alveoli with each breath.

42. Ans.— C. Respiratory Distress Syndrome (RDS) in children

Surfactant is surface tension lowering phospholipoprotein complex produced by Type-II epithelial cells or granular pneumocytes.

43. Ans.— A. Diffusion

Diffusion is the process involved in CO2 entering the capillaries.

44. Ans.— C. Transferrin

Carbon monoxide is toxic because it reacts with hemoglobin to form carbon monoxyhemoglobin (carboxyhemoglobin) and COHb cannot take up oxygen. It leads to anemic hypoxia (deficiency of Hb that carry O_2).

45. Ans.— A. Lung elasticity
46. Ans.— B. Carbon dioxide washout

Physiologically, pO2 of the arterial blood may be reduced in residents at high altitude (over 10,000 ft).

47. Ans.— D. Respiring in dead space
48. Ans.— D. None of the above
49. Ans.— B. 125-170
50. Ans.— D. Respiratory centre

51. Ans.— B 4.2

Alveolar ventilation (VA) is 4.2L/min and is equal to VA = Respiratory rate X (Vt-Vd) (Vt=Tidal volume and Vd = Dead space volume)

52. Ans.— C. 500 ml

53. Ans.— A. 3000 ml

54. Ans.— B. 4600 ml

55. Ans.— D. 3500 ml

56. Ans.— D. All of the above

57. Ans.— C. Volume of air present after normal expiration

Functional residual capacity (RC) is the volume of air left in the lungs at the end of natural passive expiration. It is sum of residual volume and ERV.

Normal values are

Pulm. vol/capacity	Volume (L)
Tidal vol.	0.5
IRV	3.0
ERV	1.0
RV	1.2
TLC	5.7
VC	4.6
FRC	2.2
MVV	125

58. Ans.— B. Pneumocyte-II

59. Ans.— D. None of the above

60. Ans.— B. 80%

61. Ans.— B. 5, 3

62. Ans.— B. 60 mm Hg

63. Ans.— B. PO_2 Decrease and PCO Decrease

64. Ans.— B. Abnormal dullness to percussion of the affected side

65. Ans.— A. Less than 1 sec

66. Ans.— D. Isoproternol

67. Ans.— C. 1500 ml

68. Ans.— A. Asthma

69. Ans.— D. All of the above

70. Ans.— C. 20

It is about 25 ml/min/mmHg. Mean oxygen pressure difference across the respiratory membrane under quiet breathing is about 11 mmHg.

71. Ans.— D. Equal

72. Ans.— B. Decreased

73. Ans.— B. IRV + TV

74. Ans.— C. 2.4 litres in women

75. Ans.— D. 2. 2 litres

76. Ans.— B. 83%

77. Ans.— C. 0.5 Kg-m/min

78. Ans.— D. 10kg-m/breath

79. Ans.— B. Tidal volume

80. Ans.— B. 4.8 litres

Vital capacity is IRV + TV+ ERV and is 3.1 L in women.

81. Ans.— C. 300 million alveoli in man

82. Ans.— C. 70 sq. m

83. Ans.— B. 500 ml

84. Ans.— C. 97%

85. Ans.— D. All of the above

86. Ans.— B. 2%

87. Ans.— D. 400 ml in a normal individual when he lies down

88. Ans.— D. Acetylcholine

89. Ans.— B. 0.95-0.99

90. Ans.— C. 500 ml of air per breath

91. Ans.— C. 200 ml

About 280 L of CO2 is formed in 24 hours

92. Ans.— C. 330 litres

93. Ans.— D. 97

94. Ans.— D. Total lung capacity

95. Ans.— C. 10-30 ml/min/mmHg

96. Ans.— C. 94%

97. Ans.— B. 100-250 ml

98. Ans.— A. Initiates the rhythmicity of normal breathing

Hering Breuer initiation reflex is an increase in duration of expiration produced by steady lung inflation and Hering Breuer deflation reflex is a decrease in duration of expiration produced by marked deflation of lung.

99. Ans.— B. Increased sensitivity of resp. center

100. Ans.— B. Compression of airway

101. Ans.— A. Respiratory Alkalosis

102. Ans.— A. PO_2 normal, $\dot{O}_2$ saturation less

103. Ans.— D. Nitrous oxide

104. Ans.— D. 400-500 L/mt

Peak expiratory flow rate (PEFR) is defined as the maximum rate of air flow which can be achieved during a sudden forced expiration.

105. Ans.— A. Decreased

106. Ans.— B. PO2

107. Ans.— D. Abdominals

108. Ans.— A. Stimulation of the respiratory centre by the cerebral cortex and the joint proprioception.

109. Ans.— C. 2700 ml/min

110. Ans.— B. Arterial PCO2

It affects by CSF H+ concentration.

111. Ans.— D. Increased blood glucose

112. Ans.— A. Hypoxia

113. Ans.— B. 3000 ml/min.

114. Ans.— B. Vital capacity

Tidal volume is 0.5 L in both men and women.

115. Ans.— D. Some portions of the lungs are perfused but not ventilated

116. Ans.— C. Of the order of 100 mmHg

117. Ans.— A. The plasma bicarbonate concentration is either low or normal

118. Ans.— B. It averages 4-5 litres in a 70-kg adult male

119. Ans.— B.& Jugular venous pressure tends to fall
C. Muscles of the anterior abdominal wall relax

120. Ans.— B. FEV1

121. Ans.— D. 100 mm Hg

122. Ans.— C. 45 mm Hg

123. Ans.— B. 40 mm Hg

124. Ans.— B. Is relatively constant with changes in altitude

125. Ans.— A. Protective function

126. Ans.— B. Hypoxaemia

127. Ans.— A. 60 mm Hg

128. Ans.— B. Respiratory alkalosis

129. Ans.— A. 600-800 ml

130. Ans.— C. Left atrial pressure

Pulmonary capillary pressure is about 10 mm Hg whereas the oncotic pressure is 25 mm Hg so that there is an inward directed pressure gradient of about 15 mm which keeps the alveoli free of fluid.

131. Ans.— A. 4500 ml

132. Ans.— A. Stops during swallowing

133. Ans.— B. Pneumotoxic

Pneumotaxic centre is located bilaterally in the upper pons. These neurones have an inhibitory influence on the dorsal respiratory group of neurones. Strong pneumotoxic discharge may cut down the respiratory phase to 0.5 sec.

134. Ans.— A. Emphysema

135. Ans.— C. Response to O_2 therapy

136. Ans.— A. Tidal volume

137. Ans.— C. Is often evidenced by an increase in lactic concentration in the blood.

At the end of treadmill exercise, O2 consumption does not return to pre-work level immediately. O2 consumption may remain elevated for a period upto 30 min or more after the end of exercise. The excess of O2 consumed during recovery phase is called O2 debt.

138. Ans.— D. Surface tension of the alveolar fluid

139. Ans.— E. Histotoxic hypoxia due to cyanide poisoning

140. Ans.— B. Carbon dioxide

141. Ans.— D. Emphysema

142. Ans.— D. Some portions of the lungs are perfused but not ventilated.

143. Ans.— D. An increase in glycolysis by H+ activation of phosphofructokinase.

144. Ans.— B. End of expiration

145. Ans.— D. All of the above

146 Ans.— D. Obstructed air passages

147. Ans.— B. 80%

Cyanosis is seen in when reduced Hb concentration of blood in capillaries is more than 5g/dL. It is most easily seen in nail beds and mucous membranes. It does not occur in anemic hypoxia because total Hb is low; in carbon monoxide poisoning, because color of reduced Hb is obscured by cherry red color of carbonmonoxy-hemoglobin or in histotoxic hypoxia, because blood gas content is normal.

148. Ans.— C. Pressure of the gas

149. Ans.— C. 80-100 mmHg

150. Ans.— B. 95-98%

151. Ans.— D. Excessive ventilation

152. Ans.— B. ↑ pCO_2, ↓ pH

153. Ans.— A. Vital capacity

154. Ans.— A. Emphysema

155. Ans.— D. Anemia

A decrease in pH of blood increase in PCO2 and increase in temperature and 2-3 DPG shift oxygen dissociation curve to right.

156. Ans.— D. Cardiac failure

157. Ans.— D. All of the above

158. Ans.— C. Inhibited by swallowing and vomiting

159. Ans.— A. Regular 3 months exercise

160. Ans.— C. Residual volume

161. Ans.— C. CO poisoning

162. Ans.— B. Low arterial O_2 content

It is seen in carbon monoxide poisoning.

163. Ans.— A. BP rise

164. Ans.— A. $\frac{\text{MMV-RMV}}{\text{MVV}} \times 100$

165. Ans.— D. Cool extremities

166. Ans.— C. Lower residual volume and total lung capacity

167. Ans.— B. Vitalograph

168. Ans.— E. Bicarbonate

CO2 is mainly transported as bicarbonate. It is 20 times more soluble than O2

169. Ans.— C. 300-400 gms

170. Ans.— C. Vertebral fractures

171. Ans.— A. Dorsal respiratory group

172. Ans.— C. 60-80

173. Ans.— C. More negative

174. Ans.— B. 50

175. Ans.— A. Apical region

The ratio of pulmonary ventilation to pulmonary blood flow for the whole lung at rest is about 0.8 (4.2 L/m divided by 5.5 L/min) blood flow.

176. Ans.— B. 20

177. Ans.— C. 2

178. Ans.— B. CO

179. Ans.— D. Bronchial Dilatation

180. Ans.— C. Diffusion decreases

181. Ans.— D. Breaking action of inspiratory airways

182. Ans.— C. ↑ respiratory minute volume

183. Ans.— C. Tachypnoea

184. Ans.— D. MBC is the largest volume of gas can be moved into and out of lungs in one second by effort.

185. Ans.— A. 80

186. Ans.— C. <40

187. Ans.— B. Increased pulmonary capillary pressure

188. Ans.— C. More negative

189. Ans.— C. Medullary chemoreceptors

190. Ans.— C. In smokers with deficiency have increased destruction of lungs.

It may lead to emphysema.

191. Ans.— B. VC

192. Ans.— D. FRC

193. Ans.— D. FEFR

194. Ans.— A. Binding with oxygen

195. Ans.— A. Dynamic compression of airway

196. Ans.— A. Sympathetic stimulation cause release of acetylcholine at neuromuscular junction.

197. Ans.— B. Arterial Na+ concentration

198. Ans.— C. Cheyne-Stokes breathing

199. Ans.— A. 4.5 litre/min

200. Ans.— A. Slow and deep

201. Ans.— A. Carbon dioxide wash out

Ascent to high altitude triggers a substantial rise in 2,3 DPG concentration in red cells. CO_2 is washed out due to hyperventilation.

202. Ans.— A. 4900 ml

203. Ans.— D. ETA epithelial receptor

204. Ans.— C. Decreased Ca++ ions

205. Ans.— D. EERV

206. Ans.— B. Humidifies air

207. Ans.— B. Type-II pneumocytes

"Surfactant is produced by type-II alveolar epithelial cells".

208. Ans.— D. 97%

209. Ans.— D. 1 : 1

210. Ans.— B. 280 L

211. Ans.— A. 1 and 2 are correct

212. Ans.— D. Diaphragm and external intercostals

213. Ans.— B K+ ions

The concentration of some ions inside and outside motor neuron.

Ion	Concentration (mmol/L of H2O) Inside cell	Outside cell	Equilibrium Potential (mV)
Na+	15.40	150.0	+60
K+	950.0	5.5	-90
Cl-	9.0	25.0	-70

214. Ans. — C Makes the apillary surface hydrophillic

Surfactant : The low surface tension when the alveoli are small is due to the presence in the fluid lining the alveoli of surfactant, a lipid surface - tension lowering agent. Surfactant is a mixture of DPPC, other lipids, and proteins. If the surface tension is not kept low when the alveoli become smaller during expiration, they collapse in accordance with the law of Laplace. In spherical structures like the alveoli, the distending pressure equals 2 times the tension divided by the radius (P=2T/r); if T is not reduced, the tension overcomes the distending pressure.

215. Ans. — C Vasoconstriction in response to hyper-capnia

* **"Effect of Diminished Alveolar Oxygen on Local Alveolar Blood Flow—Automatic Control of Pulmonary Blood Flow Distribution.**

216. Ans. C. Body plethysmography

* **A plethysmograph is instrument for measuring changes in volume within an organ.**
* **Pulmonary plethysmographys ar commonly used to measure the functional residual capacity (FRC) of the lungs - the volume in the lungs when the muscle sof respiration are relaxed —and total lung capacity.**

4.

IMPORTANT TEXT OF KIDNEY

STIMULI WHICH INCREASE RENIN SECRETION

Sodium depletion
Diuretics
Hypotension
Haemorrhage
Upright posture
Dehydration
Constriction of renal artery or aorta
Cardiac failure
Cirrhosis

ACTIVE TRANSPORT OF SUBSTANCES BY THE INTESTINE AND LOCATION OF MAXIMUM ABSORPTION OR SECRETION*

	Location of Absorptive Capacity			
	Small Intestine			*Colon*
	Upper†	*Mid*	*Lower*	
Gamma globulin (newborn animals)	+	++	+++	?
Pyrimidines (thymine and uracil)	+	+	?	?
Triglycerides	++	++	+	?
Fatty acid absorption and conversion to triglyceride	+++	++	+	0
Bile salts	0	+	+++	
Vitamin B_{12}	0	+	+++	0
Na^+	+++	++	+++	+++
H^+ (and/or HCO_3^- secretion)	0	+	++	++
Ca^{++}	+++	++	+	?
Fe^{++}	+++	++	+	?
Cl^-	+++	++	+	0
$SO_4^=$	++	+	0	?
Secretion				
K^+	0	0	+	++
H^+ (and/or HCO_3^- absorption)	++	+	0	0
Sr^{++}	0	0	+	?
Cl^- (under special conditions)	+	?	?	?
I^-	0	+	0	0

* Saunders, 1962. Amount of absorption or secretion is graded + to +++.

* † Upper small intestine refers primarily to jejunum, although the duodenum is similar in most cases studied (with the notable exception that the duodenum secretes HCO_3^- and shows little absorption or secretion of NaCl).

RELATIVE CONCENTRATIONS OF SUBSTANCES IN THE GLOMERULAR FILTRATE AND IN THE URINE

	Glomerular Filtrate (125 ml./min.)		*Urine (1 ml./min.)*		*Conc. Urine/ Conc. Plasma (Plasma Clearance per Minute)*
	Quantity/min.	*Concentration*	*Quantity/min.*	*Concentration*	
Na+	17.7 mEq.	142 mEq./L	0.128 mEq/L	128 mEq./L	0.9
K+	0.63	5	0.06	60	12
Ca++	0.5	4	0.0048	4.8	1.2
Mg++	0.38	3	0.015	15	5.0
Cl-	12.9	103	0.134	134	1.3
HCO_3^-	3.5	28	0.014	14	0.5
$H2PO_4^-$					
HPO_4^-}	0.25	2	0.05	50	25
SO_4^-	0.09	0.7	0.033	33	47
Glucose	125 mg.	100 mg.%	0 mg.	0 mg.%	0.0
Urea	33	26	18.2	1820	70
Uric acid	3.8	3	0.42	42	14
Creatinine	1.4	1.1	1.96	196	140
Inulin	...	...	...	...	125
Diodrast	...	...	...	...	560
PAH	...	...	...	...	585

CHARACTERISTICS OF A SUBSTANCE SUITABLE FOR MEASURING THE GFR BY DETERMINING ITS CLEARANCE

Freely filtered
Not reabsorbed or secreted by tubules
Not metabolized
Not stored in kidney
Not protein-bound (substances bound to albumin and globulin not filtered)
Not toxic
Has no effect on filtration rate
Preferably easy to measure in plasma and urine

FACTORS AFFECTING THE GLOMERULAR FILTRATION RATE

1. Changes in renal blood flow
2. Changes in glomerular capillary hydrostatic pressure
   a. Changes in systemic blood pressure
   b. Afferent or efferent arteriolar constriction
3. Changes in hydrostatic pressure in Bowman's capsule
   a. Ureteral obstruction
   b. Edema of kidney inside tight renal capsule
4. Changes in concentration of plasma proteins: dehydration, hypoproteinemia, etc. (minor factors)

5. Increased permeability of glomerular filter; various diseases
6. Decrease in total area of glimerular capillary bed
   a. Diseases which destroy glomeruli with or without destruction of tubules
   b. Partial nephrectomy

QUANTITATIVE ASPECTS OF Na^+ REABSORPTION IN A NORMAL MAN

GFR = 125 ml/minute
Plasma HCO_3 = 27 mEq/liter
Plasma Na^+ = 145 mEq/liter

Na^+ filtered per minute	18, 125 mEq
Reabsorbed with Cl^-	14, 585 mEq
Reabsorbed while reabsorbing 3375 $mEqHCO3^-$	3,375 mEq
Reabsorbed in association with formation of titrable acidity and ammonia	50 mEq
Reabsorbed in association with secretion of K^+	50 mEq
Total Na^+ reabsorbed per minute	18,060 mEq

MCQ's OF KIDNEY

What is important in Kidney

Kidney function tests, Structure and Physiology of a nephron

1. **Factors affecting GRF are : PGI 1981**
   A. Changes in renal blood flow
   B. Changes in glomerular capillary hydrostatic pressure
   C. Ureteric obstruction
   D. All of the above
2. **The following is the minor factor affecting GFR : AIIMS 1982, 84**
   A. Partial nephrectomy B. Ureteric obstruction
   C. Diabetes insipidus D. Hypoproteinemia
3. **The following are the characteristics of substance suitable for measuring GFR except : AMC 1984, 94**
   A. Freely filtered
   B. Stored in kidney
   C. Not reabsorbed or excreted by tubules
   D. Not protein bound
4. **Which of the following is not true about inulin : AMC 1982,99**
   A. A polymer of fructose
   B. Molecular weight 5200
   C. Found in dahlia tubers
   D. None of the above
5. **Oxygen consumption of renal cortex and inner medulla are ml/100g/min respectively : AIIMS 1983, 99**
   A. 9, 4 B. 4, 9
   C. 9, 0.4 D. 0.4, 6
6. **Creatinine is not ideal to measure GFR in humans because : AMU 1986, 99**
   A. It is toxic
   B. It is secreted by tubules and some may be reabsorbed
   C. Not freely filtered
   D. Affects filtration rate
7. **Oxygen consumption of human kidney is about ——— ml/min : AIIMS 1986, 99**
   A. 9 B. 12
   C. 18 D. 62
8. **A-V O2 difference in kidney is ——ml/L of blood : AMU 1985, 95**
   A. 14 B. 18
   C. 62 D. 114
9. **In humans, effective renal blood flow is : AIIMS 1983, 86**
   A. 425 B. 525
   C. 625 D. 725
10. **Renal blood flow is : AIIMS 1983**
    A. 0.8-1.2 L/min. B. 1.2-1.3 L/min.
    C. 1.5-2.0 L/min. D. 2.0-2.5 L/min.
11. **The volume of blood in the renal capillaries at any given time is :**
    A. 30-40 ml B. 70-100 ml
    C. 100-300 ml D. 300-450 ml
12. **Total length of nephrons including the collecting ducts ranges from : AIIMS 1981, 92**
    A. 5-10 mm B. 25-45 mm
    C. 45-65 mm D. 65-100 mm
13. **The length of distal convulated tubule is : AIIMS 1980, 95**
    A. 2 mm B. 5 mm
    C. 8 mm D. 12 mm
14. **In humans, —— of the nephrons having long loops: AMC 1985, 96**
    A. 5% B. 15%
    C. 35% D. 65%
15. **Urine/Plasma ratio of glucose in mg/dl is : PGI 1986, 97**
    A. 0 B. 1
    C. 10 D. 100
16. **Urine/Plasma ratio of Na+ (meq/L) is : CMC 1987**
    A. 0 meq/L B. 1 meq/L
    C. 10 meq/L D. 100 meq/L
17. **Total area of glomerular capillary endothelium across which filtration occurs in humans is : AIIMS 1980, 98**
    A. 0.1 sq. m B. 0.4 sq. m
    C. 0.8 sq. m D. 1.2 sq. m

Ans.	1. D	2. D	3. B	4. D	5. C	6. B	7. C	8. A	9. C	10. B
	11. A	12. C	13. B	14. B	15. A	16. B	17. C			

18. Renal blood flow is about what % cardiac output : AP 1985, 96

A. 10% B. 15%
C. 18% D. 25%

19. Urine plasma ratio of creatinine (mg/dl) is : AMU 1987, 98

A. 0 B. 1
C. 60 D. 150

20. One of the following does not form filtration barrier in nephron : AI 1995, 96

A. Mesangium B. Hypopnea
C. Endothelial cell D. Basement membrane

21. Which of the following pressure changes leads to an increased GFR : Rajasthan 1992

A. ↑ arterial plasma colloid osmotic pressure
B. ↑ glomerular capillary hydrostatic pressure
C. ↑ hydrostatic pressure in Bowman's capsule
D. ↑ net filtration pressure

22. A substance commonly used to measure renal blood flow is : DNB 1989, 95

A. Glucose
B. Cobalt labelled red cells
C. Inulin
D. Para-aminohippuric acid

23. Active reabsorption of glucose appears to occur in: AIIMS 1981, 84

A. Distal tubuleB. Loop of Henle
C. Proximal tubuleD. All of the above

24. In renal glycosuria, the renal threshold for glucose is : AIIMS 1986; PGI 1986

A. Low B. High
C. Same D. Greatly increased

25. Each kidney contains ab‹ —— nephrons : Delhi 1948, 86

A. One million B. Two million
C. Four million D. 1/2 million

26. Two substances that can probably be used to determine filtration fraction are : PGI 1987, 98

A. Inulin and mannitol B. Urea and diodrast
C. PAH and phenol red D. Inulin and PAH

27. In a normal adult the desire for micturition is felt : AMC 1987, 98

A. When about 100-200 cc of urine has collected in the bladder.
B. When about 300-400 cc of urine has collected in the bladder.
C. When about 600-800 cc of urine has collected in the bladder.
D. When about 1000 cc of urine has collected in the bladder .

28. Where in the kidney, does active reabsorption of sodium ions occur ? **Delhi 1987**

A. Collecting duct
B. Distal tubule
C. Ascending limb of Henle
D. Only B and C

29. Which of the following is minimally excreted in urine : AMU 1984

A. Urea B. Creatinine
C. Uric acid D. Chloride

W.30. Which of the following ion is not handled at loop of Henle : Rohtak 1987

A. Na B. K+
C. Cl- D. Urea

31. The following inhibits Cl- reabsorption in the loop of Henle except : AMC 1985

A. Thiazide B. Furosemide
C. Ethacrynic acid D. Triamterene

32. When GFR falls, the sodium excretion will : Delhi 1981

A. Increase
B. Fall
C. Fall followed by increased
D. No change

33. Ethyl Alcohol produces diuresis by : AIIMS 1982,97

A. Producing osmotic diuresis
B. Inhibiting vasopressin secretion
C. Decreases tubular absorption of Na+
D. Inhibits Cl- reabsorption

34. Sodium filtered per minute (micro-equivalents) is : AIIMS 1983

A. 21825 B. 18125
C. 18060 D. 14585

35. Which substance is actively transported by the tubular cells but has not been shown to have a Tm? Delhi 1986

A. Albumin
B. Haemoglobin
C. Both albumin and haemoglobin
D. Sodium ions

36. Which of the following has no Tm value ? Delhi 1987

A. Albumin, arginine
B. Betahydroxybutyrate,· glucose
C. Glucose haemoglobin, phosphate
D. Urea

37. GFR is increased when : AIIMS 1983, 87

A. Plasma oncotic pressure is increased
B. Glomorular hydrostatic pressure is decreased
C. Tubular hydrostatic pressure is increased
D. Increased renal blood flow

Ans.	18. D	19. D	20. A	21. B	22. D	23. C	24. A	25. A	26. D	27. B
	28. D	29. C	30. NONE	31. D	32. B	33. B	34. B	35. D	36. D	37. D

38. **Normal kidney does not allow passage of : PGI 1984, 87**
A. β-globuli B. Lysozyme
C. IgG D. Albumin

39. **Tubular membrane is Maximum permeable to : AIIMS 1984; Delhi 1987**
A. Creatinine B. Inulin
C. Urea D. Sucrose

40. **Glomerular filtration rate can be increased by : AIIMS 1985, 99**
A. Increasing arterial blood pressure
B. Increasing the plasma protein concentration
C. Efferent arteriolar dilation
D. Afferent arteriolar constriction

Following test results were obtained from a person over a 24 hour period : AIIMS 1986, 99
I. Urine flow rate : 1.0 ml/mt
II. Urine inulin : 100 mg/100 ml
III. Plasma inulin : 1.0 mg/100 ml
IV. Urine urea : 200 mmol/L
V. Plasma urea : 5 mmol/L

41. **What is the glomerular filtration rate ?**
A. 100 ml/min B. 125 ml/min
C. 150 ml/min D. 175 ml/min
E. 200 ml/min

42. **What is the urea clearance ? AIIMS 1989, 98**
A. 4.4 ml/min B. 88 ml/min
C. 440 ml/min D. 44 ml/min

43. **All of the following are actively reabsorbed from the proximal tubules except : PGI 1986, 96**
A. Sodium B. Urea
C. Amino acids D. Urea and water

44. **The acute control response to increased extracellular fluid volume involves or is associated with all of the following except : AMU 1985, 96**
A. Increased urine osmolarity
B. Stretch of the two atria
C. Decreased sympathetic stimulation of kidneys
D. Decreased secretion of antidiuretic hormone

45. **GFR is : Delhi 1996, 97**
A. Plasma filtered through microtubules
B. Serum filtered through microtubules
C. Arterial blood filtered through microtubules
D. Venous blood filtered through microtubules

46. **Active reabsorption of glucose occurs in : AIIMS 1983, 98**
A. Proximal tubule B. Loop of Henle
C. Distal tubule D. All of the above

47. **The hypersomolarity of the renal medulla is due to increased content of : AIIMS 1987**
A. K+ B. Na+ and urea
C. Glucose D. Na+

48. **Sodium movement in PCT from lumen to tubular cells is : AIIMS 1981, 96**
A. Active process B. Passive process
C. Filteration D. Associated with H_2O

49. **Normal creatinine clearance (in L/24 hours) : AMU 1985**
A. 46-76 B. 76-116
C. 116-148 D. 148-168

50. **Addis test is used for : AP 1985, 96**
A. Urinary sugar B. Urinary sediment
C. Blood lactate D. Serum magnesium

51. **Which of the following substances has the lowest clearance in the human kidney : Rajasthan 1992; PGI 1996**
A. Creatinine B. K+
C. Cl- D. Glucose

52. **Potassium is : AI 1993**
A. Entirely absorbed in the PCT
B. Competes with Na^+ absorption
C. Absorption depends upon aldosterone
D. Mainly absorbed in the DCT

53. **True is : AI 1993**
A. Creatine measure GFR most accurately.
B. Creatine clearance is 70 ml/mt.
C. Creatinine is a sensitive endogenous index of renal function.
D. Creatine has no relation to blood urea.

54. **Which is true regarding Renin secretion : AI 1993**
A. ↑ K+ in PCT, - Renin secretion
B. ↓ Na+ in DCT, - Renin Secretion
C. Inversely proportional to the potassium levels
D. Directly proportional to the ADH levels

55. **Water is not freely permeable but sodium and pottasium are in which portion of nephron : Delhi 1993, 98**
A. Thick ascending limb
B. Descending limb
C. DCT
D. Collecting tubules

56. **Juxtamedullary nephrons in kidney are what percentage of total nephrons : Delhi 1992, 94**
A. 15 B. 50
C. 70 D. 90

57. **Inulin clearance closely resembles : Delhi 1992; PGI 1999**
A. G.F.R. B. Renal plasma flow
C. Creatinine clearance D. P.A.H. clearance

58. **Which of the following is truly physiological ? AIIMS 1992, 98**
A. Mild pedal edema B. Increased GFR
C. Albuminuria D. Increased BP

Ans. 38. A 39. B 40. A 41. B 42. D 43. D 44. A 45. A 46. A 47. B 48. A 49. C 50. B 51. D 52. A 53. C 54. B 55. A 56. D 57. A 58. B

59. **Normal urinary protein excretion is : PGI 1993, 94**
A. 50-150 mg% B. 150-250 mg%
C. 250-500 mg% D. Nil

60. **Site of action of ADH is : AMU 1986, 99**
A. Glomerulus of nephron
B. Proximal convoluted tubule
C. Distal convoluted tubule
D. Collecting duct

61. **A substance which has a renal clearance 20 times that of inulin is probably : AIIMS 1988, 98**
A. Only filtered at the glomeruli
B. Only secreted by tubules
C. Filtered and reabsorbed
D. Synthesized in tubules and secreted

62. **Which of the following changes would not occur, under steady-state conditions in a normal person as a result of a 50 percent decrease in sodium intake : Delhi 1988, 98**
A. Increased plasma concentrationof angiotensin-II.
B. Increased plasma Aldosterone concentration.
C. Approximately a 50 per cent decrease in sodium excretion.
D. A large (greater than 10 per cent) decrease in plasma sodium concentration.

63. **Following is least absorbable in tubules : Rajasthan 1992, 98**
A. Creatinine B. Glucose
C. Urea D. Sucrose

64. **All of the following factors stimulate the release or Renin following trauma except : AIIMS 1993, 98**
A. Vasopressin release
B. Decreased renal perfusion pressure
C. Fall in circulating blood volume
D. Increased sympathetic stimulation of adrenals

65. **The daily loss of nitrogen in urine is approximately: Karnataka 1994, 99**
A. 2-5 g B. 5-10 g
C. 10-20 g D. 25-50 g

66. **Maximal urine acidity is : DNB 1992, 97**
A. 0.0003 B. 0.003
C. 0.03 D. 3.0

67. **Glucose is transported through : AIIMS 1994, 95; AI 1995**
A. Na anteport B. Na co-transport
C. K anteport D. K symport

68. **In DCT, following are absorbed except : AIIMS 1997, 98**
A. Na+ B. K+
C. Water D. Cl-

69. **Renin secretion is increased by following except : AIIMS 1997, 98**
A. Hypovolemia
B. Hyponatremia in PCT
C. Hyponatremia in DCT
D. Sympathetic stimulation

70. **Which one of the following is not responsible for concentration of urine in the kidneys ? UPSC 1997**
A. Aldosterone B. Angiotensin-II
C. Vasopressin D. Epinephrine

71. **Loop of Henle handles the following except : PGI 1997, 99**
A. Na+ B. K+
C. Cl- D. Urea

72. **Sertoli cells secrete following except : Bihar 1998, 99**
A. Mullerian inhibiting substance
B. Somatomedin
C. Inhibin
D. Androgen binding protein

73. **True statement regarding oxygen consumption in the kidney is : JIPMER 1998, 99**
A. Oxygen consumption decreases as blood flow increases.
B. O2 consumption is maximum in renal medulla.
C. O2 consumption in ml/min is maximum as compared to any organ in the body.
D. Consumption is equal in both cortex & medulla.

74. **Match List-I (Tubular function) with List-II (Substance) and select the correct answer : CSE 1997, 98**

List-I	List-II
A. Active reabsorption	1. Urea
B. Passive diffusion	2. Phenol red
C. Secretion	3. Glucose
D. Neither reabsorption nor secretion	4. Inulin

	A	B	C	D
A.	3	1	4	2
B.	1	3	2	4
C.	3	1	2	4
D.	1	3	2	4

75. **Counter current mechanism of the kidney consists of : CSE 1997, 99**
A. Proximal tubule and collecting tubule
B. Loop of Henle and vasa recta
C. Collecting tubule and vasa recta
D. Proximal tubule and loop of Henle

76. **In the nephron, reabsorption of most of the filtered water occurs in the : Manipal 1992, 95**
A. Proximal convoluted tubule
B. Loope of Henle
C. Distal convoluted tubule
D. Collecting duct

Ans.									
59. A	60. D	61. D	62. D	63. A	64. D	65. D	66. C	67. B	68. B
69. B	70. D	71. B	72. B	73. A	74. C	75. B	76. A		

77. **The renal threshold value for complete tubular reabsorption of glucose is : CSE 1996, 99**
A. 70-80 mg% blood glucose
B. 120-140 mg% blood glucose
C. 170-180 mg% blood glucose
D. 220-240 mg% blood glucose

78. **Diluting segment of a nephron is : Kerala 1999**
A. Thin ascending limb of loop of Henle
B. Thick ascending limb of loop of Henle
C. Cortical collecting duct
D. Medullary collecting duct

79. **Acidification of urine takes place in : AI-2000**
A. PCT B. DCT
C. Collecting duct D. Asc. Loop of Henle

80. **Amino acids are completely absorbed in : PGI 2000**
A. PCT B. DCT
C. CT D. All of the above

81. **Which is true about renin : PGI 2000**
A. It helps to convert angiotensinogen ------> Angiotensin - I
B. Secreted by PCT
C. ↑ GFR ↑ secretion of renin
D. ↓ plasma Na+ & H2O

82. **The sodium content of the filtrate in renal medulla is very high because : AIIMS 2000**
A. At the loop of Henle, there is counter-current mechanism.
B. Increased blood flow to vasa recta.
C. Increased absorption of sodium from PCT.
D. Increased excretion of Na+ from PCT.

83. **Max absorption of glucose is : DNB 2001**
A. 370 B. 150
C. 180 D. 120

84. **Renin activity in elderly is : JIPMER 2001**
A. High B. Low
C. No change D. A or B

85. **A dye is injected. (i) The concentration in renal artery is 2U/min. (ii) In renal vein the concentration is IU/min. (iii) Amount excreted in mine is 2U/min. Which of the following aptly describes the substance: AIIMS 2002**
A. Freely filtered in the glomerulus
B. Plasma protein bound
C. Not absorbed in the renal tubules
D. Secreted into the cortical nephrons

86. **Following cells are responsible for acid secretion in kidney : JIPMER 2002**
A. T-cells B. P-cells
C. Mesangial cells D. Pericytes

87. **Relaxation of Mesangial cells of kidney is brought about by : JIPMER 2002**
A. cAMP B. Endothelin
C. PGF2 D. Vasopressin

88. **All the following are true about uric acid excretion except : SGPGI 2002**
A. It is filtered at the glomerulus
B. It is completely reabsorbed in PCT
C. It is resecreted in the loop of Henle
D. Effectively 50% of the filtered uric acid is excreted

89. **Normal urine flow & voiding pressure is : BHU-2002**
A. 15 ml/min & < 60 mm Hg
B. 10-15 ml/min & 60-80 mm Hg
C. < 10 ml/min & > 60 mm Hg
D. 15 ml/min & > 60 mm Hg

90. **The Renal plasma flow (RPF) of a patient was to be estimated through the measurement of para amino hippuric acid (PAH) clearance. The technician observed the procedures correctly but due to an error in the weighing inadvertently used thrice the recommended dose of PAH. The RPF estimated is likely to be : AI 2003**
A. False-high
B. False-low
C. False high or false low depending on the GFR
D. Correct and is unaffected by the PAH overdose

91. **The diuretic group that does not require access to the tubular lumen to induce diuresis is : AIIMS 2003**
A. Carbonic anhydrase inhibitor.
B. Na-Cl symport inhibitor.
C. Mineralocorticoid antagonist.
D. Na-K symport inhibitor.

92. **The main site of bicarbonate reabsorption is : AI 2005**
A. Proximal convoluted tubule
B. Distal convoluted tubule
C. Cortical collecting duct
D. Medullary collecting duct

93. **Urinary concentrating ability of the kidney is increased by : AI 2005**
A. ECF volume contraction
B. Increase in RBF
C. Reduction of medullary hypersomolarity
D. Increase in GFR

94. **Which one of the following statements regarding water reabsorption in the tubules ? AI 2005**
A. The bulk of water reabsorption occurs secondary to Na+ reabsorption.
B. Majority of facultative reabsorption occurs in proximal tubule.
C. Obligatory reabsorption is ADH dependent.
D. 20% of water is always reabsorbed irrespective of water balance.

Ans.	77. C	78. B	79. B	80. A	81. A	82. A	83. A	84. A	85. A	86. A
	87. A	88. A	89. A	90. D	91. C	92. A	93. A	94. A		

95. According to myogenic hypothesis of renal autoregulation, the afferent arterioles contract in response to stretch induced by : AIIMS-2005

A. NO release
B. Noradrenaline release
C. Opening of Ca2+ channels
D. Adenosine release

96. Bicarbonate is maximally absorbed in : AIIMS 2007

A. PCT
B. DCT
C. Collecting duct
D. Thick ascending loop of Henle

97. Which of the following hormone is not secreted by the kidney : AI 2007

A. Renin B. Angiotensin I
C. Erythropoietin D. 1, 25 DHCC

98. The status of fluid in distal convoluted tuble is all except : AI 2009

A. Lean body mass B. Adipose tissue
C. Heart rate D. None of the above

99. About renal physiology all are true except : AI 2009

A. DCT always receive hypo-osmotic solution
B. Afferent artery supplies glomerulus
C. GFR is controlled by afferent and efferent arteriole
D. 5% cardiac output is received by kidney

Ans.	95. C	96. A	97. B	98. A	99. D

EXPLANATIONS OF KIDNEY

1. Ans.— D. All of the above
2. Ans.— D. Hypoproteinemia
3. Ans.— B. Stored in kidney
4. Ans.— D. None of the above
5. Ans.— C. 9, 0.4
6. Ans.— B. It is secreted by tubules and some may be reabsorbed
7. Ans.— C. 18
8. Ans.— A. 14
9. Ans.— C. 625
10. Ans.— B. 1.2-1.3 L/min.
11. Ans.— A. 30-40 ml
12. Ans.— C. 45-65 mm

    These are with glomeruli in the juxtamedullary region of cortex (juxtamedullary nephrons)
13. Ans.— B. 5 mm

    Proximal convoluted tubule is about 15 mm long and 55 μm in diameter. Total length of thin segment of loop is 2-14 mm. Ascending limb is 12 mm in length. DCT is 5 mm long and CT is 20 mm long. Total length of nephrons, including collecting ducts, ranges from 45 to 65 mm.
14. Ans.— B. 15%
15. Ans.— A. 0
16. Ans.— B. 1 meq/L
17. Ans.— C. 0.8 sq. m
18. Ans.— D. 25%

    Mass of kidneys is 0.3 Kg and blood flow is 1260 mL/min (or 420 mL/100g/min) and A-V oxygen difference is 14 and percentage of total cardiac output is 23.3 and oxygen consumption is 7.2.
19. Ans.-- D. 150
20. Ans.— A. Mesangium
21. Ans.— B. ↑ glomerular capillary hydrostatic pressure
22. Ans.— D. Para-aminohippuric acid

    Average PAH extraction ration is 0.9, Effective renal plasma flow (ERPF) is 625 mL/min. WHen PAH is infused in low doses, 90% of the PAH in arterial blood is removed in a single circulation through the kidney.

$$\frac{\text{ERPF} = \text{UPAH V}}{\text{om4 min)}} = \text{Clearance of PAH (PAH) C} = 63$$

Average PAH extraction ratio is 0.9

$$\text{Actual RPF} = \frac{630}{0.9} = 700 \text{ mL/min}$$

$$\text{Renal blood flo} = \frac{\text{RPF x 1}}{\text{1-H ematocrit (i.e. 45\%)}}$$

$$= 700\text{x}\frac{1}{0.55} = 1273 \text{ mL/min}$$

23. Ans.— C. Proximal tubule
24. Ans.— A. Low
25. Ans.— A. One million

    There are 1.3 million nephrons in each kidney. The glomerus is about 200 mm in diameter. PCT is 15 mm long and 55 mm in diameter. 15% of nephrons have longer loops.
26. Ans.— D. Inulin and PAH
27. Ans.— B. When about 300-400 cc of urine has collected in the bladder
28. Ans.— D. Only B and C
29. Ans.— C. Uric acid
30. Ans.— NONE

    Question is wrongly framed
31. Ans.— D. Triamterene
32. Ans.— B. Fall
33. Ans.— B. Inhibiting vasopressin secretion

34. Ans.— B. 18125

Sodium filtered is 26000 (meq/d) and 25,850 (meq/d) is reabsorbed. Excreted is only 150 meq/d. Percentage reabsorbed is 99.4 and location is P,L, D,C.

35. Ans.— D. Sodium ions

Transport maximum (Tm) is the maximal rate at which the transport systems can transport a particular solute. Tm for glucose is 180 mg/dL after which glycosuria occurs. Glucose is transported at the rate of 100mg/min (80 mg/dL of plasma X 125 mL/min). Urea also does not has Tm value.

36. Ans.— D. Urea

37. Ans.— D. Increased renal blood flow

38. Ans.— A. β-globuli

39. Ans.— B. Inulin

Inulin is neither absorbed nor metabolised. It is a polymer of fructose with Mol. Wt. 5200 that is found in dahlia tubers.

40. Ans.— A. Increasing arterial blood pressure

41. Ans.— B. 125 ml/min

42. Ans.— D. 44 ml/min

43. Ans.— D. Urea and water

44. Ans.— A. Increased urine osmolarity

45. Ans.— A. Plasma filtered through microtubules

Normal GFR is 125 ml/min

46. Ans.— A. Proximal tubule

47. Ans.— B. Na+ and urea

48. Ans.— A. Active process

49. Ans.— C. 116-148

50. Ans.— B. Urinary sediment

51. Ans.— D. Glucose

Glucose is 100% reabsorbed. The other substances absorbed are :

Substance	Per 24 hours Filtered	Reabsorbed	Secreted	Excreted	Percentage reabsorbed	
Na+ (meq)	26000	25850		150	99.4	P,L,D,C
K+ (meq)	600	5602	502	90	93.3	"
Cl- (meq)	180000	17850		150	99.2	"
HCO3- (meq)	4900	4900		0	100	P,D
Urea (mmol)	870	4603	410	53	P,L,D,C	
Creatine (mmol)	12	14	14	12		
Uricacid (mmol)	50	49	4	5	98	P
Glucose (mmol)	800	800		0	100	P
Total solute (mosm)	54,000	53,4000	100	700	98.9	P,L,D,C
Water (mL)	180,000	179,000	1000	99.4	P.K.D.C	

1. P-Proximal Tubules ' L- Loops of Henle, D- distal tuble, C-Collect ducts
2. K+ is reabsorbed and secreted
3. Urea moves into as well as out of some portions of the nephron
4. Valuable secretion and probable reabsorption of creatinine in humans

52. Ans.— A. Entirely absorbed in the PCT

53. Ans.— C. Creatinine is a sensitive endogenous index of renal function

54. Ans.— B. ↓Na+ in DCT, - Renin Secretion

The conditions which increase renin secretion are sodium depletion, diuretics, hypotension, haemorrhage, upright posture, dehydration, cardiac failure, cirrhosis, constriction of renal artery or aorta and various psychologic stimuli.

55. Ans.— A. Thick ascending limb

56. Ans.— D. 90

57. Ans.— A. G.F.R.

Normal GFR is approximately 125 mL/min or 7.5 L/h or 180 L/d. 99% or more of filtrate is normally reabsorbed. In a day, kidney filter an amount of fluid which is 4 times the total body water, 15 times the ECF volume and 60 times the plasma volume.

58. Ans.— B. Increased GFR

59. Ans.— A. 50-150 mg%

60. Ans.— D. Collecting duct

61. Ans.— D. Synthesized in tubules and secreted

62. Ans.— D. A large (greater than 10 per cent) decrease in plasma sodium concentration

63. Ans.— A. Creatinine

64. Ans.— D. Increased sympathetic stimulation of adrenals

65. Ans.— D. 25-50 g

66. Ans.— C. 0.03

67. Ans.— B. Na co-transport

68. Ans.— B. K+

69. Ans.— B. Hyponatremia in PCT

70. Ans.— D. Epinephrine

71. Ans.— B. K+

PCT handles Na/glucose CT, Na+/Pi CT, Na+ amino acid CT, Na+/Lactate CT, Na+ H+ exchanger, Cl- base exchanger. Thick ascending limb is Na+, 2 Cl-, KCT, Na+/H+ exchanger, K+ channels. DCT is NaCl CT whereas CT is Na+ channel transporter.

72. Ans.— B. Somatomedin

73. Ans.— A. Oxygen consumption decreases as blood flow increases.

74. Ans.— C. 3 1 2 4

75. Ans.— B. Loop of Henle and vasa recta

76. Ans.— A. Proximal convoluted tubule

77. Ans.— C. 170-180 mg% blood glucose

78. Ans.— B. Thick ascending limb of loop of Henle

79. Ans.— B. DCT

80. Ans.— A. PCT

81. Ans.— A. It helps to convert angiotensinogen ----> Angiotensin - I

82. Ans.— A. At the loop of Henle, there is counter-current mechanism

83. Ans.— A. 370

84. Ans.— A. High

This may lead to hypertension

85. Ans.— A. Freely filtered in the glomerulus

86. Ans.— A. T-cells

87. Ans.— A. cAMP

88. Ans.— A. It is filtered at the glomerulous

89. Ans.— A. 15 ml/min & < 60 mm Hg

90. Ans.— D. Correct and is unaffected by the PAH overdose

Renal plasma flow (RPF) can be measured by infusing pera-aminohippuric acid (PAH) and determining its urine and plasma concentration.

PAH is infused at low dose 90% of the PAH in anterial blood is removed in a single circulation through the kidney.

It is commonly used to calculate the renal plasma flow by dividing the amount of PAH in the urine by the plasma PAH level (hence ignoring amount of PAH given).

91. Ans.— C. Mineralocorticoid antagonist.

92. Ans.— A. Proximal convoluted tubule

"About 90% of the Filtered bicarbonate is reabsorbed in the proximal tubule".

- * In the proximal tubule, most of the secreted H+ react with HCO3- to form H2CO3.
- * The H2CO3 breaks down to form CO2 and H2O
- * In the proximal (but not in the distal) tubule, there is carbonic anhydrase in the brush border of the cell. This facilitates the formation of CO2 and H2O in the tubular fluid.
- * The CO2 which diffuses readily across all biologial membrane, enters the tubular cell, where it adds to the pool of CO2 available to form HCO3.

93.

Water deficity or ECF volume contraction
↓
↑ Extracellular osmolarity
↓ osmoreceptors
↓
↑ ADH secretion from posterior pituitary
↓
↑ Plasma ADH
↓
↑ HO permeability in Distal Tubular & collecting Ducts
↓
↑ H.O. Reabsorption
↓
↓ H.O Excrected
or
Urinary concentration

93. Ans.— A. ECF volume contraction

94. Ans.— A. The bulk of water reabsorption occurs secondary to Na+ reabsorption

* **This question is incomplete on reading and analysing all 4 options, one can came to a conclusion that they intended to ask to choose the correct option.**

Facts

- **Passive water reabsorption by osmosis is completed mainly to sodium reabsorption**
- **Water permeability of the proximal-tubule epithelium to water is so high, the osmolity gradient needed to generate the observed passive reabsorption of water is only 2 to 3 mOsm.**
- **65% of water is reabsorbed in PCT.**
- **Facultative reabsorption of water in collecting duct depend on principal cell response to ADH and aldosterone.**

95. Ans.— C Opening of Ca2+ channels

Autoregulation of GFR and renal blood flow occurs via two mechanisms :

a. **Tubuloglomerular feedback**

b. **Myogenic autoregulation**

* **Myogenic autoregulation refers to the ability of individual bloods vessels to resist stretching during increased arterial pressure.**

* **Studies of individual blood vessels (especially small arterioles) throughout the body have shown that the respond to increased wall tension or wall stretch by contraction of smooth muscle.**

* **Stretching of the vascular wall allows increased movement of calcium ions from the extracellular fluid into the cells through the calcium channels.**

The entry of calcium ions in the cells through calcium channel causes :

- **Development of action potential of smooth muscle**
- **Contraction of smooth muscle (calcium acts directly on the smooth muscle and cause its contraction).**

How does this mechanism helps in autoregulation?

* **The contraction of vessels prevent over distension of the vessel and at the same time by raising vascular resistance helps to prevent excessive increase in renal blood flow and GFR when arterial pressure increases.**

Also know :

Also know :

Tubuloglomerular feedback

* **This feed back mechanism links changes in sodium chloride concentration at the macula densa with the control of renal arteriolar resistance.**
* **This feedback ensures a relatively constant delivery of sodium chloride to the distal tubule and helps to prevent spurious fluctuation in renal excretion that would otherwise occur.**

96. Ans.— A PCT

The PCT reabsorbs about 65% of the filtered sodium, chloride, bicarbonate, and potassium and essentially all the filtered glucose and amino acids. About two-thirds of water is also reabsorbed in the PCT so that the fluid leaving the PCT is isotonic.

Amount of bicarbonate filtered per day in a normal adult on an average diet—4900mEq

Amount reabsorbed per day—4900 mEq

Amount secreted—0

Amount excreted—0

Percentage reabsorbed—100

Location of reabsorption —PCT (65%), DCT.

97. Ans.— B Angiotensin—IL

The kidneys produce three hormones, 1, 25 Dihydrochole calciferol, Renin and Erythropoetin

Angiotensin-I is not secreted by any organ. It is formed by the action of Renin (secreted by kidney) on Angiotensinogen (secreted by Liver).

Hormones produced kidney

* **Renin**
* **Erythropoetin**
* **1, 25 Dihydrocholecalciferol**

98. Ans.— A. Loan body mass

So energy expenditur in resting state would depend very much on body weight, thereby lean body mass which is around 80-85% of total body weight is the correct answer.

99. Ans.— D. 5% cardiac output is received by kidney

In a resting adult, the kidneys receive 1.2-1.3 L of blood per minute, or just under 25% of the cardiac output.

5.

IMPORTANT TEXT OF GIT

PRINCIPLE DIGESTIVE ENZYMES, THE CORRESPONDING PROENZYMES ARE SHOWN IN PARENTHESIS

Source	*Enzyme*	*Activator*	*Substrate*	*Catalytic Function or Products*
Salivary glands	Salivary a-amylase	...	Starch	Hydrolyzes 1,4a linkages, producing a-limit dextrins, malto--triose, and maltose
Stomach	Pepsins (pepsinogens)	HCl	Proteins and polypeptides	Cleave peptide bonds adjacent to aromatic amino acids
	Trypsin (trypsinogen)	Enterokinase	Proteins and polypeptides	Cleave peptide bonds adjacent to arginine or lysine
	Chymotrypsins (chymotrypsinogens)	Trypsin	Proteins and polypeptides	Cleave peptide bonds adjacent to aromatic, large hydrophobic amino acids
	Elastase (proelastase)	Trypsin	Elastin, some other proteins	Cleaves bonds adjacents to alanine, glycine, or serine
Exocrine pancreas	Carboxypeptidase-A (procarboxypeptidase-A)	Trypsin	Proteins and polypeptides	Cleaves carboxy terminal amino acids with basic side chains
	Carboxypeptidase-B (procarboxypeptidase-B)	Trypsin	Proteins and polypeptides	Cleaves carboxy terminal amino acids with basic side chains
	Pancreatic lipase	Emulsifying agents	Triglycerides	Di- and monoglycerides and fatty acids
	Pancreatic a-amylase	Cl-	Starch	Same as salivary a-amylase
	Ribonuclease	...	RNA	Nucleotides
	Deoxyribonuclease	...	DNA	Nucleotides
	Phospholipase-A (prophospholipase-A)	Trypsin	Lecithin	Lysolecithin
Intestinal mucosa	Enterokinase	...	Trypsinogen	Trypsin
	Aminopeptidases	...	Polypeptides	Cleave N-terminal amino acid from peptide
	Dipeptidases	...	Dipeptides	Two amino acids
	Glucoamylase	...	Maltose, maltotriose	Glucose
	Lactase	...	Lactose	Galactose and glucose
	Sucrase*	...	Sucrose	Fructose and glucose
	a-Dextrinase	...	a-Limit dextrins	Glucose
	Nuclease and related enzymes	...	Nucleic acids	Pentoses and purine and pyrimidine bases
	Intestinal lipase	...	Monoglycerides	Glycerol, fatty acids

* Sucrase and a-dextrinase are actually 2 parts of a single hybrid molecule.

MCQ's OF GIT

What is important in GIT

Functional types of movements, Digestion of food, Important local hormones and Enzymes

1. **All of the following enzymes are active within a cell except: AIIMS 2005, 2008**
   A. Trypsin
   B. Fumerase
   C. Hexokinase
   D. Alcohol dehydrogenase
2. **Pepsinogen-I is secreted from : AIIMS 1985, 88, 89; AI 1988; AMC 1985, 90**
   A. Parietal cells B. Chief cells
   C. G-cells D. Mucous cells
3. **Calcium absorption is controlled by : AMC 1986, 87, 99**
   A. Vitamin-D B. Parathormone
   C. Both D. None of the above
4. **Cation more in gastric secretion than in blood is : AMC 1986, 89; ESI 1987, 92**
   A. Sodium B. Potassium
   C. Calcium D. Magnesium
5. **Cephalic phase of gastric secretion is mediated by: AIIMS 1985; AI 1990, 99**
   A. Neurohormones B. Parasympathetic
   C. Sympathetic D. Gastrin
6. **In severe diarrhea : PGI 1986, 94, 95**
   A. Serum K+ level declines
   B. Intravenous infusion should be given rapidly
   C. Blood pressure declines and pulse rate increase
   D. All of the above
7. **Vitamin-B12 is absorbed from : AI 1996, 98**
   A. Jejunum B. Proximal ileum
   C. Terminal ileum D. Stomach
8. **Pancreatic juice rich in water and electrolytes but poor in enzymes is secreted in response to : PGI 1992**
   A. Pancreatozymin B. Cholecystokinin
   C. Secretin D. Proteins
9. **Gastric secretion is not influenced by : PGI 1984; Delhi 1986, 98**
   A. Diet B. Gastrin
   C. Secretin D. Cholecystokinin
   E. None of the above
10. **Milk is first acted by : Delhi 1986,93**
    A. Rennin B. Pepsin
    C. Trypsin D. Renin
11. **The most important stimulus for secretion of secretin is : AMU 1988, 98**
    A. Vagal stimulation
    B. Mechanical duodenal distension
    C. Acidic chyme reaching duodenum
    D. Fat reaching the duodenum
12. **Sphincter of Oddi is located in : AIIMS 1985, 95**
    A. Gastrium B. Urinary bladder
    C. Biliary system D. Central nervous system
13. **Water absorption is mainly a function of : PGI 1982, 93**
    A. Colon B. Intestine
    C. Gastrium D. Appendix
14. **Total Gastrectomy may lead to : AIIMS 1983, 98**
    A. Indigestion
    B. Severe anaemia
    C. Giddiness
    D. Dizziness, pallor and swelling after meals
15. **Process of normal swallowing involves all except : PGI 1985, 99**
    A. Vocal cords approximation
    B. Soft palate elevation
    C. Palatopharyngeal folds
    D. Tracheal valves
16. **Daily secretions of gastrointestinal tract amount to : AIIMS 1985; Delhi 1987, 99**
    A. 8000 ml B. 4000 ml
    C. 2000 ml D. 2 to 4 liters

Ans.	1. B	2. B	3. C	4. A	5. B	6. D	7. C	8. C	9. E	10. C
	11. C	12. C	13. B	14. A	15. D	16. A				

17. **There are about ——acini in human liver : AIIMS 1983, 93**
A. 10,000 B. 1 lac
C. 10 lacs D. 50 lacs

18. **Hepatic failure : AIIMS 1984, 94**
A. Results in low A : G ratio
B. Results in high A : G ratio
C. Results in high serum albumin
D. Always is associated with jaundice

19. **False about ileum and jejunal resection : AIIMS 1985, 95**
A. Results in pale bulky stools
B. Osteomalacia
C. Steatorrhoea
D. Rise in prothrombin time

20. **True about Gastrin : AIIMS 1988, 98**
A. Marked secretion of pepsinogen
B. Decreased gastric motility
C. Acid stimulates gastrin secretion
D. Is a polypeptide

21. **Exocrine secretion of pancreas is controlled by : AMU 1985, 96**
A. Secretin
B. Cholecystokinin
C. N-benzyol L-tytesyl amino benzoic acid
D. All of the above

22. **Intestinal Juice contains : AIIMS 1983, 89**
A. Enzymes responding to vagal activity
B. Saccharidase
C. Potassium equal in concentration to extracellular fluid
D. A substance which activates trypsinogen activity

23. **The type of taste is most sensitive to minute concentrations of the substance to be tasted is : Rohtak 1984, 94**
A. The sour taste B. The salty taste
C. The sweet taste D. The bitter taste

24. **What hormone causes contraction of the gall bladder : UPSC 1984, 94**
A. Secretin B. Gastrin
C. Villikinin D. Cholecystokinin

25. **What of the following enzymes requires an acid pH of approximately 2.0 to function optimally : AMU 1985, 97**
A. Trypsin B. Chymotrypsin
C. Pepsin D. Pancreatic lipase

26. **What is the usual cause of megacolon (also called Hirschsprung's disease) : Delhi 1983, 93**
A. Infection in the colon
B. Excessive parasympathetic stimulation
C. Excessive sympathetic stimulation
D. Congenital absence of the myenteric

27. **Approximately what proportions of the bile salts is normally reabsorbed and then rasecreted by the liver : DNB 1989, 98**
A. 5 per cent B. 15 per cent
C. 40 per cent D. 95 per cent

28. **What substance in gallstones causes them to be sometimes opaque : AIIMS 1985, 99**
A. Bile salts B. Bilirubin
C. Cholesterol D. Calcium

29. **Duodenal mucosa is protected from the action of acid and pepsin by : TNPSC 1997, 99**
A. Reduced secretion of bicarbonate
B. Secretion of Brunner's glands
C. Hyperplasia of duodenal mucosa
D. Stimulation of sympathetics

30. **Sympathectomy—mucus secretion by the intestine: AIIMS 1982, 96**
A. Decreases B. Increases
C. Has no effect D. A or B

31. **Hydrochloric acid is secreted by the : AIIMS 1984, 86**
A. Paneth cells B. Goblet cells
C. Chief cells D. Parietal cells

32. **The three phases of gastric secretion are : AIIMS 1986, 87, 88**
A. First, Second and Third
B. Cephalic, gastric and intestinal
C. Ptylin, gastrin, secretion
D. Gastric, intestinal, colonic

33. **Ingestion of a meal containing only protein would result in : JIPMER 1998, 99**
A. Hypoglycemia
B. Increased insulin release
C. Decreased insulin release
D. Decreased hepatic glycogen

34. **Most potent stimulus for bile secretion is : AMC 1985; AIIMS 1987; AI 1999**
A. Cholecystokinin B. Gastrin
C. Secretin D. Bile salts

35. **Which of the following is fastest to be absorbed from stomach : DNB 1992, 99**
A. Carbohydrates B. Proteins
C. Fats D. Water

36. **Maximum absorption of bile occurs at : Delhi 1990; AMC 1987, 97**
A. Jejunum B. Duodenum
C. Ileu D. Colon

37. **After absorption, iron in blood is : AIIMS 1983, 93**
A. Apoferritin B. Ferritin
C. Transferrin D. Ceruloplasmin

Ans.									
17. B	18. A	19. D	20. D	21. D	22. D	23. D	24. D	25. C	26. D
27. D	28. D	29. B	30. B	31. D	32. B	33. C	34. D	35. D	36. C
37. C									

38. Failure to absorb Vitamin-B12 from the gastro-intestinal tract results in a syndrome called : AMC 1984; UPSC 1985, 87
A. Pernicious anemia B. Hemolytic anemia
C. Polycythemia D. Thalassemia

39. Gastrocolic reflex causes : Orissa 1998
A. Pendular movement B. Mass peristasis
C. Colonic disease D. All of the above

40. One of the following is not a constituent of saliva : Delhi 1983, 93
A. Glucose B. Bicarbonate
C. Lysozyme D. Phosphate

41. Basal migrating motor complex in gut originates in the : Delhi 1998, 99
A. Pyloric end of stomach
B. Longitudinal muscle layer of small intestine
C. Circular muscle layer in small intestine
D. All of the above

42. Which of the following is lower in Gall blader bile in comparison to hepatic bile : DNB 1991, 97
A. Water B. Fatty acids
C. Bile pigments D. pH

43. The first part of test meal reaches the caeum in about —hours, the hepatic flexure in —hours, the splenic flexure in — hours and sigmoid colon in — hours : AIIMS 1987, 99
A. 4,6,9,12 B. 6,9,12,16
C. 2,4,6,8 D. 2,6,8,12

44. Iron is absorbed almost entirely in : UPSC 1984, 86, 90; Delhi 1988; TN 1993
A. Stomach B. Duodenum
C. Jejunum D. Ileum

45. All of the following are sources of Liver glycogen except : PGI 1988, 95
A. Glycerol B. Fructose
C. Lactic acid D. Triglycerides

46. Lipase is not present in : AMC 1986, 98
A. Saliva B. Pancreatic juice
C. Succus entericus D. Gastric juice

47. Liver has the maximum O2 consumption (51 ml/mt), the next organ to have the maximum O2 oxygen (ml/mt) is : AIIMS 1985, 97
A. Heart B. Brain
C. Skeletal muscle D. Kidney

48. Of total hepatic blood flow, hepatic artery supplies: AMU 1985, 98
A. 15-20% B. 25-30%
C. 35-50 D. 50-65%

49. Salivary amylase digests starch in : AIIMS 1985, 92
A. Mouth B. Stomach
C. Duodenum D. Jejunum

50. Prolonged vomiting may result in : UPSC 1985, 96
A. Metabolic acidosis B. Metabolic alkalosis
C. Respiratory acidosis D. Respiratory alkalosis

51. The only sugar normally absorbed by the intestine against a concentration gradient is : AIIMS 1984, 99
A. Xylose B. Mannose
C. Glucose D. Ribose

52. Surface protection is given by following except : Kerala 1997, 99
A. Mucin B. IgA
C. Pepsin D. All of the above

53. In distal ileum resection, following are seen except: AIIMS 1997, 99
A. B12 deficiency
B. Fe deficiency
C. ↓ absorption of bile salts
D. None

54. Surgical removal of about 90% of the ileum and jejunum tends to cause all, except : AIIMS 1982, 92
A. An increase in fat content of stool
B. Deminalisation of bones
C. A fall in extracellular fluid volume
D. Anaemia

55. All is true for cells of liver, except : AIIMS 1982, 94
A. Are important site for synthesis of plasma albumin.
B. Are the only important site for synthesis of plasma globulins.
C. Can store vitamin B12.
D. Release glucose when blood glucose level tends to fall below normal.

56. The duodenum secretes a hormone which has following effects except : DNB 1991, 99
A. Causes copious pancreatic juice rich in bicarbonate and poor in enzymes.
B. Increases gastric motility.
C. Causes gall bladder to contract and sphincter of Oddi to relax.
D. Leads to meagre flow of pancreatic juice rich in enzymes.

57. Two basic types of electrical waves in smooth muscle of the gastrointestinal tract are : Delhi 1984, 99
A. Fast waves and spikes
B. Short and long spikes
C. Slow waves and spikes
D. Slow waves and fast waves

58. The usual stimulus of peristalsis is : PGI 1984, 86
A. Distention
B. Sympathetic stimulation
C. Acid chyme
D. Alkaline chyme

Ans.									
38. A	39. B	40. A	41. A	42. A	43. A	44. B	45. C	46. D	47. C
48. B	49. D	50. B	51. C	52. C	53. B	54. C	55. B	56. B	57. C
58. A									

59. **The principal function of the gastro-esophageal sphincter is : AIIMS 1982, 95**
A. To allow stomach acid into the esophagus
B. To maintain food in the esophagus for digestion
C. To prevent reflux of stomach contents
D. Non existent

60. **Which of the following is not present in the pancreatic juice : AI 1993**
A. Aminopeptidase B. Elastase
C. Colipase D. Ribonuclease

61. **Which converts chymotrypsin to trypsinogen : AI 1993**
A. Trypsin B Low pH
C. Chymosin D. Pepsinogen

62. **False about Pancreatic secretion is : AIIMS 1997**
A. 1 L/day
B. Osmolality 1/2 of plasma
C. Secretin-produces HCO3 rich
D. Pancreozymin-enzyme rich

63. **The following are hormones secreted locally in gut except : Delhi 1993, 94**
A. Gastrin B. Enterogastrone
C. Secretin D. None of the above

64. **Gastric emptying is decreased by all the following except : AIIMS 1989, 92**
A. Distention of duodenum
B. Alkaline pH in duodenum
C. Fatty meal
D. Hypersomality in duodenum

65. **Vagal stimulation following intake of food does not affect secretion of : JIPMER 1993, 98**
A. Pancreas B. Gastric mucosa
C. Gall bladder D. Parotid

66. **The normal portal venous pressure is : JIPMER 1993, 99**
A. 4-6 mm Hg B. 8-12 mm Hg
C. 25-30 mm Hg D. 12-16 mm Saline

67. **The normal basal acid output is : AP 1990, Jipmer 1993**
A. 2-3 mmol/hour B. 5-10 mmol/hour
C. 15-20 mmol/hour D. 20-25 mmol/hour

68. **The Mechanism which causes maximum gastric by secretion is : Rajasthan 1994, 99**
A. Cholinergic receptor stimulation
B. H2 receptor stimulation
C. Neurogenic
D. Na+K+-ATPase Pump

69. **An adult human pancreas has about : DNB 1990, 99**
A. 1000-2000 islets
B. 100,000-200,000 islets
C. 250,000-750,000 islets
D. Above 1000,000 islets

Match the following (Qs. 70-73) : AIIMS 1984, 87
A. Cholagogue B. Choleretic
C. Hydrocholeretic D. Cholecystokinin

70. **Increases bile flow by contracting gall bladder :**
71. **Increases the output of bile from liver :**
72. **Increases flow of bile into intestine :**
73. **Increases the volume of bile but not necessarily the amount of bile solid :**

Match the following (74 to 78): AI 1993
A. Myenteric reflex B. Gastrocolic reflex
C. Mass movement D. Segmentation
E. Law of intestine

74. **Local, non-propagated contraction and relaxation of the intestine.**
75. **Single, vigrous peristaltic contraction and relaxation of the intestine.**
76. **A dilatation of intestinal lumen causes contraction above and relaxation below that point.**
77. **Peristalsis travels from the oral to the aboral end of the intestine.**
78. **Ingestion of food causes an increase in motility of large intestine.**

79. **Amino acids are transported in the blood mainly in the form of : DNB 1988, 92**
A. Plasma proteins
B. Lipoproteins
C. In combination with a carbohydrate carrier
D. In combination with phospholipid carrier
E. Amino acids themselves

80. **An average 70 Kg man has— Kg glycogen in liver: DNB 1988, 96**
A. 0. B. 0.4
C. 0.8 D. 1.0

81. **Peristalsis may be initiated by or affected directly by all of the following except : AIIMS 1984**
A. Inhibitors of striated muscle contraction
B. The myenteric plexus
C. Distension of the gut wall
D. Irritation of mucous
E. The composition of the chyme

82. **Following are translatory movements of intestine except : WB 1998**
A. Peristalsis B. Segmentation
C. Antiperistalsis D. Mass peristalsis

83. **Maximum Na+ concentration is found in : UP 1998, 99**
A. Pancreatic Juice B. Gastric Juice
C. Bile Juice D. Intestinal Juice

84. **Saliva differs from plasma in : UP 1998, 99**
A. Hypotonicity B. HCO3- concentration
C. Protease enzyme D. Aldosterone decreases

Ans.									
59. C	60. A	61. B	62. B	63. D	64. B	65. D	66. A	67. B	68. B
69. C	70. D	71. B	72. A	73. C	74. D	75. C	76. A	77. E	78. B
79. E	80. B	81. A	82. B	83. C	84. D				

85. In which of the following situations is the secretion of saliva increased? Manipal 1995, 98
A. When the touch receptors in the mouth are stimulated
B. Just before vomiting
C. When bitter food is placed on the tongue
D. All of the above

86. When excess amounts of carbohydrates or proteins are consumed, they are stored in the body as : PGI 1987, 99
A. Glucose B. Glucogen
C. Protein D. Triglycerides

87. Stored fat is usually transported from one part of the body to another in the form of : AIIMS 1987, 98
A. Triglycerides B. Free fatty acids
C. Glycerol D. Neutral fat

88. The hormone generally considered to be the major stimulus for enzyme secretion by the pancreas is : PGI 1986
A. Cholecystokinin B. Secretin
C. Trypsin D. Gastrin

89. Failure to absorb bile salts in the distal ileum causes: AMC 1984, 92
A. Constipation B. No effect
C. Diarrhea D. Dysentry

90. The absence of lactate in the intestine would cause failure to digest completely : AMC 1986; UPSC 1983
A. Steak B. Beer
C. Milk D. Peptones

91. A large greasy smelly stool usually indicates failure of digestion of : Delhi 1983, 85
A. Carbohydrates B. Fats
C. Proteins D. Peptones

92. Na+ content of gastric juice is : PGI 1994, 99
A. 30-40 meq/L B. 50-60 meq/L
C. 60-80 meq/L D. 100 meq/L

93. Raised gastrin levels without associated increase in gastric acid secretin is seen in : AIIMS 1994
A. Gastrinoma B. G-cell hyperplasia
C. Pernicious anaemia D. Ca stomach

94. 'D' cells of pancreas secrete : AI 1995
A. Insulin B. Glucagon
C. VIP D. Somatostatin

95. The gas present in the fundus of the stomach is mostly due to : AP 1993, 98
A. Fermentation B. Putrefaction
C. Swallowing D. Diffusion

96. The function of vasoactive intestinal peptide is : AP 1993, 99
A. Inhibits gastric acid secretion
B. Inhibits the motility of the stomach and gallbladder
C. Stimulates pancreatic and intestinal secretions
D. All of the above

97. Maximum secretory glands in stomach are : AP 1994
A. Fundic glands B. Pylorus
C. Gastric glands D. Brunner's glands

98. Cholagogues are the substances which causes : AP 1995, 99
A. Contraction of the gallbladder
B. Increase concentration of bile
C. Increase secretion of bile
D. Favour acidification of bile

99. Severe irritation of the mucosal lining of small intestine may cause : Rajasthan 1989, 90
A. A stop in the propulsion of chyme.
B. Intestinal obstruction.
C. The chyme to move more slowly to reduce the irritation.
D. A "peristaltic rush" quickly move the chyme into the colon.

100. Which enzyme is secreted by intestine : UP 1995
A. Phospholipase B. Dipeptidase
C. Trypsin D. Elastase

101. Pepsinogen is converted to pepsin by : UP 1995, 98
A. Low pH B. Trypsinogen
C. Chymotrypsin D. Enterokinase

102. Small intestinal peristalsis is controlled by : Kerala 1994, 99
A. Myenteric plexus B. Meissner's plexus
C. Sympathetic system D. Parasympathetic system

103. Enterogastic reflex may be stimulated by all of the following except : Karnataka 1987
A. Distension of duodenum
B. Alkaline duodenal contents
C. Presence of protein breakdown products
D. Hyperosmolarity of chyme

104. Bicarbonate rich secretion is by : Delhi 1994, 99
A. Cholecystokini B. Secretin
C. Pancreozymin D. Gastrin

105. For calcium metabolism, all of the following are required except : Delhi 1994, 99
A. Vitamin-D B. Parathyroid hormone
C. Calcitonin D. Thyroxine

106. Iron absorption is increased by : AIIMS 1994, 97
A. Vitamin-C B. Phytic acid
C. Fibre diet D. Phosphates

107. Man is unable to digest dietary : AMU 1992
A. Glycoge B. Dextrin
C. Saccharose D. Cellulose

108. Oxyntic or parietal cells secrete : AMU 1993
A. Zymogen granules B. Intrinsic factor
C. Pepsinogen D. HCl

109. Which of the following GIT glands do not secrete mucin : AI 1994
A. Pareth cell B. Crypts of Lieberkuhn
C. Goblet cells D. Brunner's glands

Ans.									
85. D	86. D	87. B	88. A	89. C	90. C	91. B	92. A	93. C	94. D
95. C	96. D	97. C	98. A	99. D	100. B	101. A	102. D	103. B	104. B
105. D	106. A	107. D	108. D	109. A					

110. Bile acids are derived from : AI 1994
A. Cholesterol B. Galactose
C. Glycogen D. Ketone bodies

111. SI unit of enzymatic activity is defined as : AI 1994
A. International unit
B. Available enzymes
C. Most often used
D. Has totally replaced traditional ones

112. Following stimulate HCl secretion except : AI 1994
A. Gastrin B. Ethanol
C. Aspirin D. Prostaglandin

113. Function of HCl is : PGI 1995
A. Secretion of secretin B. ↑ gastrin release
C. Secretion of CCK D. Secretion of glucagon

114. Gastro-colic reflex is related to : Orissa 1998
A. Mass peristalsis B. Segmental movement
C. Pendular movement D. Colonic disorder

115. Which of the following has the highest pH? Karnataka 1999
A. Gastric juic B. Pancreatic juice
C. Bile D. Saliva

116. Brunner's gland is concerned with a: Kerala 1999
A. Mucus production to protect intestine from acid
B. Water and electrolyte secretion
C. Secretion of enzymes
D. All of the above

117. Oesophageal peristalsis begins : Kerala 1999
A. During swallowing.
B. When food is present in upper part of oesophagus.
C. By closure of upper oesophageal sphincter.
D. By opening of lower oesophageal sphincter.

118. True about secretin is : AI 1988; PGI 1999
A. Increased gall-bladder contraction and HCO3 rich pancreatic fluid.
B. Increased gastrin secretion.
C. Gastric hypermotility.
D. Increased HCO_3 rich pancreatic fluid.

119. Fat in duodenum : AI-2000
A. Contracts gallbladder
B. Inhibits CCK
C. Increases gastric emptying
D. Inhibits gastrin

120. Actions of cholecystokinin include all of the following except : Kerala 2000
A. Contraction of the gall bladder
B. Secretion of pancreatic juice rich in enzymes
C. Increases the secretion of enterokinase
D. Augments the action of secretin
E. Stimulates gastric emptying

121. Maximum contraction of gall bladder is seen with : PGI 2000
A. CCK B. Secretin
C. Gastrin D. Enterogastrone

122. Physiological gastrectomy : PGI 2000
A. Ligate all major arteries
B. Antrectomy
C. Upper 1/3 of stoma resected
D. Ligation of 4-out of five arteries

123. Max. blood supply to liver is by : PGI 2000
A. Portal-V. B. Hepatic-A.
C. Splenic-A. D. Mesenteric-A.

124. Bile acids are not required for the absorption of : Kerala 2001
A. Vit-C B. Vit-B6
C. Vit-B1 D. Vit-K

125. Intestinal peristalsis affected by : Rohtak 2001
A. Vagus B. Sympathetic
C. Neissner D. Mysenteric

126. Iron is transported adluminally into sertoli cells by: AIIMS 2002
A. Transferrin
B. Androgen binding protein
C. Alpha-2 glycoprotein
D. Glycosylated sulphoprotein

127. Short chain fatty acid produced by bacteria are maximally absorbed in : JIPMER 2002
A. Duodenum B. Colon
C. Ileum D. Jejunum

128. Which of the following hormone decreases intestinal motility ? UP-2002
A. Glucagon B. CCK
C. Serotonin D. Gastrin

129. Which of the following is not required for calcium absorption : AIIMS 1984, 87; PGI 1983, 88
A. Parathyroid hormone
B. Calcitonin
C. Vitamin-D
D. Bile salts

130. Which pair is correct ? AIIMS 2007
A. G-cell-gastrin B. Alpha cell-insulin
C. D-cell-Glucagon D. Beta cell-Somatostatin

131. True about secretin includes all of the following except : AI 2008
A. It increases the acidity of biliary and pancreatic secretions.
B. It decreases gastric acid secretion.
C. It decreases gastrin secretion and gastric emptying.
D. Increases flow and velocity of bile.

132. Post prandial maximal contractility is in : AIIMS 2008
A. Ascending colon B. Descending colon
C. Transverse colon D. Sigmoid colon

Ans.									
110. A	111. A	112. D	113. A	114. A	115. C	116. A	117. B	118. A	119. A
120. B	121. A	122. A	123. A	124. A	125. A	126. B	127. C	128. A	129. B
130. A	131. A	132. D							

EXPLANATIONS OF GIT

1. Ans.— A Trypsin
   * Trypsin is a powerful pancreatic proteolytic enzyme which would digest the pancreatic cell that produced it, if any have been produce as a proenzyme (-its inactive form known as trypsinogen). Trypsinogen is activated in the intestinal tract by enzyme calledenterokinase.
   * Pancreas has additional protective mechanism against self-digestion by Trypsin-Secretion of trypsin inhibitor.
   * All other options are enzymes of the glycolytic pathway which are in their active form within the cells.
2. Ans.— B. Chief cells
3. Ans.— C. Both
4. Ans.— A. Sodium
5. Ans.— B. Parasympathetic
6. Ans.— D. All of the above
7. Ans.— C. Terminal ileum
8. Ans.— C. Secretin
9. Ans.— E. None of the above
10. Ans.— C. Trypsin
11. Ans.— C. Acidic chyme reaching duodenum
12. Ans.— C. Biliary system
13. Ans.— B. Intestine

Intestine is presented each day with about 200 ml of digested fluid plus 70000 me L of secretions from mucosa of GIT and associated glands. 98% of this is absorbed with a daily fluid loss of about 200 ml in the stools. Daily water turnover is :

	Ingested	2000
A)	Endogenous secretions	7000
	Salivary glands	2500
	Bile	500
	Pancreas	1500
	Intestine	1000
	Total input	9000
B)	Reabsorbed	
	Jejunum	5500
	Ileum	2000
	Colon	1300
C)	Total	8800

14. Ans.— A. Indigestion
15. Ans.— D. Tracheal valves
16. Ans.— A. 8000 ml
17. Ans.— B. 1 lac

The average transit time for blood across liver lobule from portal venule to central hepatic vein is about 8.4 seconds. Numerous macrophages (Kupffer cells) are anchored to the endothelium of sinusoids and project into lumen.

18. Ans.— A. Results in low A : G ratio
19. Ans.— D. Rise in prothrombin time
20. Ans.— D. Is a polypeptide
21. Ans.— D. All of the above
22. Ans.— D. A substance which activates trypsinogen activity
23. Ans.— D. The bitter taste
24. Ans.— D. Cholecystokinin

Cholecystokinin causes contraction of GB and panereozymic increases secretion of pancreatic juice rich in enzymes. It is secreted by upper small intestine.

25. Ans.— C. Pepsin
26. Ans.— D. Congenital absence of the myenteric
27. Ans.— D. 95 per cent

About 500 ml of bile is secreted per day. Some of the components of bile are reabsorbed in intestine and then excreted again by liver via enterohepatic circulation.

28. Ans.— D. Calcium
29. Ans.— B. Secretion of Brunner's glands
30. Ans.— B. Increases
31. Ans.— D. Parietal cells

Parietal cells are also called oxyntic cells. They secreted HCL and intrinsic factor whereas chief cells secrete pepsinogens.

32. Ans.— B. Cephalic, gastric and intestinal
33. Ans.— C. Decreased insulin release
34. Ans.— D. Bile salts

35. Ans.— D. Water

36. Ans.— C. Ileu

37. Ans.— C. Transferrin

Transferrin, as name indicates, transports iron in blood

38. Ans.— A. Pernicious anemia

39. Ans.— B. Mass peristasis

40. Ans.— A. Glucose

41. Ans.— A. Pyloric end of stomach

42. Ans.— A. Water

43. Ans.— A. 4,6,9,12

44. Ans.— B. Duodenum

Iron absorption is facilitated by acidic pH and vitamin-C whereas inhibited by oxalates and phylates.

45. Ans.— C. Lactic acid

46. Ans.— D. Gastric juice

47. Ans.— C. Skeletal muscle

48. Ans.— B. 25-30%

49. Ans.— D. Jejunum

50. Ans.— B. Metabolic alkalosis

51. Ans.— C. Glucose

Glucose is actively absorbed against a concentration gradient.

52. Ans.— C. Pepsin

See Ques. 31

53. Ans.— B. Fe deficiency

54. Ans.— C. A fall in extra-cellular fluid volume

55. Ans.— B. Are the only important site for synthesis of plasma globulins

Plasma globulins are formed by β-lymphocytes

56. Ans.— B. Increases gastric motility

57. Ans.— C. Slow waves and spikes

58. Ans.— A. Distention

Peristalsis is a reflex response that is initiated when the gut wall is stretched by the contents of the lumen and it occurs in all parts of GIT from oseophagus to rectum. The waves of contraction moves in an oral to caudal direction propelling the contents of lumen forward at rates from 2 to 25 cm/s.

59. Ans.— C. To prevent reflux of stomach contents

60. Ans.— A. Aminopeptidase

Aminopeptidase is secreted by intestinal mucosa and are polypeptides which cleave amino terminal amino acid from peptide. The other enzymes are enteropeptidase, carboxypeptidases dipeptidases, maltase, lactase, sucrase, alpha dextrinase, trehalase and nuclease.

61. Ans.— B. Low pH

62. Ans.— B. Osmolality 1/2 of plasma

63. Ans.— D. None of the above

64. Ans.— B. Alkaline pH in duodenum

65. Ans.— D. Parotid

Parotid is not supplied by this nerve

66. Ans.— A. 4-6 mm Hg

67. Ans.— B. 5-10 mmol/hour

68. Ans.— B. H2 receptor stimulation

69. Ans.— C. 250,000-750,000 islets

The islets of Langerhans are ovoid, 76 x 175 mm collections of cells scattered throughout pancreas. They make up about 2% of volume of gland whereas exocrine part constitutes 80% and rest are blood vessels. There are 1-2 million islets.

70. Ans.— D. Cholecystokinin

71. Ans.— B. Choleretic

72. Ans.— A. Cholagogue

73. Ans.— C. Hydrochleretic

74. Ans.— D. Segmentation

75. Ans.— C. Mass movement

76. Ans.— A. Myenteric reflex

77. Ans.— E. Law of intestine

78. Ans.— B. Gastrocolic reflex

79. Ans.— E. Amino acids themselves

80. Ans.— B. 0.4

81. Ans.— A. Inhibitors of striated muscle contraction

82. Ans.— B. Segmentation

83. Ans.— C. Bile Juice

84. Ans.— D. Aldosterone decreases

85. Ans.— D. All of the above

86. Ans.— D. Triglycerides

They are converted in liver

87. Ans.— B. Free fatty acids

88. Ans.— A. Cholecystokinin

89. Ans. C. Diarrhea

90. Ans. C. Milk
91. Ans.— B. Fats
92. Ans.— A. 30-40 meq/L
Contents of normal gastric juice are cations Na+, K+, Mg++, H+ (pH=1.0), anions - Cl+, HPO4⁻, SO_4^{-2}, Pepsins, lipase, mucus, intrinsic factor.
93. Ans.— C. Pernicious anaemia
94. Ans.— D. Somatostatin
95. Ans.— C. Swallowing
96. Ans.— D. All of the above
97. Ans.— C. Gastric glands
98. Ans.— A. Contraction of the gallbladder
99. Ans.— D. A "peristaltic rush" quickly move the chyme into the colon.
100. Ans.— B. Dipeptidase
101. Ans.— A. Low pH
102. Ans.— D. Parasympathetic system
103. Ans.— B. Alkaline duodenal contents
104. Ans.— B. Secretin
105. Ans.— D. Thyroxine
106. Ans.— A. Vitamin-C
Whereas phylates and oxalates decreases iron absorption
107. Ans.— D. Cellulose
108. Ans.— D. HCl
109. Ans.— A. Pareth cell
110. Ans.— A. Cholesterol
111. Ans.— A. International unit
112. Ans.— D. Prostaglandin
Prostagland has no role
113. Ans.— A. Secretion of secretin
114. Ans.— A. Mass peristalsis
In mass action contractions, there is simultaneous contraction of smooth muscle over large confluent areas. The other contractions are segmentation and peristaltic type.
115. Ans.— C. Bile
116. Ans.— A. Mucus production to protect intestine from acid.
117. Ans.— B. When food is present in upper part of oesophagus.
118. Ans.— A. Increased gall-bladder contraction and HCO3 rich pancreatic fluld.
Increased pancreatic cholecystokin causes contraction of GB.
119. Ans.— A. Contracts gallbladder
120. Ans.— B. Secretion of pancreatic juice rich in enzymes
121. Ans.— A. CCK
122. Ans.— A. Ligate all major arteries
123. Ans.— A. Portal V.B.
The central portion of acinus is well oxygenated (zone 1), intermediate zone is moderately well oxygenated (zone 2) and peripheral zone is least well oxygenated (zone 3) and most susceptible to anoxic injury. Normal portal pressure is 10 mmHg and hepatic venous pressure is 5 mmHg.
124. Ans.— A. Vit-C
125. Ans.— A. Vagus
126. Ans.— B. Androgen binding protein
127. Ans.— C. Ileum
Ileum is the site for absorption.
128. Ans.— A. Glucagon
129. Ans.— B. Calcitonin
130. Ans. — A G-cell-gastrin
G-cell (antral mucosa)—Gastrin
T-cell (upper small intestine)—Cholecystokinin
S-cells (upper small intestine)—Secretin
K-cells (duodenal and jejunal mucosa—GIP
Mo-cells (stomach, small intestine, colon) Motilin
D/delta cells (pancreatic islets, GI mucosa—Somatostatin
A/alpha cells (pancreatic islets, GI mucosa—Glucagon
B/beta cells (pancreatic islets)—Insulin
F-cells (pancreatic islets)—Pancreatic polypeptide
131. Ans.— A It increases the acidity of biliary and pancreatic secretions
* Secretin increases the secretion of bicarbonate by the duct cells of the pancreas and biliary tract. It thus causes the secretion of a watery, alkaline pancreatic juice.
132. Ans.— D. Sigmoid colon (Nearest answer to the explanation)
* Distension of the stomach by food initiates contraction of the rectum and frequently, a desire to defaecate. the response is called Gastrocolic Reflex, although there is some evidence that it is due to an action of gastrin on the colon and is nto neurally mediated. Because of this response defaecation after meals is the rule in children.

6.

IMPORTANT TEXT OF CIRCULATION

METABOLIC CHANGES IN SHOCK

Plasma/blood	Cells	Urine
↑ Glucose	↓ O2 consumption	↑ Ketones
↓ pH	↓ Glucose oxidation	↑ N2
↑ Lactate	Glycogen depletion	
↑ FFA	Mobilization of fat	
↑ Glycerol	Depletion of ATP	
↑ NPN	↓ Membrane Potential	
	↑ Gluconeogenosis	

* In hypovolemic shock, grading is also done by fall in BP—— mild (upto ↓ 20%), moderate (upto ↓ 40%) and severe (↓ above 40%)
* Diisopropyl flurophosphate is called nerve gas
* Acidosis means fall of pH below 7.35 and alkalosis pH above 7.45
* Tm of important substances :
  Glucose - 320 mg/min, Urate - 15 mg/min.
  Hemoglobin - 1.2 mg/min, plasma protein 25-30 mg/min.
  Amino acid - 1.4 mg/min
* Total amount of fluid filtered by both, kidneys per min is called **'Tubular Load'**
* Normal glomerular pressure is 60 mm Hg
* Normal capsular pressure in 18 mm Hg
* Normal colloid osmotic pressure is 32 mmHg
* Normal filtration pressure is 10 mmHg

GAS CONTENT OF BLOOD

ml/dl of Blood Containing 15g of Hemoglobin

Gas	Arterial Blood (PO_2 95 mm Hg; PCO_2 40 mm Hg; Hb 97% Saturated)		Venous Blood (PO_2 40 mm Hg; PCO_2 46 mm Hg; Hb75% Saturated)	
	Dissolved	*Combined*	*Dissolved*	*Combined*
O_2	0.29	19.5	0.12	15.1
CO_2	2.62	46.4	2.98	49.7
N_2	0.98	0	0.98	0

FATE OF CO_2 IN BLOOD

In plasma

1. Dissolved
2. Formation of carbamino compounds with plasma protein
3. Hydration, H^+ buffered, HCO_3^- in plasma

In red blood cells

1. Dissolved
2. Formation of carbamino-Hb
3. Hydration, H^+ buffered, 70% of HCO_3^- diffuses into plasma
4. Cl^- shifts into cells; mOsm/liter in cells increases

MCQ's OF CIRCULATION

What is important in Circulation

Hemodynamics of blood flow (especially to heart, lungs, kidney etc.), Dynamics of shock

1. **Which of the following favours filtration in the arteriolar end of the capillary bed ?** **AIIMS 2006, 2007**
   A. Increased oncotic pressure in the capillaries
   B. Decreased hydrostatic pressure in capillaries
   C. Decreased oncotic pressure in capillaries
   D. Increased oncotic pressure in the interstitium
2. **Arterial blood gas of a 5 year old child done at sea level gives the following results : pH 7.41, PaO2 100 mmHg, and PaCO2 to mm Hg. This child is being ventilated with 80% oxygen. What is the (A-a) PO2- :** **AIIMS 2005**
   A. 570.4 mm Hg B. 520.4 mm Hg
   C. 470.4 mm Hg D. 420.4 mm Hg
3. **Which of the following situation will lead to increased viscosity of blood :** **AIIMS 2005, 2006**
   A. Fasting state B. Hypoglycemia
   C. Multiple myeloma D. Amyloidogenesis
4. **The velocity of blood is maximum in the :** **AIIMS-2005**
   A. Large veins B. Small veins
   C. Venules D. Capillaries
5. **Which of the following conditions lead to tissue hypoxia without alteration of oxygen content of blood ?** **AIIMS 2005**
   A. CO poisoning B. Met Hb
   C. Cyanide poisoning D. Respiratory acidosis
6. **Vasoconstriction is exhibited by all except :** **AMC 1984, 92**
   A. Valsalva manoeuvre B. Asphyxia
   C. Haemorrhage D. Lying down

Directions for Questions (below) (Ques. 7 to 10) for each type of blood vessel listed below, choose the characteristic with which it is usually associated : **AIIMS 1982, 89**

A. Arteries B. Arterioles
C. Capillaries D. Venules
E. Veins

7. **Slowest pulmonary compliance :**
8. **Lowest hydrostatic pressure :**
9. **Least resistance to blood flow :**
10. **Largest surface area :**
11. **Blood flow in carotid body in ml/100g of tissue :** **AMU 1987, 97**
    A. 500 B. 1000
    C. 2000 D. 4000
12. **Which of the following is most fatal complication of increased barometric pressure :** **AMC 1983, 93**
    A. Oxygen toxicity
    B. Nitrogen narcosis
    C. Air embolism
    D. Decompensation sickness
13. **Administration of oxygen rich gas mixtures is of value in all except :** **PGI 1982, 98**
    A. Histotoxic hypoxia B. Stagnant hypoxia
    C. Anemic hypoxia D. Hypoxic hypoxia
14. **Carbon monoxide reacts with hemoglobin to form:** **UPSC 1985, 98**
    A. Carboxy hemoglobin
    B. Reduced hemoglobin
    C. Cyanmethemoglobin
    D. Any of the above
15. **Hemoglobin has ——— times affinity for carbon monoxide than oxygen :** **AMC 1985, 95**
    A. 50 B. 100
    C. 210 D. 320
16. **The most common form of hypoxia is :** **AIIMS 1996**
    A. Hypoxic B. Stagnant
    C. Anemic D. Histotoxic
17. **Causes of hypoxic hypoxia include all except :** **Rohtak 1988, 93**
    A. Kyphoscoliosis
    B. Emphysema
    C. Pulmonary fibrosis
    D. Carbon monoxide poisoning

Ans.									
1. C	**2. D**	**3. C**	**4. A**	**5. C**	**6. D**	**7. C**	**8. E**	**9. C**	**10. C**
11. C	**12. C**	**13. A**	**14. A**	**15. C**	**16. A**	**17. D**			

18. **The carotid bodies have all the features, except : PGI 1980, 90**
A. Have blood flow rate similar to that of brain.
B. More influenced by arterial PO2 than by arterial oxygen content.
C. Stimulated by a rise in blood hydrogen ion concentration.
D. Along with aortic bodies are wholly responsible for stimulation of ventilation in response to hypoxia.

19. **All of the following statements about the monocytes are true except: Manipal 1995, 98**
A. They originate from precursors in the bone marrow.
B. They can ingest dead granulocytes.
C. They may migrate from the blood into the tissues.
D. They can manufacture immunoglobulins.

20. **Oxygen dissociation curve is sigmoid in shape because of : JIPMER 1986, 99**
A. Shifting affinity for oxygen
B. Shifting affinity for CO_2
C. Blood pH
D. All of the above

21. **Direct Fick method of measuring cardiac output requires estimation of : DNB 1989, 96**
A. O2 content of arterial blood
B. O2 consumption per unit time
C. Arteriovenous O2 difference
D. O2 content of blood from right ventricle

22. **A shift of the oxygen dissociation curve of blood to the right a feature not found : PGI 1986, 99**
A. In pulmonary capillaries
B. With rise in temperature
C. When foetal blood is replaced by adult blood
D. In all of the above

23. **Select the statement which best characterises lymph capillaries : Rohtak 1986, 99**
A. Have smaller diameter than blood capillaries
B. Less permeable than blood capillaries
C. Have no endothelial lining
D. Have a discontinuous basement membrane

24. **What best characterises the sinusoids ? AMU 1986, 99**
A. Have smaller diameter than lymph capillaries
B. Are not found in sketetal muscle
C. Have a continuous endothelial lining
D. Have a continuous basement membrane

25. **A substance on I.V. injection was found to be distributed through thirty percent of body water. It probably : DNB 1988, 98**
A. Did not pass freely through blood capillaries
B. Was distributed evenly throughout body water
C. Did not enter cells of body
D. Was excluded from CSF

26. **To estimate cardiac output by dye-dilution technique, dye concentration is measured in : DNB 1989, 94**
A. Sample from peripheral artery
B. Sample from right atrium
C. Sample from aorta
D. Sample from pulmonary artery continuously

Match the following (27-33) : AIIMS 1986, 96
A. Anaemic anoxia B. Anoxic anoxia
C. Histotoxic anoxia D. Stagnant anoxia

27. **Venous pO_2 higher than normal:**
28. **Mercury poisoning of respiratory enzymes :**
29. **Thromboembolism occluding a leg vein**
30. **Breathing atmospheric air at high altitude :**
31. **Drowning :**
32. **Excessive blood loss :**
33. **Carbon monoxide poisoning of Hb :**

34. **Following are increased during exercise except : AP 1997, 99**
A. Cardiac output
B. Venous rectum
C. Coronary blood flow
D. Peripheral vascular resistance

35. **The prime regulator of blood flow through exercising muscles is : AIIMS 1983, 87**
A. Venous tone
B. Sympathetic control
C. Vasodilator metabolites
D. Parasympathetic control

36. **The law relating distending pressure and tension in a blood vessels wall is called : AIIMS 1985, 98**
A. Frank Starling's law B. Einthoven's law
C. Law of Laplace D. Mary's law

37. **Vascular distensibility is least for the following vascular segment : DNB 1989, 95**
A. Pulmonary artery B. Systemic artery
C. Systemic vein D. Pulmonary vein

38. **At a constant pressure gradient across the ends of a vessel, the laminar flow through the vessel is proportional to : AIIMS 1993, 98**
A. Square of the redius (R)
B. 1/R2
C. 1/R4
D. R4

39. **Turbulant blood flow is produced by : Delhi 1988, 99**
A. Decreased velocity of circulation
B. Decreased cardiac output
C. Decreased haematocrit
D. All of the above

Ans.									
18. A	19. D	20. A	21. D	22. A	23. D	24. B	25. C	26. A	27. D
28. C	29. D	30. B	31. B	32. A	33. A	34. D	35. C	36. C	37. B
38. D	39. C								

40. **Factors which increase the hardness of arterial walls : AMC 1984, 98**
A. Decrease in the velocity of arterial pulse
B. Increase in peripheral resistance
C. Raised systolic blood pressure
D. Raised diastolic blood pressure

41. **Venoconstriction is exhibited by all, except : Delhi 1990, 91**
A. Valsalva manoeuvre B. Asphyxia
C. Haemorrhage D. Lying down
E. Carotid artery occlusion

42. **Blood flow is largely regulated by local metabolic effects in : AI 1991**
A. Kidney B. Muscle
C. Bone D. Skin

43. **The arterial pulse pressure in the femoral artery is normally : PGI 1980, 99**
A. Less than the pulse pressure in the upper aorta
B. Less than 20 mmHg
C. Greater than the pulse pressure in the upper aorta
D. Equal to the pulse pressure in the upper aorta

44. **The most dializable anion in RBC is : Bihar 1998, 99**
A. Hemoglobin B. Cl-
C. HCO3- D. PO43-

45. **What is the correct sequence of the following events that lead to regulation of blood volume by the kidney when the blood volume is raised ? CSE 1997**
1. Increase in GFR and urine output
2. Increase in arterial blood pressure
3. Increase in cardiac output
4. Decrease in blood volume

Select the correct answer using the codes given below:
A. 3,1,2,4 B. 1,3,2,4
C. 3,2,1,4 D. 1,2,3,4

46. **The pressure at one end of an artery is 60 mm Hg, the pressure at the other end of the artery is 20 mm Hg, and the flow through the artery of 200 ml/min. What is the resistance of the artery expressed in the above units ? PGI 1982, 99**
A. 0.05 B. 0.1
C. 0.2 D. 0.4

47. **Oncotic pressure is measured by : Rajasthan 1995, 96**
A. Osmal B. Joule
C. mm of Hg D. Kg/m2

48. **Pulse pressure is lowest in : AIIMS 1993, 98**
A. Capillaries B. Arterioles
C. Radial artery D. Femoral artery

49. **Which causes a left shift of the oxygen dissociation curve : AI 1993, Delhi 1988, 97; PGI 2000**
A. ↓ Diphosphoglycerate
B. ↑ 2,3 DPG
C. ↓ Lactate
D. ↑ Lactate

50. **A Rt. sided shift of the oxygen dissociation curve is caused by : AI 1993, Delhi 1987, 97**
A. ↓ 2, 3DPG B. Hyperthermia
C. Hypothermia D. Low Altitudes

51. **In cellular hypoxia, following are seen except : Delhi 1992, 99**
A. Cellular swelling B. Loss of ATP
C. Extrusion of Na D. None of the above

52. **Autoregulation of blood flow is caried out by : AP 1991, JIPMER 1992**
A. Muscles B. Pottassium
C. Substance-P D. Kinins

53. **Shift in Oxygen dissociation curve to the right is caused by : JIPMER 1990, 92**
A. Raised 2-3 DPG B. Raised pH
C. Raised PO2 D. Low PCO2

54. **'J' receptors stimulation causes : AIIMS 1992, 99**
A. Tachycardia B. Hypertension
C. Apnoea D. Tachynoea

55. **The pressure required to occlude blood flow with a tourniquet exceeds systolic pressure by : JIPMER 1992, 98**
A. 4 mm Hg
B. 25-50 mm Hg
C. Twice systolic pressure
D. None of the above

56. **The amount of O2 in blood is determined by the : AMC 1985, 99**
A. Amount of dissolved O2
B. Amount of hemoglobin in blood
C. Affinity of hemoglobin for oxygen
D. All of the above

57. **In arterial blood, hemoglobin which is satured with O2 is : AMU 1987, 99**
A. 100% B. 97%
C. 87% D. 75%

58. **Which of the following is true about composition of venous blood : AIIMS 1982, 99**

	PO_2 (mmHg)	PCO_2 (mmHg)	Hb saturated (%)
A.	95	40	75
B.	40	40	75
C.	40	46	75
D.	46	40	75

Ans.	40. C	41. D	42. B	43. C	44. C	45. B	46. C	47. A	48. A	49. C
	50. B	51. C	52. B	53. A	54. D	55. B	56. D	57. B	58. C	

59. The presence of hemoglobin increase the oxygen carrying capacity of the blood : Delhi 1982, 99
A. 30 fold B. 50 fold
C. 70 fold D. 100 fold

60. Heart receives about : UPSC 1983, 93
A. 1% of cardiac output
B. 2% of cardiac output
C. 5% of cardiac output
D. 10% of cardiac output

61. The commonest cause of sustained diastolic hypertension is : UPSC 1984, 94
A. Unknown B. Conn's syndrome
C. Renal disease D. Phaeochromocytoma

62. Hepatic venous pressure is : Delhi 1983, 93
A. 22 mmHg in man B. 3 mmHg in man
C. 5 mmHg in man D. 10 mmHg in man

63. Hepatic blood flow is : AMC 1987, 98
A. 500 ml/min B. 800 ml/min
C. 1200 ml/min D. 1500 ml/min

64. Blood flow reaching the liver via portal versus hepatic artery is : AMU 1986, 98
A. 2 : 1 B. 3 : 1
C. 4 : 1 D. 6 : 1

65. The most important response to the stimulation of beta adrenergic receptors is : AIIMS 1980, 99
A. Cerebral vasodilation
B. Splanchnic vasoconstriction
C. Decreased blood sugar
D. Increased cardiac activity

66. Major part of total peripheral resistance is : DNB 1989, 95
A. Medium and small arteries
B. Venules
C. Capillaries
D. Arterioles

67. Which of the following has the maximum oxygen consumption (ml/min) : AMC 1982, 89
A. Brain B. Skeletal muscle
C. Heart muscle D. Kidneys

68. A-V oxygen difference is maximum in : AMU 1986, 89
A. Skeletal muscle B. Brain
C. Heart muscle D. Liver

69. After liver and kidneys, the blood flow is maximum in : TN 1986,87, 99
A. Brain B. Skeletal muscle
C. Skin D. Heart muscle

70. Which of the following shows the maximum absolute resistance in : AMU 1986, 99
A. Skin B. Brain
C. Heart D. Liver

71. In capillaries, blood flow at the rate of —— cm/sec: Delhi 1996, 98
A. 0.007 B. 0.07
C. 0.15 D. 1.0

72. Which of the following organ has the maximum weight : AMC 1985, 95
A. Liver B. Kidneys
C. Brain D. Heart

73. Blood flow in ml/100g/min is maximum in : Delhi 1980, 99
A. Kidneys B. Liver
C. Heart D. Skin

74. Blood pressure is not reliable in : Rohtak 1985, 99
A. Coarctation of aorta B. Pulmonary stenosis
C. Atrial fibrillation D. Polyarteritis nodosa

75. Plasma CO2 content is : UPSC 1989, 99
A. 10-12 mm/L B. 15-18 mm/L
C. 25-28 mm/L D. 32-35 mm/L

76. The avarage normal arm to tongue circulation time is : AMU 1984, 94
A. 5 sec B. 10 sec
C. 15 sec D. 30 sec

77. Normal A-V O2 difference at rest is : UPSC 1980, 94
A. 2.1 ml B. 3.4 ml
C. 4.3 ml D. 5.6 ml

78. Caliber of the arterioles is increased by following except : AMU 1985, 98
A. Circulating angiotensin-II
B. Kinins
C. Increased PCO_2
D. Decreased pH

79. "Axon reflex"—the arteriole : AMU 1984, 95
A. Dilate B. Constricts
C. A or B D. Does not affect

80. On Poiseuille Hagen formula, the relationship is calculated between following except : AMU 1984, 96
A. Flow in a long narrow tube
B. Viscosity of fluid
C. Radius of tube
D. pH of blood

81. Dopamine is used in the treatment of shock because it is : AIIMS 1982, 83, 85; AMC 1986, 89
A. Strongly ionotropic
B. Strongly chronotropic
C. Increased renal arterial blood flow
D. All of the above

82. Which of the following changes would tend to cause accumulation of fluid (edema) in the tissues : AIIMS 1985, 94
A. Increased precapillary vascular resistance
B. Decreased postcapillary vascular resistance
C. Increased plasma colloid osmotic pressure
D. Increased venous pressure

Ans.									
59. C	60. C	61. A	62. C	63. A	64. A	65. D	66. D	67. B	68. C
69. B	70. C	71. B	72. A	73. A	74. C	75. C	76. C	77. C	78. A
79. A	80. D	81. C	82. D						

83. **Which of the following change would probably occur as a result of two fold increase in the net filtration of fluid into the tissue : AIIMS 1984, 94**
A. A marked increase in lymph flow rate
B. Approximately a two-fold increase in interstitial fluid volume
C. A decrease intertstitial fluid colloid osmotic pressure
D. a and b
E. a and c

W.84. **Which of the following would not be expected to cause hypoxia : AIIMS 1984, 96**
A. Hypoventilation
B. Abnormal ventilation to perfusion ratio
C. Diminished diffusing capacity for O2
D. Excessive blood flow through venous to arterial shunt

85. **Maximum surface area of circulating system is seen in : PGI 1985, 88**
A. Arteries B. Vein
C. Arterioles D. Capillaries

86. **Which of the following statements about erythropoietin is false ? Manipal 1996**
A. It is a glycoprotein
B. It has been isolated in the pure form
C. It is mainly produced by the bone marrow
D. It can be measured by radioimmunoassay

87. **Following acute failure of the left ventricle is the heart in man, pulmonary edema generally begins to appear when left atrial pressure approaches : AIIMS 1980, 98**
A. 7 mm Hg B. 15 mm Hg
C. 20 mm Hg D. 30 mm Hg

88. **When a normal person suddenly changes from recumbent to standing posture : AIIMS 1981, 98**
A. Blood pressure falls dramatically
B. Renin secretion is suppressed
C. Blood pools in the jugular vein
D. Heart rate increase

89. **Vasovagal syncope is called : AIIMS 1985; Delhi 1986, 98**
A. Hypovolemic shock B. Anaphylactic shock
C. Emotional shock D. Septicemic shock

90. **Dilatation of capillaries may result due to : Delhi 1984, 89, 94**
A. 5-HT B. Norepinephrine
C. Low temperature D. Axon reflex

91. **Coronary blood flow stops during : Delhi 1989; UPSC 1991, 95**
A. Protodiastole
B. End of diastole
C. Isometric contraction
D. Isovolumetric contraction

92. **After haemorrhage, restoration of blood volume is due to : AIIMS 1985, 95**
A. Arterial constriction
B. Shift of intracellular fluid to extracellular space
C. Venous return increases
D. Intravenous infusion

93. **Consider the following statements : Complete compensation for acid-base disturbances within a short time is characteristic of regulation by: CSE 1997, 99**
1. Chemical buffers
2. Respiratory regulatory system
3. Renal regulatory system
Of these statements
A. 1,2 and 3 are correct
B. 2 and 3 are correct
C. 3 alone is correct
D. 1 alone is correct

94. **Which one of the following is the correct sequence in increasing order of their basal blood supply (ml/min/100g of tissue)? CSE 1998, 99**
A. Heart, brain, kidney B. Brain, kidney, heart
C. Kidney, heart, brain D. Brain, heart, kidney

95. **Hypoxia is characterised by : AIIMS 1984, 85, 90**
A. Low arterial PO_2
B. Intense chemoreceptor response
C. Favourable response to 100% oxygen
D. All of the above

96. **Which of the following statements is incorrect : AMU 1986, 98**
A. Blood velocity in capillary is greater than in large vein.
B. Total surface area of the capillary is much greater than large veins.
C. Reduced O_2 tension in the tissue tend to relax pre-capillary sphincters.
D. Increased sympathetic nervous stimulation would tend to constrict the small arterioles.

97. **Peripheral chemoreceptors are not stimulated in which type of hypoxia : AI 1995; AIIMS 1995**
A. Hypoxic hypoxia B. Anaemic hypoxia
C. Stagnant hypoxia D. Histotoxic hypoxia

98. **In cyanide poisoning, there is : Delhi 1995, 99**
A. ↓ Cellular respiration
B. Cyanosis
C. ↓ O_2 transport
D. All of the above

99. **The arteriovenous oxygen difference (ml/L) is minimum in the following organ : AI 1995, 99**
A. Skin B. Skeletal muscle
C. Kidneys D. Liver

Ans.	83. E	84. NONE	85. D	86. C	87. D	88. D	89. C	90. D	91. D	92. B
	93. D	94. D	95. D	96. A	97. D	98. A	99. C			

100. Difference of pulmonary microcirculation from systemic one is : AI 1995, 99

A. Resistance low, pulsatile flow
B. Resistance low, capillary pressure low
C. Capillary pressure high, pulsatile flow
D. Resistance high, capillary pressure high

101. During exercise, blood does not decrease in : AI 1995

A. Cutaneous circulation
B. Hepatosplanchinic circulation
C. Coronary circulation
D. Renal circulation

102. Oxygen affinity is increased by following except : AI 1995

A. Alkalosis B. Hypopnea
C. Increased HbF D. Hyperthermia

103. The amount of blood in capillaries is : Rajasthan 1990, 94

A. 30-50 ml B. 500-600 ml
C. 2-2.5 Litres D. 4-4.5 Litres

104. Which of the following would not be expected to occur during sternuous physical exercise : AIIMS 1987, 99

A. Large $\uparrow$ Pulm. blood flow
B. Large $\uparrow$ Pulm. Artery pressure
C. Large $\downarrow$ Pulm. vascular resistance
D. Pulm. capillary distension
E. Pulm. capillary recruitment

105. Splanchnic vessels and venules contain —— % of blood volume : AMC 1986, 87

A. 10-20 B. 20-30
C. 40-50 D. 60-70

106. If the baroreceptor reflexes are fully functional when upright posture is assumed : AIIMS 1980, 90

A. Blood vessels of arm will be vasodilated
B. Arterial pressure in foot maintained at 120/80 mmHg
C. Bradycardia
D. Cerebral blood flow will not change appreciably

107. In a person who stands suddenly from lying posture, there is : Delhi 1997, 99

A. Increased different discharge from IX nerve
B. Increased tone of capacitance veins
C. Decreased HR
D. None of the above

108. A substance which has a distribution of 30-35% in body water is injected intravenously. True statement is : Rajasthan 1995

A. Distributed evenly through body water
B. Does not pass freely through capillary water
C. Distributed in cells only
D. Does not enter the body cells

109. Autoregulation of blood flow is seen in: AIIMS 1999; JIPMER 2000

A. Cardiac muscle B. Splanchnic blood flow
C. Cerebrum D. Spleen

110. The cardiac output can be determined by all except: PGI 1999

A. Fick's principle B. V/Q ratio
C. Angiocardiography D. Thermodilution

111. True about blood flow in various organs is : PGI 1999

A. Liver>Kidney>brain>heart
B. Liver>brain>kidney>heart
C. Kidney>brain>heart>liver
D. Liver>heart>brain>kidney

112. Pressure on carotid sinus causes : PGI 1999

A. Reflex bradycardia
B. Tachycardia
C. Bainbridge reflex
D. $\uparrow$ BP

113. Consider the following statements regarding nitric oxide : UPSC 2000

1. It is synthesized from L. Arginine
2. It is a vasodilator
3. It modifies platelet neutrophil interaction
4. It modifies release of prostaglandins.

Which of the statements are correct ?

A. 1, 2 and 3 B. 2, 3 and 4
C. 1, 3 and 4 D. 1, 2 and 4

114. Endothelium derived relaxing factor (EDRF) is : JIPMER 2000

A. Nitric oxide B. Thromboxane A2
C. Bradykinin D. Angiotensin

115. In which of the following organs will the rate of blood flow change the least during exercise ? TNPSC 1998

A. Skin B. Brain
C. Intestine D. Heart

116. True about Nitric oxide is : UP 2000

A. Synthesized from arginine
B. Spontaneous production from NO2
C. Vasoconstriction
D. Released from mitochondria

117. A 0.5 litre blood loss in 30 minutes will lead to : AI 2001

A. Increase in HR, decrease in BP
B. Slight increase in HR, normal BP
C. Decrease in HR and BP
D. Prominent increase in HR

Ans. **100. B** **101. C** **102. D** **103. B** **104. B** **105. B** **106. D** **107. B** **108. D** **109. C** **110. B** **111. A** **112. A** **113. A** **114. A** **115. C** **116. A** **117. B**

118. **Albumin contributes maximum to oncotic pressure because of its : AI 2001**
A. High mol wt., low concentration
B. Low mol wt., low concentration
C. High mol wt., high concentration
D. Low mol wt., high concentration

119. **Increased radius of resistance vessels lead to : Delhi 2001**
A. Increased systolic blood pressure
B. Increased diastolic blood pressure
C. Increased rate of blood flow
D. None of the above

120. **Velocity of blood in capillaries is : Delhi 2001**
A. 0.1 mm/sec B. 1 mm/sec
C. 5 mm/sec D. 10 mm/sec

121. **Cyanosis with normal arterial O2 concentration cause : DNB 2001**
A. Anaemic hypoxia B. Stagnant hypoxia
C. Histotoxic hypoxia D. Hypoxic hypoxia

122. **Mechanism of restoration of blood volume in acute hemorrhage is by : Kerala 2001**
A. Vasoconstriction
B. Redistribution of body fluids
C. Heart rate increase
D. Heart rate decrease

123. **In hypercarbia, which of the following is seen : AIIMS 2001**
A. Hypertension B. Bradycardia
C. Cold clammy skin D. Miosis

124. **A low lander lands at an attitude of 6500 m with an atmospheric pressure of 347 mm, the partial pressure of 0_2 is : AIIMS 2002**
A. 53 B. 63
C. 73 D. 83

125. **True about closed homeostatic treatment is : AIIMS 2002**
A. Value of controlled variable is compared to the reference value
B. Positive feedback stabilizes system
C. Negative feedback
D. Oscillates around set point

126. **Albumin does not pass through the glomerulus because of the presence of : Maharashtra -2000**
A. Proteoglycans B. Glycolipid
C. Phospholipid D. Carbohydrates

127. **Structure with richest blood supply is : CMC 2001**
A. Retina B. Renal cortex
C. Heart D. Carotid body

128. **Maximum pressure drop occurs at the level of : A.P.-2002**
A. Capillaries B. Small arteries
C. Large arteries D. Veins

129. **One intern calculated the concentration of O_2 in blood as 0.0025 ml/ml of blood. Considering atmospheric pressure as 760 mm Hg, how much approx. O_2 tension could have been in the blood? AI 2004**
A. 40 mm Hg B. 60 mm Hg
C. 80 mm Hg D. 100 mm Hg

130. **The blood in the vessels normally does not clot because? AI 2004**
A. Vitamin-K antagonists are present in plasma.
B. Thrombin has a positive feedback on plasminogen.
C. Sodium citrate in plasma chelates calcium ions.
D. Vascular endothelium is smooth and coated with glycocalyx.

131. **In which of the following a reduction in arterial oxygen tension occurs ? AI 2005**
A. Anaemia B. CO poisoning
C. Moderate exercise D. Hypoventilation

132. **The vasodilatation produced by carbon dioxide is maximum in one of the following : AI 2005**
A. Kidney B. Brain
C. Liver D. Heart

133. **Distribution of blood flow is mainly regulated by the : AI 2005**
A. Arteries B. Arterioles
C. Capillaries D. Venules

134. **CO2 is primarily transported in the arterial blood as : AI 2005**
A. Dissolved CO2
B. Carbonic Acid
C. Carbamino-hemoglobin
D. Bicarbonate

135. **The normal plasma oncotic pressure is : Kerala 1997**
A. 10 mmHg B. 15 mmHg
C. 20 mmHg D. 30 mmHg

136. **All of the following increase the interstitial pressure except : Delhi 1996**
A. ↓ Capillary permeability
B. ↑ Capillary permeability
C. a+b
D. None of the above

137. **Blood volume is equal to : UPSC 1983**
A. Plasma Volume $\times \frac{100}{100-0.87 \text{ haematocrit}}$
B. Plasma Volume $\times \frac{100-0.87 \text{ haematocrit}}{100}$
C. Plasma Volume $\div \frac{100}{100-0.87 \text{ haematocrit}}$
D. Plasma Volume $\div \frac{100-0.87 \text{ haematocrit}}{100}$

Ans.									
118. D	119. C	120. C	121. A	122. B	123. A	124. A	125. B	126. A	127. D
128. B	129. D	130. D	131. D	132. B	133. B	134. D	135. D	136. A	137. A

138. Blood flow is largely regulated by local metabolic effects in : AIIMS 1983

A. Skin B. Brain
C. Kidney D. Muscle

139. Velocity of blood is ——— times that of urine : AIIMS 1982

A. Same as of ECF
B. 10 times of urine
C. 5-6 times more that of water
D. 5-6 times less that of water

140. When a person changes position from standing to lying down leads to : AIIMS 2007

A. Heart rate increases and settles at a higher level.
B. Venous return to the heart rises immediately.
C. Cerebral blood flow becomes more than in the standing position and settles at a higher level.
D. Decrease in blood flow to the lung apex.

141. O2 delivery to tissues depends on all/except : AIIMS 2007

A. Cardiac output
B. Type of fluid administered
C. Hemoglobin concentration
D. Affinity of hemoglobin for O2

142. Lymph flow from the foot is : AI 2008

A. Increased when an individual rises from the supine to standing position.
B. Increased by massaging the foot.
C. Increased when capillary permeability is decreased.
D. Decreased when the valves of the leg veins are incompetent.

143. Venous flow in the lower limb veins in the standing position depends upon all except : AIIMS 2008

A. Arterial blood pressure
B. Presence of deep facial planes
C. Compressin of calf muscles
D. Presence of perforators

144. Mean circulatory filling pressure is : AIIMS 2008

A. Differences between systemic arterial pressure and pulmonary artery pressure
B. It is pressure everywhere in the ciruclation when heart is suddenly stopped
C. Pressure in the atrium during the filling
D. Signifies the pulmonary and aortic pressure

145. Diastolic pressure in aorta is maintained by : AI 2009

A. Elastic recoil of aorta
B. Muscular artery
C. Resistance in arterioles
D. Capillaries

146. A person sits from standing position, change seen in : AI 2009

A. Immediate increase in venous return
B. Increase in heart rate
C. Increase epinephrine
D. Increased cerebral blood flow

Ans.	138. D	139. C	140. B	141. B	142. B	143. B	144. B	145. A	146. A

EXPLANATIONS OF CIRCULATION

1. Ans.— C **Decreased oncotic pressure in capillaries**

* **The rate of filtration at any point along a capillary depends on a balance of forces sometimes called the Starling forces after the physiologist who first described their operation in detail.**
* **One of these forces is the hydrostatic pressure gradient (the hydrostatic pressure in the capillary minus the hydrostatic pressure of the interstitial fluid) at the point. The interstitial fluid pressure varies from one organ to another, and there is considerable evidence that it is subatmospheric (about - 2 mmHg) in subcutaneous tissue. It is positive in the liver and kidneys and is as high as 6 mm Hg in the brain.**
* **The other force is the osmotic pressure gradient across the capillary wall (colloid osmotic pressure of plasma minus colloid osmotic pressure of interstitial fluid). This component is directed inward. Thus :**

k = capillary filtration coefficient

pc= capillary hydrostatic pressure

p1 = interstitial hydrostatic pressure

c = capillary colloid osmotic pressure

Pie1 = interstitial colloid osmotic pressure

pi is usually negligible, so the osmotic pressure gradient (pc-p1) usually equals the oncotic pressure.

* **The capillary filtration coefficient takes into account, and is proportionate to the permeability of the capillary wall and the area available for filtration.**
* **Fluid moves into the interstitial space at the arteriolar end of the capillary, where the filtration pressure across its wall exceeds the oncotic pressure, and into the capillary at the venular end, where the oncotic pressure exceeds the filtration pressure.**
* **In other capillaries, the balance of Starling force is different and, for example, fluid moves out of almost the entire length of the capillaries in the renal glomeruli. On the other hand, fluid moves into the capillaries through almost their entire length in the intestines.**

2. Ans.— D **420.4 mm Hg**

The data provided in the question is :

* **PaO2 —> 100 mm Hg**
* **PaCO2 —> 40 mm Hg**
* **FiO2 —> 8 mm Hg**

What is FiO2?

FiO is the fraction of oxygen in inspired air.

At sea level (760 mm Hg pressure), the composition of the air is roughly :

O2 —>20%

N2 —>80%

So FiO2 is $\frac{20}{100} = .2$

In the question, the child is being ventilated with 80% Oxygen

So the FiO2 will be = $\frac{80}{100}$ **.8**

Now, PAO2 can be calculated by Alveolar gas equation :

$$PAO2 = FIO2 \times (Ps - PH2O) - \frac{PaCO2}{R}$$

Where

* **PAO2 —> PO2 of the alveolar air**
* **FiO2 —> Fraction of O2 in the air**
* **PB—> Barometric pressure (N is 760 mm Hg)**
* **PH2O—> Water vapour pressure (N is 47 mm H2O)**
* **PaCO2 —> 40**

Substituting these values

PAO2 = .8 x (760-47) - 40/.8

= 520.4 mm Hg

* **Therefore, PAO2 - PaO2 = (520.4 mm/Hg - 100 mm Hg) = 420.4 mm Hg**

3. Ans.— C Multiple Myeloma

In Multiple myeloma M proteins increase in the blood, this may cause cryoglobulinemia which leads to increase in viscosity of the blood.

Viscosity of the blood depends upon :

a) Hematocrit
b) Composition of the plasma

a) Hematocrit - (percentage of the volume of the blood occupied by red blood cells).

* Increase in hematocrit
(e.g. Polycythemia)—>Increase in viscosity
* Decrease in hematocrit
(e.g) Anemia—> Decrease in viscosity

b) Composition of the plasma - Composition of the plasma depends upon the presence of plasma proteins such as immunoglobulins and the resistance of the cells to deformation.

* Increase in plasma protein
(immunoglobulin) —> Increase in viscosity e.g. multiple myeloma.
* Increase in resistance of cells to :
deformation—> Increase in viscosity e.g. hereditary spherocytosis.

4. Ans.— A Large veins

* The velocity of blood is inversely proportional to the total cross-sectional area at that point.
* Thus, the velocity of blood is high in aorta, declines steadily in the smaller arteries and is lowest in the capillaries. (The capillaries have 1000 times the total cross-sectional area of the aorta). The velocity of blood flow increases again as the blood enter the veins and is relatively high again in the vena cava, although not so high as in the aorta.

5. Ans.— C Cyanide poisoning

* This type of hypoxia where the oxygen content of blood is normal, but the tissue is unable to utilizes the oxygen due to failure of its cellular metabolic processes is known as histotoxic hypoxia.
* The best known cause of histotoxic hypoxia is cyanide poisoning, which inhibits cytochrome oxidase.
* Another example of histotoxic hypoxia is beri-beri, where several important steps in tissue utilization of oxygen are compromised because of vitamin-B Deficiency.

Other Types of Hypoxia :

a. Hypoxic hypoxia.
— When there is poor availability of O2 for diffusion to the pulmonary capillaries.
— There is inadequate PO2 in arterial blood.

b. Anemic hypoxia
— When the hypoxia is due to quantitative or qualitative deficiency of Hb.
— The oxygen content of arterial blood is almost all bound to Hb. In the presence of severe anemia or CO poisoning, the oxygen content of blood will fall, even though the PO2 of arterial blood will remain normal.

c. Stagnant or circulatory hypoxia.
— When the hypoxia is due to poor velocity of blood.
— In cases of circulatory failure even though the oxygen content of arterial blood may be adequate, delivery to the tissue is not.

6. Ans.— D. Lying down
7. Ans.— C. Capillaries
8. Ans.— E. Veins
9. Ans.— C. Capillaries
10. Ans.— C. Capillaries
11. Ans.— C. 2000

The rate of flow ($F=P_1-P_2$) depends upon the resistance

$$Fa\frac{1}{R}$$

12. Ans.— C. Air embolism
13. Ans.— A. Histotoxic hypoxia
14. Ans.— A. Carboxy hemoglobin
15. Ans.— C. 210
16. Ans.— A. Hypoxic
17. Ans.— D. Carbon monoxide poisoning
18. Ans.— A. Have blood flow rate similar to that of brain
19. Ans.— D. They can manufacture immunoglobulins
20. Ans.— A. Shifting affinity for oxygen

21. Ans.— D. O2 content of blood from right ventricle
22. Ans.— A. In pulmonary capillaries
23. Ans.— D. Have a discontinuous basement membrane
24. Ans.— B. Are not found in skeletal muscle
25. Ans.— C. Did not enter cells of body
26. Ans.— A. Sample from peripheral artery

    Pulse pressure is the difference between the systolic and diastolic pressures, is normally about 50 mmHg.
27. Ans.— D. Stagnant anoxia
28. Ans.— C. Histotoxic anoxia
29. Ans.— D. Stagnant anoxia
30. Ans.— B. Anoxic anoxia
31. Ans.— B. Anoxic anoxia
32. Ans.— A. Anaemic anoxia
33. Ans.— A. Anaemic anoxia
34. Ans.— D. Peripheral vascular resistance
35. Ans.— C. Vasodilator metabolites

    Lactate is important
36. Ans.— C. Law of Laplace

    Law of Laplace states that tension in the wall of a cylinder (T) is equal to the product of the transmural pressure (P) and the radius (r) divided by wall thickness (w) i.e. (T= Pr/w).
37. Ans.— B. Systemic artery
38. Ans.— D. R4
39. Ans.— C. Decreased haematocrit
40. Ans.— C. Raised systolic blood pressure
41. Ans.— D. Lying down
42. Ans.— B. Muscle
43. Ans.— C. Greater than the pulse pressure in the upper aorta
44. Ans.— C. HCO3-
45. Ans.— B. 1,3,2,4
46. Ans.— C. 0.2
47. Ans.— A. Osmal
48. Ans.— A. Capillaries
49. Ans.— C. ↓ Lactate

    A fall in temperature or a rise in pH also shifts the curve to the left. Fall in 2, 3 DPG concentration also shifts the curve to left.
50. Ans.— B. Hyperthermia

    It is forms carboxyhemoglobin
51. Ans.— C. Extrusion of Na
52. Ans.— B. Pottassium
53. Ans.— A. Raised 2-3 DPG

    A rise of temperature or a fall in pH also shifts the oxygen dissociation curve to right.
54. Ans.— D. Tachynoea
55. Ans.— B. 25-50 mm Hg
56. Ans.— D. All of the above
57. Ans.— B. 97%
58. Ans.— C. 40 46 and 75
59. Ans.— C. 70 fold
60. Ans.— C. 5% of cardiac output

    Heart muscle has mass of 0.3 Kg and blood flow of 250 mL/min or 84 mL/100g/min. It receives 4.7% of cardiac output and 11.6% of total oxygen consumption.
61. Ans.— A. Unknown
62. Ans.— A. 22 mmHg in man
63. Ans.— A. 500 ml/min
64. Ans.— A. 2 : 1
65. Ans.— D. Increased cardiac activity
66. Ans.— D. Arterioles
67. Ans.— B. Skeletal muscle
68. Ans.— C. Heart muscle
69. Ans.— B. Skeletal muscle
70. Ans.— C. Heart
71. Ans.— B. 0.07
72. Ans.— A. Liver

    Weight of liver is 1.2 -1.5 kg
73. Ans.— A. Kidneys
74. Ans.— C. Atrial fibrillation
75. Ans.— C. 25-28 mm/L
76. Ans.— C. 15 sec
77. Ans.— C. 4.3 ml
78. Ans.— A. Circulating angiotensin-II
79. Ans.— A. Dilate

    'Axon reflex' is a response in which impulse initiated in sensory nerves by the injury are relayed antidromically down other branches of the sensory nerve fibres.
80. Ans.— D. pH of blood
81. Ans.— C. Increased renal arterial blood flow

    Surface area of capillaries is maximum

82. Ans.— D. Increased venous pressure

83. Ans.— E. a and c

84. Ans.— NONE

85. Ans.— D. Capillaries

86. Ans.— C. It is mainly produced by the bone marrow

87. Ans.— D. 30 mm Hg

88. Ans.— D. Heart rate increase

89. Ans.— C. Emotional shock

90. Ans.— D. Axon reflex

91. Ans.— D. Isovolumetric contraction

At the start of ventricular systole, the mitral and tricuspid valves close, ventricular muscle initially shortens relatively little but intraventricular pressure rises sharply as the myocardium presses on the blood in the ventricle. This period of isovolumetric (isovolumic, isometric) ventricular contraction lasts about 0.05 sec until the pressures in the left and right ventricles exceed the pressures in the aortic and pulmonary valves open.

92. Ans.— B. Shift of intracellular fluid to extracellular space

93. Ans.— D. 1 alone is correct

94. Ans.— D. Brain, heart, kidney

95. Ans.— D. All of the above

96. Ans.— A. Blood velocity in capillary is greater than in large vein

97. Ans.— D. Histotoxic hypoxia

98. Ans.— A. Cellular respiration

99. Ans.— C. Kidneys

100. Ans.— B. Resistance low, capillary pressure low

101. Ans.— C. Coronary circulation

Coronary circulation is not affected in exercise in a normal person

102. Ans.— D. Hyperthermia

103. Ans.— B. 500-600 ml

104. Ans.— B. Large ↑ Pulm. Artery pressure

105. Ans.— B. 20-30

106. Ans.— D. Cerebral blood flow will not change appreciably

107. Ans.— B. Increased tone of capacitance veins

108. Ans.— D. Does not enter the body cells

109. Ans.— C. Cerebrum.

Autoregulation of blood flow is typically seen in brain

110. Ans.— B. V/Q ratio

According to Fick's principle, the blood flow of any organ can be measured by determining the amount of a given substance (Qx) removed from the blood stream by the organ per unit of time and dividing that value by the difference between the concentration of the substance in arterial blow and concentration in venous blood from organ.

111. Ans.— A. Liver>Kidney>brain>heart

112. Ans.— A. Reflex bradycardia

113. Ans.— A. 1, 2 and 3

114. Ans.— A. Nitric oxide

115. Ans.— C. Intestine

116. Ans.— A. Synthesized from arginine

117. Ans.— B. Slight increase in HR, normal BP

118. Ans.— D. Low mol wt., high concentration

119. Ans.— C. Increased rate of blood flow

120. Ans.— C. 5 mm/sec

Velocity of blood is v = Q/A

121. Ans.— A. Anaemic hypoxia

122. Ans.— B. Redistribution of body fluids

123. Ans.— A. Hypertension

124. Ans.— A. 53

125. Ans.— B. Positive feedback stabilizes system

126. Ans.— A. Proteoglycans

127. Ans.— D. Carotid body

The blood flow in each 2 mg of carotid body about 0.04 mL/min or 2000 mL/100 gm of tissue/min compared to 100 g/min of 54 ml in brain and 420 mL in the kidneys.

128. Ans.— B. Small arteries

129. Ans.— D. 100 mm Hg

$$\text{Pressure} = \frac{\text{Concentration of dissolved gas}}{\text{Solubility coefficients}}$$

When pressure is expressed in atmospheric (1 atmospheric = 760 mmHg) and conc. is expressed in volume of gas dissolved in each volume of water, the solubility coefficient for gases at body temperature.

Gases	Solubility coefficient
O_2	0.025
CO_2	0.57
CO	0.018
N_2	0.012
He	0.008

In these question –

Conc. of O_2 in blood = 0.0025 ml/ml

= 2.5 ml/L

$$O_2 \text{ tension} = \frac{\text{Conc. of } O_2}{\text{Solubility coefficient}} = \frac{2.5}{0.025} = 100 \text{ mmHg}$$

130. Ans.— D. Vascular endothelium is smooth and coated with glycocalyx

- Intact endothelial cells serves primarily to inhibit platelet adherence and blood clotting.
- Injury or activation of endothelial cells, however, results in a procoagulant phenotype that augments local clot formation.

Role of vascular endothelium in hemostasis

- The vascular endothelium acts as a barrier between the thrombogenic subendothelial tissue and the blood.
- The smoothness of endothelial cells hinder platelet aggregation.
- They manufactures heparan and a_2 macroglobulin which are coagulation inhibitors.
- These cells manufactures PHI_2 (prostacyclin) which opposes platelet aggregation.

Factors opposing coagulation, existing clots and platelets plugging and occurring naturally

A. Opposing coagulation	B. Causing lysis of existing clot	C. Opposing platelet aggregation
• Antithrombin-III • Heparin • Heparan • a_2 macroglobulin • Protein-C	• Plasminogen activators	• Endoperoxidase from platelets • Prostacyclin

Note

- Vit-K dependent factor 2, 7, 9, 10, CS
- Factor-II (prothrombin), VII, IX, and X
- Protein-C and Protein-S
- Factors synthesis by liver 2, 7, 9, 10, CS + 1, 5, 11
- Factor-I (fibrinogen), II (Prothrombin), V, VII, IX, X, XI
- Protein-C and protein-S
- Antithrombin-III and heparin

131. Ans.— D. Hypoventilation

DISORDER WHICH LOWERS ARTERIAL PO2

1. Hypoventilation
2. Diffusion defects
3. Low ventilation perfusion ratio
4. Arteriovenous shunts
5. Pump failure (ventilatory failure)
   - Fatigue
   - Mechanical defects
   - Depression of respiratory controller in Brain

* Anemic hypoxia : Arterial PO2 is normal

* CO poisoning : PO2 remains normal

* Moderate excercise : Almost normal PO2 (Due to increase in pulmonary ventilation, perfusion and diffusion).

132. Ans.— B. Brain

"Exposure to high concentration of CO2 is associated with marked cutaneous and cerebral vasodilatation but there is vasoconstriction elsewhere and usually a slow rise in blood pressure".

133. Ans.— B. Arterioles

"Arterioles, metarterioles and precapillary sphincters are rich in smooth muscle, contraction of which is subject of REGULATORY MECHANISM."

* The smooth muscle of these segments respond to stretch, temperature and other neurohumoral and chemical factors. (given in the previous ques.)

* Response to these factors help in matching blood flow to organs with their requirement.

Pressure gradient	Diameter of vessel	Flow rate
P= 100 mm Hg	1 mm	1ml/min
P= 100 mm Hg	2 mm	16 ml/min
P= 100 mmHg	4 mm	256 ml/min

This is determined by Poiseuille's law

137. Ans.— A. Plasma Volume x $\frac{100}{100-0.87 \text{ haematocrit}}$

138. Ans.— D. Muscle

139. Ans.— C. 5-6 times more that of water

Velocity (V) is proportionate to flow (Q) divided by the area of conduit (A) i.e. V=Q/A. Therefore Q=AV, and if flow stays constant, in A.

140. Ans.— B Venous return to the heart rises immediately

On changing position from standing to lying, there is an increase in venous return to the heart and an increase in the B.P. in the carotid sinus and aortic arch. This leads to decrease in heart rate. There is an increase in arterial pressure at head level but because of prominent autoregulation in the brain blood flow remains relatively normal. In the lying down position blood flow to the apices increase.

141. Ans.— B Type of fluid administered

O2 delivery to a particular tissue depends on :

* amount of O2 entering the lungs
* the adequacy of pulmonary gas exchange
* the blood flow to the tissues
* - cardiac output
  - degree of constriction of the vascular bed in the tissue
* the capacity of blood of carry O2
  - the amount of dissolved O2 in plasma
  - the amount of hemoglobin
  - the affinity of the hemoglobin for O2

142. Ans.— B Increased by massaging the foot

As evident, when an individual rises from the supine to standing position the lymphatic flow from the foot will decrease and not increase, due to gravity.

If we massage the foot we will force the lymphatic flow (as well as venous return), by forcing the lymph to enter the lymphatic vessels.

143. Ans.— B. Presence of deep facial planes (most probably)

* So the factors which keeps blood flowing in the veins towards the heart are :

1. Pumping action of the heart (arterial blood pressure).
2. Heartbeat (also contributes to the arterial blood pressure).
3. The increase in the negative intrathoracic pressure during each inspiration.
4. Contractions of skeletal muscles that compress the veins (muscle pump).

144. Ans. B. It is pressure everywhere in the circulation when heart is suddenly stopped

* Mean circulatory filling pressure a measure of the average (arterial and venous) pressure necessary to cause filling of the circulation with blood;
* It varies with blood volume and is directly proportional to the rate of venous return and thus to cardiac ourput.
* The mean circulatory filling pressure is also defined as the mean vascular pressure that exists after a stop in cardiac output and redistribution of blood, so that all pressures are the same throughout the system.

145. Ans. A. Elastic recoil of aorta

Due to presence of elastic fibers in the Windkessel vessels there is a elastic recoil during the diastole (they are stretched during systole), which results in a forward flow and a aortic pressure wave called as diastolic pressure.

146. Ans. A. Immediate increase in venous return

In the standing position, as a result of the effect of gravity on the blood, the mean arterial blood pressure in the feet of a normal adult is 180-200 mm Hg and venous pressure is 85-90 mm Hg. The arterial pressure at head level is 60-75 mm Hg, and the venous pressure in zero. If the individual does not move, 300-500 mL of blood pools in the venosu capacitance vessels of the lower extremities, fluid begins to accumulate in the interstitial spaces because of increased hydrostatic pressure in the capillaries, and stroke volume is decreased.

7.

IMPORTANT TEXT OF ENDOCRINOLOGY

HYPOTHALAMIC REGULATORY MECHANISMS

Function	*Afferents From*	*Integrating Areas*
Temperature regulation	Cutaneous cold receptors; temperature-sensitive cells in hypothalamus	Anterior hypothalamus, response to heat; posterior hypothalamus, response to cold
Neuroendocrine control of:		
Catecholamines	Emotional stimuli, probably via limbic system	Dorsomedial and posterior hypothalamus
Vasopressin	Osmoreceptors, "volume receptors", others	Supraoptic and paraventricular nuclei
Oxytocin	Touch receptors in breast, uterus, genitalia	Supraoptic and paraventricular nuclei
Thyroid-stimulating hormone	Temperature receptors, perhaps others	Anterior median eminence (TSH) and anterior hypothalamus
Adrenocorticotropic hormone (ACTH)	Limbic system (emotional stimuli); reticular formation ("systemic" stimuli); hypothalamic or anterior pituitary cells sensitive to circulating blood cortisol level; others (?)	Ventral hypothalamus
Follicle-stimulating hormone luteinizing hormone (LH)	Hypothalamic cells sensitive to estrogens; eyes, touch receptors in skin and genitalia of reflex ovulating species	Anterior hypothalamus, (FSH) and other areas
Prolactin	Touch receptors in breasts, other unknown receptors	Arcuate nucleus, median eminence (hypothalamus inhibits secretion)
Growth hormone	Unknown receptors	Anterior median eminence
"Appetitive" behaviour		
Thirst	Osmoreceptors	Lateral superior hypothalamus
Hunger	"Glucostat" cells sensitive to rate of glucose utilization also limbic components	Ventromedial satiety center, lateral hunger center,
Sexual behavior	Cells sensitive to circulating estrogen and androgen, others cortex	Anterior ventral hypothalamus, plus in the male, piriform
Defensive reactions		
Fear, rage	Sense organs and neocortex, paths unknown	Diffuse, in limbic system and hypothalamus
Control of various endocrine and activity rhythms	Retina via retinohypothalamic fibers	Suprachiasmatic nuclei

EFFECT OF VARIATIONS IN THE CONCENTRATIONS OF THYROID HORMONE-BINDING PROTEINS IN THE PLASMA ON VARIOUS PARAMETERS OF THYROID FUNCTION

	Concentrations of Binding Proteins	*Total Plasma T3 and T4*	*Free Plasma T3 and T4*	*Clinical State*
Hyperthyroidism	Normal	High	High	Hyperthyroid
Hypothyroidism	Normal	Low	Low	Hypothyroid
Pregnancy, estrogen treatment, congenital elevation of TBG	High	High	Normal	Euthyroid

(Contd....)

EFFECT OF VARIATIONS IN THE CONCENTRATIONS OF THYROID HORMONE-BINDING PROTEINS IN THE PLASMA ON VARIOUS PARAMETERS OF THYROID FUNCTION. (Contd..)

	Concentrations of Binding Proteins	*Total Plasma T3 and T4*	*Free Plasma T3 and T4*	*Clinical State*
Nephrosis, methyltestosterone, phenytoin, congenital depression of TBG	Low	Low	Normal	Euthyroid

Relative potencies of corticosteroids. Values are approximations based on liver glucagon depletion or anti-inflammatory assays for glucocorticoid activity, and effect on urinary Na+/K+ or maintenance of adrenalectomized animals for mineralocorticoid activity. The last 3 steroids listed are synthetic compounds that do not occur naturally.

	Glucocorticoid Activity	*Mineralocorticoid Activity*
Cortisol	1.0	1.0
Corticosterone	0.3	15
Aldosterone	0.3	3000
Deoxycorticosterone	0.2	100
Cortisone	0.7	1.0
Prednisolone	4	0.8
9α-Fluorocortisol	10	125
Dexamethasone	25	~0

STIMULI WHICH INCREASE ALDOSTERONE SECRETION

Glucocorticoid secretion also increased

- Surgery
- Anxiety
- Physical trauma
- Hemorrhage

Glucocorticoid secretion unaffected

- High potassium intake
- Low sodium intake
- Constriction of inferior vena cava in thorax
- Standing
- Secondary hyperaldosteronism (in some cases of congestive heart failure, cirrohosis, and nephrosis)

STIMULI THAT AFFECT GROWTH HORMONE SECRETION IN HUMANS

Stimuli that increase secretion

Deficiency of energy substrate

- Hypoglycemia
- 2-Deoxyglucose
- Exercise
- Fasting

Increase in circulating levels of certain amino acids

- Protein meal
- Infusion of arginine and some other amino acids
- Glucagon
- Stressful stimuli
- Pyrogen
- Lysine vasopressin
- Various psychologic stresses
- Going to sleep
- L-Dopa
- Apomorphine

Stimuli that decrease secretion

- REM sleep
- Glucose
- Cortisol
- Free fatty acids
- Medroxyprogesterone
- Growth hormone

Stimuli that affect gastrin secretion

Stimuli that increase gastrin secretion

Luminal

- Peptides and amino acids
- Distention

Neural

- Increased vagal (cholinergic) discharge

Blood-borne

- Calcium
- Epinephrine

Stimuli-that inhibit gastrin secretion

Luminal

- Acid

Blood-borne

- Secretin, GIP, VIP, glucagon, calcitonin

FACTORS AFFECTING INSULIN SECRETION

Stimulators	*Inhibitors*
Glucose	2-Deoxyglucose
Mannose	Mannoheptulose
Amino acids (leucine, arginine, others)	Ò-Adrenergic stimulating agents (norepinephrine, epinephrine)
Ò-Adrenergic blocking agents	Ò-Adrenergic stimulating agents (propranolol)
Acetylcholine	Diazoxide
Glucagon	Thiazide diurètics
Cyclic AMP and various cyclic AMP-generating substances	Phenytoin
	Alloxan
Theophylline	Microtubule inhibitors
Sulfonylureas	Somatostatin
Intestinal hormones (GIP, gastrin, secretin, CCK, glucagon, others?)	

FACTORS AFFECTING GLUCAGON SECRETION

Stimulators	*Inhibitors*
Amino acids (particularly the glucogenic amino acids : alanine, serine, glycine, cysteine and threonine)	Glucose Secretin FFA Ketones
CCK, gastrin	Phenytoin
Ò-Adrenergic Stimulation	a-Adrenergic stimulators
Theophylline	Somatostatin
Cortisol	
Exercise	
Infections	
Other stresses	

SUMMARY OF STIMULI AFFECTING VASOPRESSIN SECRETION.

Vasopressin Secretion Increased	*Vasopressin Secretion Decreased*
Increased effective osmotic pressure of plasma	Decreased effective osmotic pressure of plasma
Decreased extracellular fluid volume	Increased extracellular fluid volume
Morphine, nicotine, barbiturates	Alcohol
Pain, emotion, "stress", exercise.	

SOME HORMONES AND NEUROTRANSMITTERS THAT APPEAR TO EXERT THEIR EFFECTS BY INCREASING INTRACELLULAR CYCLIC AMP

Catecholamines	Activation of phosphorylase in liver, heart, and skeletal muscle Lipolysis Positive inotropic response in heart Increased renin secretion Inhibition of Purkinje cell discharge in cerebellum

Glucagon	Activation of phosphorylase in liver Lipolysis Positive inotropic effect Stimulation of insulin secretion
Vasopressin	Increased water permeability of renal collecting duct epithelium
ACTH	Steroidogenesis in adrenal cortex
LH	Steroidogenesis in ovary and testis
TSH	Increased secretion of thyroid hormones
TRH and some other hypothalamic hormones	Increased secretion of anterior pituitary hormones
Parathyroid hormone	Increased Ca^{++} mobilization from bone Increased renal tubular reabsorption of Ca^{++}; increased PO_4^- excretion Increased intestinal absorption of Ca^{++}
Gastrin	Increased gastric secretion of hydrochloric acid
FSH	Actions on seminiferous tubules

CHIEF ACTIONS OF INSULIN

Adipose tissue

1. Increased glucose entry
2. Increased fatty acid synthesis
3. Increased glycerol phosphate synthesis
4. Increased triglyceride deposition
5. Activation of lipoprotein lipase
6. Inhibition of hormone-sensitive lipase
7. Increased potassium uptake

Muscle

1. Increased glucose entry
2. Increased glycogen synthesis
3. Increased amino acid uptake
4. Increased protein synthesis in ribosomes
5. Decreased protein catabolism
6. Decreased release of gluconeogenic amino acids
7. Increased ketone uptake
8. Increased potassium uptake

Liver

1. Decreased cyclic AMP
2. Decreased ketogenesis
3. Increased protein synthesis
4. Increased lipid synthesis
5. Decreased glucose output due to decreased gluconge-nesis and increased glycogen synthesis

STIMULI WHICH INCREASE ALDOSTERONE SECRETION

Glucocorticoid secretion also increased

Surgery
Anxiety
Physical trauma
Hemorrhage

Glucocorticoid secretion unaffected

High potassium intake
Low sodium intake
Constriction of inferior vena cava in thorax
Standing
Secondary hyperaldosteronism (in some cases of congestive heart failure, cirrhosis, and nephrosis)

MCQ's OF ENDOCRINOLOGY

What is important in Endocrinology

Pituitary, Hypophysis, Thyroid, Pancreas, Parathyroid, Sexual function

1. **Follicular stimulating hormone receptors are present on : AIIMS 2006**
   A. Theca cells
   B. Granulosa cells
   C. Leydig cells
   D. Basement membrane of ovarian follicle
2. **In a foetus the insulin secretion begins by : AIIMS 2005**
   A. 3rd month B. 5th month
   C. 7th month D. 9th month
3. **Which of the following hormones is an example of a peptide hormone ? AIIMS 2005**
   A. Parathormone B. Adrenaline
   C. Cortisol D. Throxine
4. **Ovulation is associated with sudden rise in : AIIMS 2004**
   A. Prolactin B. Testosterone
   C. LH D. Oxytocin
5. **Hypercalcemia associated with malignancy is most often mediated by : AI 2005**
   A. Parathyroid hormone (PTH)
   B. Parathyroid hormone related protien (PTHRP)
   C. Interleukin - 6 (IL-6)
   D. Calcitonin
6. **Which of the following statements can be regarded as primary action of Inhibin ? AI 2005**
   A. It inhibits secretion of prolactin
   B. It stimulates synthesis of estradiol
   C. It stimulates secretion of TSH
   D. It inhibits secretion of FSH
7. **Sertoli cells have receptors for : AI 2004**
   A. Inhibin
   B. Luteinizing hormone
   C. Follicle stimulating hormone
   D. Melatonin
8. **The enzyme associated with the conversion of androgen to oestrogen in the growing ovarian follicle is : AI 2004**
   A. Desmolase B. Isomerase
   C. Aromatase D. Hydroxylase
9. **Before the onset of puberty, the GnRH neurons are under the inhibitory control of : AI 2004**
   A. Glycine
   B. Glutamate
   C. Gamma amino butyric acid (GABA)
   D. Beta-endorphin
10. **In which of the following form the Anti-diuretic hormone (ADH) is circulated in plasma : AI 2004**
    A. Bound to neurophysin-I
    B. Bound to neurophysin-II
    C. Bound to plasma albumin
    D. Free form
11. **Experimental diabetes is caused by : AIIMS 1984, 87, 98**
    A. Alloxan B. PgE1
    C. Radioactive yitrium D. Gold chloride
12. **Which of the following statements is not correct? Release of acetylcholine at the neuromuscular junction : PGI 1995, 99**
    A. Produces an end-plate potential
    B. Increase sodium movement into the muscle cell
    C. Always causes the muscle fiber to contract
    D. Is followed by rapid destruction of acetylcholine
13. **Which of the following does not act at receptors : AIIMS 1985; Delhi 1985**
    A. TRH B. Thyroxine
    C. Insulin D. Epinephrine
14. **Simmond's disease is characterized by all except : AIIMS 1984, 95**
    A. Infertility B. Increase BMR
    C. Increase Immunity D. Polyurea

Ans.	1. B	2. A	3. A	4. A	5. B	6. A	7. A	8. A	9. C	10. A
	11. A	12. C	13. B	14. B						

15. Uterine contracility is increased by hormone : UPSC 1983, 86

A. Progesterone B. LH
C. FSH D. Oestrogen

16. Gluconeogenesis requires the action of : Delhi 1983, 99

A. Growth hormone B. Insulin
C. Estradiol D. Calcitoni

17. The only hormone for which no stimulatory factor has been isolated is : JIPMER 1998, 99

A. Growth hormone B. Gonadotropin
C. Thyroxine D. Prolactin

18. Which of the following is not caused by estrogen ? AIIMS 1992, 99

A. ↓ serum Alkaline phosphatase
B. ↑ Blood sugar
C. ↓ Folate level
D. ↑ HDL

19. Menopausal hot flushes is due to : AIIMS 1992, 99

A. FSH surge
B. LH surge
C. Decreased estrogen
D. Decreased progesterone

20. Increase in Insulin receptors is seen in: AMU 1990, JIPMER 1993

A. Acromegaly B. Starvation
C. Obesity D. Diabetes

21. Which neurotransmitter controls secretion of Prolactin? JIPMER 1993

A. Dopamine B. Serotonin
C. Somatostatin D. GABA

22. Urine osmolality in Diabetes insipidus is : Kerala 1990, JIPMER 1993

A. 150 mmol/L B. 300 mmol/L
C. 600 mmol/L D. 900 mmol/L

23. Following are changes seen in SIADH except : JIPMER 1991, 93

A. Low plasma osmolality
B. Low urine osmolality
C. Hyponatremia
D. Edema

24. Insulin promotes transport of glucose in which of these : JIPMER 1993

A. Adipose tissue B. RBC
C. Muscles D. Hepatocytes

25. Steroids are synthesized by : Delhi 1995, UP 1995

A. Smooth ER B. Rough ER
C. Mitochondria D. Lysosomes

26. Deficient adrenal function leads to rise in blood : TN 1991; Kerala 1991

A. Sodium B. Glucose
C. Pressure D. Potassium

27. A patient with a secreting tumour of adrenal medulla (phaeochromocytoma) typically has : TN 1991, 92

A. Raised blood pressure transcient or constant.
B. A fine tremor of extended hand.
C. Lowering of blood pressure when alpha adrenoceptor antagonist is given.
D. Increase in BMR.
E. All of the above.

28. Growth hormone secretion is increased in normal person in all of the following except : Karnataka 1994, 98

A. Exercise
B. Hyperglycemia
C. Infusion of Levodopa
D. Infusion of Arginine

29. The likelihood of developing tetany is increased when : Delhi 1983, 99

A. Plasma HCO_3 rises
B. Plasma magnesium rises
C. Respiratory failure develops
D. Anterior pituitary removed

30. TSH is secreted at a higher rate : PGI 1983, 99

A. After removal of one lobe of thyroid
B. In warm adapted than in cold adapted persons
C. When BMR falls
D. During physical injury and emotional stress

31. In the absence of ADH (Anti-dieuritic Hormone) : Karnataka 1994, 98

A. There would not be any water absorption in renal tubules.
B. Facultative water absorption is deficient.
C. Facultative water absorption is increased.
D. Obligatory water absorption is increased.

32. Sertoli cells secrete : AI 1994

A. Testosterone B. Androstenedione
C. PG E2 D. Estrogens

33. Calcium metabolism is mainly dependent on : Delhi 1997, 98

A. Calcitonin B. Parathormone
C. Thyroxine D. Growth hormone

34. Activation of renin-angiotensin mechanism result in the following except : AIIMS 1985, 98

A. Aldosterone secretion
B. Increased arteriolar tone
C. Decrease in renal sodium excretion
D. Decrease in blood volume

Ans.	15. D	16. A	17. D	18. B	19. B	20. B	21. A	22. B	23. B	24. D
	25. A	26. D	27. E	28. B	29. A	30. A	31. B	32. D	33. B	34. D

35. Production of aldosterone under normal conditions will be influenced by all except : NIZAM'S 1991
A. Blood sodium level
B. Blood angiotensin level
C. Crystalloid osmotic pattern of blood
D. ACT

36. Which of the following is not true about calcium metabolism : Delhi 1997, 99
A. Phytates in diet increase absorption
B. Dihydroxycholecalciferol increases absorption
C. High protein diet increases absorption
D. 40% of total calcium is in ionized form

37. Aldosterone secretion is regulated by following except : Rajasthan 1995, 99
A. ACTH B. Calcium
C. Blood volume D. Potassium

38. Menopause is caused due to : Rajasthan 1995, 98
A. Endometrium becomes insensitive to oestrogen & progesterone.
B. Ovary does not produce oestrogen & progesterone.
C. Pituitary
D. Hypothalamus

39. Thyroxin causes following except : Rajasthan 1996, 99
A. Increased BMR
B. Increased cholesterol
C. Increased Beta-I-receptors
D. Increased heat production

40. Hyperthyroidism is associated with : Orissa 1991, 96
A. Positive nitrogen balance.
B. A decreased urinary excretion of calcium.
C. A rise in level of plasma protein which binds thyroxine.
D. Certain feature due to excessive beta adrenergic stimulation.

41. Hyperglycemia is associated with : TNPSC 1997, 98
A. ↓ Insulin secretion
B. ↑ Glucagon secretion
C. ↑ Insulin and glucagon secretion
D. A and B

42. The thyroid hormone stored in the lumen of follicles is in the form of : NIMHANS 1990, 91
A. Free T3
B. Free T4
C. Attached to thyroglobulin
D. Attached to thyroid binding globulin

43. All of the following pituitary hormones are derived from basophilic and acidophilic cells except : Delhi 1994, 98
A. GH B. ACTH
C. PIH D. FSH

44. All of the following are true about insulin except : Delhi 1994, 99
A. Glucose is absorbed from renal tubules
B. Short polypeptide with C-chain
C. Proinsulin is coiled and cross-linked by disulfide bonds
D. Proinsulin is inactive

45. Cortisol : DNB 1989, 98
A. Secretion increases following injury
B. Favours protein synthesis
C. Enhances effects of antigen-antibody reactions
D. Tends to lower blood pressure

46. Aldosteronism is associated with : AMU 1990, 96
A. Oedema
B. Retention of sodium
C. Retention of potassium
D. Hypotension

47. Calcitonin is responsible for : AMU 1988, 99
A. Increasing the plasma Ca^{++} level
B. Decreasing the plasma Ca^{++} level
C. Increasing parathormone level
D. Decreasing thyroxine level

48. Regarding Myxoedema the following are true except : AP 1992, 96
A. Swollen, Oedematous look of the face
B. Impotency, amenorrhoea etc.
C. B.M.R. increased by 30-45%
D. Dullness, loss of memory

49. The following features are found in hyperthyroidism except : Orissa 1992, 98
A. Enlarged thyroid
B. Exophthalamos
C. Decreased body weight
D. Decreased B.M.R.

50. Regarding parathyroid the following statements are true except : TN 1990
A. It regulates Ca and P metabolism
B. Controls the balance of inorganic ions in blood
C. It is not essential for life
D. Its cellular effects are mediated through Cyclic AMP

51. In Cushing syndrome the following features are found except : UP 1992
A. Rapidly increasing adiposity
B. Polycythaemia
C. Hypotension
D. Impotence with atrophy of testis

52. Progesterone is secreted by the following except : DNB 1990
A. Corpus luteum B. Placenta
C. Adrenal cortex D. Testis

Ans.									
35. D	36. A	37. B	38. B	39. B	40. D	41. D	42. C	43. C	44. A
45. A	46. B	47. B	48. C	49. D	50. C	51. C	52. D		

53. Epinephrine predominantly causes : AIIMS 1986, AI 1993
A. Glycogenolysis B. Gluconeogenesis
C. Glycolysis D. Glycogen storage

54. Estrogens in the post-menopausal period is metabolized mostly into : AIIMS 1989, Delhi 1993
A. Estriol B. Estrone
C. Estradiol D. Androstenedione

55. FSH is secreted by : JIPMER 1992; Rajasthan 2001
A. Chromophobes B. Acidophils
C. Basophils D. Theca internal cells

56. Transection of the Pituitary stalk leads to increase in : JIPMER 1992, 98
A. Growth Hormone B. TSH
C. Prolactin D. ACTH

57. Anabolic action on proteins is mediated by : DNB 1990, JIPMER 1992, 96
A. Growth hormone B. Insulin
C. ACTH D. Testosterone

58. Following are true of insulin except : JIPMER 1992, 99
A. Glycopeptide B. Secreted by Beta cells
C. Causes lipogenesis D. Promotes glycogenesis

59. Estrogens acts on : AIIMS 1988, 92
A. Cell membrane B. Nucleus
C. Mitochondria D. Cytoplasmic receptor

60. In diabetic ketosis, there is a decreased metabolic breakdown of : PGI 1984, 99
A. Fat B. Protein
C. Glucose D. Glycogen liver

Match the following : (Ques. 61 to 64) UPSC 1982, 99
A. Cortisol B. Androgen
C. Aldosterone D. Norepinephrine

61. Zona glomerulosa :
62. Zona relicularis :
63. Zona fasciculata :
64. Adrenal medulla :

65. Peak testosterone levels are seen at about : PGI 1984, 99
A. 7-8 PM B. 2 AM
C. 7-8 AM D. 12 PM

66. Following are the effects of testosterone except : Delhi 1986, 99
A. Increased Haemopoiesis
B. Calcium retention
C. Increased Total quantity of bone matrix
D. Increased BMR

67. Amino acid sequence of human insulin differs from porcine insulin in : PGI 1987
A. 1 amino acid B. 3 amino acids
C. 5 amino acids D. None of the above

68. Which of the following arterioles is least sensitive to epinephrine : AIIMS 1986
A. Skeletal muscle arteriole
B. Cerebral
C. Cutaneous
D. Afferent renal

69. The following hormones increase the level of intra-cellu-lar cAMP except : AIIMS 1981, AMU 1987, 99
A. Vasopressin
B. Glucagon
C. Parathyroid hormone
D. Somatostatin

70. Which of the following G-protein is associated with receptors for norepinephrine : DNB 1989, 95
A. Gt1 B. Gi1
C. Gt2 D. Go

71. Following stimuli increase aldosterone as well as glucocorticoids secretion except : DNB 1995, 99
A. Anxiety B. Cirrhosis
C. Surgery D. Hemorrhage

72. The size and number of inclusions in the type-II alveolar epithelial cells producing surfactant are increased by : AMU 1985, 99
A. Growth hormone B. Androgens
C. Thyroxine D. Insulin

73. The following is true about carbonic anhydrase except : Rohtak 1984, 99
A. A protein with a molecular weight of 30,000.
B. Contains an item of copper in each molecule.
C. Inhibited by cyanide, azide and sulfide.
D. Sulfonamides also inhibit this enzyme.

74. Islet cells of Pancreas secrete all of the following except : AIIMS 1996, 99
A. Somatostatin B. Gastrin
C. VIP D. Pancreozymin

75. Pheochromocytomas predominantly secrete : UPSC 1981, 99
A. Epinephrine B. Norepinephrine
C. 5-HT D. Renin

76. Which of the following responses is not initiated by the stimulation of adrenergic sympathetic neurons? AIIMS 1982, 99
A. Hepatic glycogenolysis
B. Skeletal muscle vasoconstriction
C. Ventricular force increase
D. Ventricular conduction time increase
E. Contraction of pyloric sphincter of stomach

Ans.									
53. A	54. B	55. C	56. C	57. D	58. A	59. B	60. C	61. C	62. B
63. A	64. D	65.C	66. A	67. A	68. B	69. D	70. C	71. B	72. C
73. B	74. D	75. A	76. D						

77. **An animal deprived of its adrenal glands : Karnataka 1987, 99**
A. Losses most of its reactions due to increased sympathetic activity, because of the lack of circulating epinephrine
B. Can still develop tachycardia and sympathetic hypertension in response to exercise
C. Has a much greater rate of glycogenolysis
D. Usually is hyperglycemic during fasting periods

78. **When a patient is treated with aldosterone antagonist there is likely to be a fall in ? PGI 1981, 99**
A. Urine volume
B. Plasma potassium level
C. Blood volume
D. Blood viscosity

79. **Increased release of aldosterone from adrenal cortex is not a feature in : AIIMS 1980, 99**
A. Increased arterial pressure
B. Hyponatremia
C. Hyperkalemia
D. Epinephrine and norepinephrine

80. **If there is a decrease in extracellular fluid volume, the body may respond by increasing the secretion of : PGI 1981, 98**
A. Epinephrine
B. Aldosterone
C. Epinephrine and aldosterone
D. Epinephrine, aldosterone and A.D.H.

81. **True about gastrin is : AIIMS 1985, 86, 89; PGI 1985, 86**
A. A peptide hormone
B. An analogue of Pentagastrin which decreases secretion of HCl
C. Secreted with HCl from parietal cells
D. Increased in Zollinger Ellison syndrome

82. **Somogyl phenomenon is : AMC 1987, 88, 99**
A. Hypoglycemia followed by hyperglycemia
B. Hyperglycemia followed by hypoglycemia
C. Glycosuria with normal blood sugar
D. Reactive hyperglycemia

83. **Pain producing substance is : Delhi 1984, 98**
A. Serotonin B. Substance-P
C. Histamine D. Acetylcholine

84. **Cyclic AMP serves as second messenger in the secretion of all except : AIIMS 1984, 88**
A. FSH B. Estrogen
C. Glucagon D. Epinephrine

85. **Function of Leutenizing hormone is : Delhi 1988,99**
A. Follicle maturation and ovulation
B. Milk secretion
C. Causes progesterone secretion during ovulation
D. Maintain placenta

86. **Precursor of testesterone is : AIIMS 1986; AI 1990**
A. Methyl testesterone B. Pregnenolone
C. Aldosterone D. Cortisone

87. **Metyrapone is useful in congenital hyperplasia because it inhibits : PGI 1984; AI 1990, 91**
A. 17-alpha hydroxylase
B. 21-alpha hydroxylase
C. 11-beta hydroxylase
D. Desmolase

88. **FSH and ICSH are secreted by : AMC 1986; Delhi 1989, 92**
A. Adenohypophysis B. Hypothalamus
C. Ovaries D. Placenta

89. **Position of estradiol/OH is at : UP 1998, 99**
A. C3 & C17 B. C & C
C. C & C D. C & C

90. **Hormones secreted by anterior pituitary lobe is/are: PGI 1987; NIMHANS 1986**
A. GH B. Prolactin
C. TSH D. All

91. **Function of acini in thyroid gland is synthesis of : Delhi 1989, 99**
A. Tyrosine B. Thyroxine
C. Mucus D. TSH

92. **Which of the following does not have natriuretic actions : PGI 1986, 88**
A. Aldosterone B. Natriuretic peptide
C. Angiotensin D. Prednisolone

93. **The hormone responsible for increased body temperature after ovulation is : AMC 1985, 99**
A. Lutenizing hormone B. Progesterone
C. Increased estrogen D. Androgens

94. **Secretion of estriol during pregnancy : AMU 1986, 95**
A. Is independent on both a viable fetus and a functioning placenta.
B. Is largely produced by the maternal ovaries.
C. Is not dependent on a viable fetus.
D. Is lower than the secretion rate of etriol is non-pregnancy body.

95. **Which is not formed in tryptophan metabolism : UP 1998, 99**
A. Melatonin B. Dopamine
C. Serotonin D. Epinephrine

96. **Beta endorphins are found in high concentration in : Delhi 1982, 95**
A. Substantia gelatinosa
B. Post-pituitary
C. Spinal cord
D. Medulla

Ans.									
77. B	78. C	79. A	80. D	81. D	82. A	83. B	84. B	85. A	86. B
87. C	88. A	89. A	90. D	91. B	92. A	93. B	94. A	95. B	96. A

97. Most potent vasopressor is : **AIIMS 1984, 86; AI 1989**

A. Angiotensin-II B. Renin
C. Aldosterone D. Cortisol

98. Levels of which of the following hormones are increased in post-menopausal women : **UPSC 1987, 88; AI 1989**

A. Estrogen B. FSH
C. Progesteron D. Cortisone

99. Blockage of the hypothalamic-hypophyseal venous portal system would be expected to cause increased secretion of : **AIIMS 1980, 98**

A. Growth hormone
B. Adrenocorticotropic hormone
C. Thyroid-stimulating hormone
D. Prolactin

100. High plasma levels of thyroxine can lead to all of the following except : **DNB 1989, 99**

A. Increased cardiac output
B. Increased plasma triglyceride concentration
C. Increased heart rate
D. Decreased body weight

101. Thyroid-stimulating hormone stimulates thyroid function in many ways, but it does not increase : **AMC 1986,96, 99**

A. Synthesis of thyroxine-binding globulin
B. Rate of synthesis of thyroglobulin
C. Iodine uptake from the blood
D. Iodination of tyrosine

102. Cortisol can cause all of the following except : **AIIMS 1986, 98**

A. Inflammation to be suppressed
B. Fat to be used for energy
C. Lysosomal membranes to become unstable
D. The blood glucose concentration to increase

103. Growth hormone increases all of the following except : **PGI 1984, 92**

A. Blood glucose concentration
B. Blood free fatty acid concentration
C. Protein synthesis
D. None of the above

104. All of the following hormones mediate their major effects without actually entering the target cell except : **PGI 1982, 93**

A. Cortisol B. Insulin
C. Growth hormone D. Glucagon

105. Increased plasma parathyroid hormone concentration tends to increase all of the following except : **AIIMS 1984, 94**

A. Number of active osteoclasts
B. Extracellular phosphate concentration
C. Absorption of calcium from the gastrointestinal tract
D. Absorption of calcium from the renal tubules

106. The active form of Vitamin-D is : **AIIMS 1983, 88, 98**

A. Calcitonin
B. 1, 25 dihydroxycholecalciferol
C. Parathyroid hormone
D. Cholecalciferol

107. Important effects of testosterone include all of the following except : **AIIMS 1988, 98**

A. Formation of the fetal penis
B. Descent of the testes into the scrotum
C. Increased muscle development
D. Initiation of ejaculation

108. Synthesis of testosterone is controlled by : **CSE 1996**

A. LH B. LHRH
C. FSH D. TSH

109. Cortisol increases the blood glucose concentration either directly or indirectly by : **PGI 1982, 99**

A. Decreasing glucose uptake by the cells
B. Decreasing the rate of gluconeogenesis
C. Decreasing the rate of glucose utilization by the cells
D. Inhibiting hormone-sensitive lipase

110. The principal estrogen found in the urine of pregnant women is : **CSE 1997, 99**

A. Estriol B. Estrone
C. Beta-estradiol D. Pregnanediol

111. Which of the following statements about thyroxine is false ? **Manipal 1994, 95**

A. Its production requires the amino acids tyrosine.
B. Its effect is slower in onset and longer in duration than that of triiodothyronine (T3).
C. It increases cerebral metabolic oxygen consumption.
D. It is essential for the production of erythrocytes.

112. Which of the following statements about androgens is false ? **Manipal 1994, 99**

A. They are formed by seminiferous tubules of the testis.
B. they are formed in greater quantities in foetal life (in the male foetus) than in childhood.
C. Are secreted in small amounts in normal adult females.
D. Their concentration in blood decreases after the age of 30 in men.

113. Which of the following statements about calcitonin is false ? **Manipal 1996, 99**

A. It reduces the number and activity of osteoclasts.
B. It reduces the renal tubular absorption of calcium.
C. It reduces the renal tubular absorption of phosphate.
D. When present in excess, it commonly causes tetany.

Ans.	97. A	98. B	99. D	100. B	101. A	102. C	103. D	104. A	105. B	106. B
	107. D	108. A	109. C	110. A	111. C	112. A	113. D			

114. In which of the following organ, glucose uptake depends on insulin : Delhi 1998, 99

A. Renal epithelium B. Heart
C. Brain D. Intestinal epithelium

115. Vitamin-D deficiency leads to : Delhi 1998, 99

A. Decreased calcium absorption by renal tubules
B. Decreased calcium absorption by intestine
C. Increased phsophate excretion by renal tubules
D. None of the above

116. The following substances cross blood brain barrier: AIIMS 1986, 95

A. Insulin B. Testosterone
C. Glucose D. All of the above

117. In the female rat, selective neutralization of follicle-stimulating hormone with anti-FSH antibodies : AIIMS 1980, 90

A. Increases estrogen and progesterone secretion by the corpus luteum.
B. Prevents early uniting of the epiphyses.
C. Prevents early follicular growth.
D. Suppresses the secretion of hypothalamic releasing factors.

118. Spontaneous hypoglycemia may be caused by : PGI 1997, 99

A. Glucagonoma
B. Chronic Pancreatitis
C. Cushing's syndrome
D. Hepatocellular carcinoma

119. 'C' cells are present in : PGI 1993, 98

A. Thyroid B. Adrenal
C. Parathyroid D. Pituitary

120. Stimulation of both glucocorticoid and mineralocorticoid secretion is seen with : Delhi 1988, 96

A. Anxiety B. Exercise
C. Hyperkalemia D. Low sodium diet

121. After drinking a large amount of hypotonic fluid and after absorption of the fluid from the gut into the blood, which of the following changes would you expect : AIIMS 1986, 99

A. Increased secretion of antidiuretic hormone
B. A decrease in distal tubular permeability to water
C. A marked decrease in glomerular filtration rate
D. A marked increase in sodium excretion

122. Overall regulating organ for neuroendocrinal system is : PGI 1993, 95

A. Hypothalamus
B. Pituitary
C. Reticulo-endothelial system
D. Pineal gland

123. Calcitonin is produced by: AIIMS 1986; PGI 1993, 99

A. Thyroid B. Parathyroid
C. Thymus D. Kidney

124. Maximum production of HCG occurs during : AIIMS 1983; AI 1989, 96

A. First trimester B. Second trimester
C. Third trimester D. Implantation

125. Melatonin is secreted by : AIIMS 1984; AI 1989, 96

A. Hypothalamus B. Adrenal cortex
C. Pineal gland D. Melanocytes

126. The excretion of estrogens and progesterone are through : AIIMS 1982, 99

A. Bile B. Sweat
C. Urine D. Faeces

127. In the testes, the cells that secrete testosterone are : Rajasthan 1991, 99

A. Germinal epithelium B. Leydig cells
C. Sertoli cells D. Sperm cells

128. Estrogen secretion by the ovary is influence of the following except : Rajasthan 1991, 95

A. Follicle stimulatory hormone
B. Luteinizing hormone
C. Sympathetic nerve activity
D. Progesterone

129. ACTH is most effective in stimulating the secretion of : Rajasthan 1991, 99

A. Hydrocortisone
B. Cortisone
C. Adrenal androgenic hormones
D. Aldosterone

130. Luteal phase of menstrual cycle is characterized by : DNB 1990, Rajasthan 1993

A. A variable length
B. Secretion of osteogen
C. Low basal body temperature
D. Secretion on progesterone

131. Which of the following hormone acts by decreasing cAMP levels : Delhi 1995, 99

A. Epinephrine (Beta 1 receptors)
B. Dopamine (D2 receptors)
C. Glucagen
D. None of the above

132. Reverse T3 is : AP 1995; MAHE 1999

A. Synthetic derivative
B. Isomerisation product of T1 and active
C. Isomerisation product of T3 and inactive
D. Reverse T1

133. Actions of insulin except : AI 2000

A. Glycolysis B. Glycogenesis
C. Lipogenesis D. Gluconeogenesis

Ans.	114. B	115. B	116. C	117. C	118. B	119. A	120. A	121. B	122. A	123. A
	124. A	125. C	126. C	127. B	128. C	129. A	130. D	131. D	132. C	133. D

134. Dopamine is inhibitor of: JIPMER 2000
A. Prolactin B. Growth hormone
C. Oxytocin D. Epinephrine

135. Spermatogenic epithelium is maintained by : Delhi 2000
A. Somatostatin B. TRH
C. FSH D. LH

136. Level of T3 indicates : UP 1999
A. Metabolic state
B. Thyroid state
C. Pituitary function state
D. Not important

137. Gonadal function is regulated by : UP 2000
A. Anterior hypothalamus
B. Posterior hypothalamus
C. Anterior pituitary
D. Posterior pituitary

138. The prohormone produced by the theca internal of the ovary is : TNPSC 2000
A. α 17- ketosteroid
B. An estrogen
C. A dehydroepiandrosterone
D. All of these

139. The hormone which diminishes the excretion of magnesium is : TNPSC 2000
A. Antidiuretic hormone (ADH)
B. Parathormone (PTH)
C. Growth hormone (G.H.)
D. Aldosterone

140. Every nucleated cell has one of the following proteins which is involved in transmission of the message of many hormones called : TNPSC 2000
A. Calcium binding protein
B. Calmodulin
C. Apotransferrin
D. Apoceruloplamin

141. A cortisol deficient individual : TNPSC 2000
A. Has reduced resistance to stress
B. Has increased ability to mobilize stored triglyceride
C. Has reduced sensitivity to insulin
D. Shows all of these

142. All of the following are the actions of glucocorticoids on blood cells except : Kerala 2000
A. Decrease in the number of Eosinophils
B. Decrease in the number of Basophils
C. Increase in the number of lymphocytes
D. Increase in the number of neutrophils and platelets
E. Increase in the number of Red blood cells

143. Which of the following statements about progesterone is not true ? Kerala 2000
A. It stimulates the development of lobules and alveoli in the breast.
B. It increases the excitability of myometrium.
C. It is thermogenic.
D. It can prevent ovulation in large doses.
E. In large doses it produces natriuresis.

144. cAMP action mediates all except : PGI 2000
A. Glucagon B. FSH
C. LH D. Estrogen

145. Thyroxine is injected to rat A/E : PGI 2000
A. ↓↓ lipolysis
B. ↑↑ O2 consumption
C. ↓ BMR
D. ↑myocardial contractility

146. FSH is produced by : PGI 2000
A. Chromphobes B. Acidophils
C. Basophils D. All of the above

147. A person who is on starvation for 5 days, Glucose is given for GTT will cause the following except : AI 2001
A. GH decrease
B. Decreased Insulin
C. Increase cortisol
D. Increased Insulin tolerance

148. Lack of which of the following hormone causes osteoporosis : Delhi 2001
A. Oestrogen B. Progesterone
C. Thyroxine D. Testosterone

149. Which of the following feature is not seen in hypopituitary state : AI 1989; Delhi 2001
A. Cachexia
B. Growth failure
C. Infertility
D. Increased sensitivity to insulin

150. Secretion does not increase in night : JIPMER 2001
A. Growth hormone B. ACTH
C. Insulin D. TSH

151. Thyroxine does not increase the metabolism in : Kerala 2001
A. Heart B. Liver
C. Pituitary D. Kidney

152. Which is produced in Cushing's syndrome in excess: Kerala 2001
A. Epinephrine B. Norepinephrine
C Cortisol D. Dopa

153. On injecting, concentrated NaCl solution into the carotid artery, there was increased production of ADH. The source of it's secretion in the hypothalamus is in the : AIIMS 2001
A. Paraventricular nucleus
B. Supraoptic nucleus
C. Anterior nucleus
D. Ventromedial nucleus

Ans.										
	134. A	135. C	136. C	137. C	138. D	139. D	140. A	141. D	142. C	143. B
	144. D	145. C	146. C	147. B	148. A	149. A	150. B	151. C	152. C	153. B

154. **FSH acts on : AIIMS 2002**
A. Theca cell B. Granulosa cell
C. Stromal cell D. Interstitial cell

W.155. **Following have both alpha and beta subunits except : JIPMER 2002**
A. TSH B. LH
C. FSH D. HCG

156. **The blood testis barrier is seen in : SGPGI 2002**
A. Leydig cells B. Spermatogonia
C. Sertoli cells D. Spermatozoa

157. **Which of the following is an endocrine organ : SGPGI 2002**
A. Lamina dura B. Small intestine
C. Ciliary body D. Breast

158. **Steroid hormones are produced by all except : Maharashtra 2000**
A. Testis B. Placenta
C. Ovaries D. Adrenal Medulla

159. **Somatostatin Inhibits all except : Maharashtra 2000**
A. GH B. ACTH
C. TSH D. Prolactin

160. **Thyrotropin release is mainly dependent on : CMC 2001**
A. Thyroid status
B. TIBG levels
C. Levels of thyroid hormones in blood
D. Catecholamine levels

161. **Circadian rhythm of ACTH is controlled by : BHU 2002**
A. Supraoptic nucleus of hypothalamus
B. Paraventricular nucleus of hypothalamus
C. Suprachiasmatic nucleus of hypothalamus
D. Lateral nucleus of hypothalamus

162. **The laboratory report shows values of gonadotropin and ovarian hormones of the blood sample taken on day 20 of the menstrual cycle of a young woman. Whether her cycle was ovulatory or not may be validly assessed by the reported serum level of : AIIMS 2002**
A. FSH B. LH
C. Oestradiol D. Progesterone

163. **Even in the presence of vasopressin the greatest fraction of filtered water is reabsorbed in which part of the nephron : AI 2003**
A. Proximal tubule B. Distal tubule
C. Loop of Henle D. Collecting duct

164. **The hormone associated with cold adaptation is : AIIMS 2003**
A Growth hormone
B Thyroxine
C Insulin
D Melanocyte Stimulating Hormone

165. **In which of the following forms the Anti-diuretic hormone (ADH) is circulated in plasma? AI 2004**
A. Bound to neurophysin-I
B. Bound to neurophysin-II
C. Bound to plasma albumin
D. Free form

166. **Sertoli cells have receptors for? AI 2004**
A. Inhibin
B. Luteinising hormone
C. Follicle stimulating hormone
D. Melatonin

167. **Before the onset of puberty, the GnRH neurons are under the inhibitory control of : AI 2004**
A. Glycine
B. Glutamate
C. Gamma amino butyric acid (GABA)
D. Beta-endorphin

168. **The enzyme associated with the conversion of androgen to oestrogen in the growing ovarian follicle is : AI 2004**
A. Desmolase B. Isomerase
C. Aromatase D. Hydroxylase

169. **Which of the following statements can be regarded as primary action of inhibin ? AI 2005**
A. It inhibits secretion of prolactin
B. It stimulates synthesis of estradiol
C. It stimulates secretion of TSH
D. It inhibits secretion of FSH

170. **Osteoclasts are inhibited by : AI 2005**
A. Parathyroid hormone
B. Calcitonin
C. 1, 25-dihydroxycholecalciferol
D. Tumor necrosis factor

171. **All of the following hormones have cell surface receptors except : AI 2005**
A. Adrenaline B. Growth Hormone
C. Insulin D. Thyroxine

172. **Which of the following hormones is not secreted by the adenohypophysis : PGI 1986**
A. ADH B. ACTH
C. TSH D. FSH

173. **The hormone with the shortest half life in the blood stream in the following list is : AIIMS 1986**
A. Epinephrine B. Acetylcholine
C. Insulin D. T3

174. **Following are local hormones except : Delhi 1992**
A. Insulin B. Heparin
C. Bradykinin D. Acetylcholine

175. **Sertoli cells have receptors for : AIIMS 2007**
A. FSH B. LH
C. Inhibin D. All of the above

Ans. 154. B 155. NONE 156. C 157. B 158. D 159. D 160. C 161. C 162. D 163. A 164. B 165. B 166. D 167. C 168. C 169. D 170. B 171. D 172. A 173. B 174. A 175. A

176. A patient is on a low calcium diet for 6 weeks. He is most likely to have : AIIMS 2007
A. Raised parathyroid hormone levels
B. Raised calcitonin levels
C. Increased phosphate levels
D. None of the above

177. True about free water clearance is : AIIMS 2007
A. Regulated by ADH
B. Regulated by aldosterone
C. Increased by furosemide
D. None of the above

178. Aldosterone receptors are present in all except : AIIMS 2007
A. Liver B. Colon
C. Hippocampus D. Distal nephron

179. Males and females show difference in the age of onset of puberty. The difference in the age of onset of puberty amongst males may be explained by : AI 2007
A. Increased Activin — A levels
B. Decreased Follistatin levels
C. Increased Inhibin levels
D. Easily releaseable FSH poolz

180. Correct sequence of sperm movement is : AI 2008
A. Rete testis-straight tubules-efferent tubules
B. Straight tubules-rete testis-efferent tubules
C. Straight tubules-efferent tubules-epididymis
D. Straight tubules-rete testis-epididymis

181. Which of the following is true regarding requirement of temperature for spermatogenesis? AI 2008
A. Requires temperature higher than core temperature
B. Required temperature should be conducive
C. Requires temperature lower than core temperature
D. Requires temperature equal to core temperature

182. Which of the following is the active form of calcium in the body ? AI 2008
A. Ionized calcium
B. Complexed with phosphate
C. Complexed with oxalates
D. Bound to albumin

183. Mineralocorticoid receptor is present in all except : AIIMS 2008
A. Liver B. Colon
C. Hippocampus D. Kidney

184. In obstructive azoospermia : AI 2009
A. FSH and LH both increase
B. FSH and LH both normal
C. FSH decrease but LH increases
D. FSH and LH both decrease

185. Paneth cells are rich in : AI 2009
A. Zinc B. Lysozyme
C. Mucus D. Intrinsic factor

186. After 48 hours of fasting insulin receptors are down regulated in : AI 2009
A. Brain B. Liver
C. RBC D. Adipocytes

Ans.	176. A	177. A	178. A	179. C	180. B	181. C	182. A	183. A	184. B
	185. A, B	186. D							

EXPLANATIONS OF ENDOCRINOLOGY

1. Ans.— B Granulosa cells :
   * FSH acts on the Granulosa cells of ovary.
   * LH acts on both theca interna and granulosa cells.
2. Ans.— A 3rd month

   "Insulin containing granules can be identified in the human fetal pancreas by 9 to 10 weeks, and insulin in fetal plasma is detectable at 12 weeks. " *Williams, Obstetrics.*

   Also Remember :
   - Glucagon secretion begins by 8th week.
   - Thyroxin secretion begins by 10th to 12th week.
3. Ans.— A Parathormone :
   * Hormones can be classified chemically into three major groups >
   1. Steroid hormones
      — Glucocorticoids
      — Mineralocorticoids
      — Estrogens
      — Progestins
      — Androgens
   2. Amino acid derivative
      — They are derived from amino acid tyrosine.
        — Catecholamines
        — Thyroid hormones
   3. Peptide / Protein Hormones.
      — Parathormone
      — Calcitonin
      — Insulin
      — Glucagon
      — Pituitary hormones.
4. Ans.— A. Prolactin
5. Ans.— B. Parathyroid hormone related protein (PTHRP)
6. Ans.— A. It inhibits secretion of prolactin
7. Ans.— A. Inhibin
8. Ans.— A. Desmolase
9. Ans.— C. Gamma amino butyric acid (GABA)
10. Ans.— A. Bound to neurophysin-I
11. Ans.— A. Alloxan
12. Ans.— C. Always causes the muscle fiber to contract
13. Ans.— B. Thyroxine
14. Ans.— B. Increase BMR

    There is fall in BMR & depression or psychosis
15. Ans.— D. Oestrogen
16. Ans.— A. Growth hormone
17. Ans.— D. Prolactin

    Prolactin releasing hormone has been postulated to exist but not yet fully identified.
18. Ans.— B. ↑ Blood sugar

    Corticosteroids and not oestrogens produce diabetes mellitus.
19. Ans.— B. LH surge
20. Ans.— B. Starvation
21. Ans.— A. Dopamine
22. Ans.— B. 300 mmol/L

    In diabetes insipidus, percentage of filtered water reabsorbed in 87.1% whereas in normal, it is 98.7% absorption. Urine volume is 23.3 L/d in diabetes insipidus whereas in normal it is 2.4 L/d. Urine concentration (mosm/Kg H2O) in diabetes insipidus is 30 whereas in normal, it is 290. There is 20.9 L/d loss of water in excess of solute.
23. Ans.— B. Low urine osmolality
24. Ans.— D. Hepatocytes
25. Ans.— A. Smooth ER
26. Ans.— D. Potassium
27. Ans.— E. All of the above
28. Ans.— B. Hyperglycemia
29. Ans.— A. Plasma HCO_3 rises

    There is hyperventilation and fall of ionized calcium.

30. Ans.— A. After removal of one lobe of thyroid

31. Ans.— B. Facultative water absorption is deficient

32. Ans.— D. Estrogens

Sertoli cells secrete androgen-binding protein (ABP), inhibin and MIS. They do not synthesize androgens but they contain aromatase (CYp 19), the enzyme responsible for conversion of androgens to estrogens. They can produce estrogens.

33. Ans.— B. Parathormone

34. Ans.— D. Decrease in blood volume

35. Ans.— D. ACT

36. Ans.— A. Phytates in diet increase absorption

37. Ans.— B. Calcium

Aldosterone secretion is increased by

Glucocorticoid secretion also - ed	*Glucocorticoid secretion unaffected*
Surgery	High potassium intake
Anxiety	Low sodium intake
Physical trauma	Constriction of IVC in thorax

Hemorrhage Standing secondary hyper-aldoseronism (in CHF, ARF, Cirrhosis)

38. Ans.— B. Ovary does not produce oestrogen & progesterone

39. Ans.— B. Increased cholesterol

Cholesterol level rises in thyroxine deficiency (in myxedema)

40. Ans.— D. Certain feature due to excessive beta adrenergic stimulation

41. Ans.— D. A and B

42. Ans.— C. Attached to thyroglobulin

43. Ans.— C. PIH

Prolactin inhibitory hormone is Dopamine.

44. Ans.— A. Glucose is absorbed from renal tubules

45. Ans.— A. Secretion increases following injury

46. Ans.— B. Retention of sodium

47. Ans.— B. Decreasing the plasma Ca^{++} level

48. Ans.— C. B.M.R. increased by 30-45%

In myxoedema, BMR falls

49. Ans.— D. Decreased B.M.R.

50. Ans.— C. It is not essential for life

51. Ans.— C. Hypotension

Cushing's syndrome is an important cause of hypertension.

52. Ans.— D. Testis

53. Ans.— A. Glycogenolysis

Hepatic glucose output is increased, producing hyperglycemia. The response to an injection of epinephrine is an initial glycogenolysis followed by a rise in hepatic glycogen content.

54. Ans.— B. Estrone

55. Ans.— C. Basophils

56. Ans.— C. Prolactin

57. Ans.— D. Testosterone

58. Ans.— A. Glycopeptide

Insulin is a polypeptide

59. Ans. B. Nucleus

60. Ans.— C. Glucose

61. Ans.— C. Aldosteron

62. Ans.— B. Androgen

63. Ans.— A. Cortisol

64. Ans.— D. Norepinephrine

65. Ans.— C. 7-8 AM

It is appropriate to check its fasting levels around this time.

66. Ans.— A. Increased Haemopoiesis

67. Ans.— A. 1 amino acid

68. Ans.— B. Cerebral

69. Ans.— D. Somatostatin

70. Ans.— C. Gt2

71. Ans.— B. Cirrhosis

72. Ans.— C. Thyroxine

73. Ans.— B. Contains an item of copper in each molecule

74. Ans.— D. Pancreozymin

Cholecystokinin-Pancreozymin is secreted by cells in the mucosa of upper small intestine.

75. Ans.— A. Epinephrine

76. Ans.— D. Ventricular conduction time increase

77. Ans.— B. Can still develop tachycardia and sympathetic hypertension in response to exercise.

78. Ans.— C. Blood volume

Spironolactone (aldosterone antagonist) is used in treatment of oedema in cirrhosis.

79. Ans.— A. Increased arterial pressure

80. Ans.— D. Epinephrine, aldosterone and A.D.H.

81. Ans.— D. Increased in Zollinger Ellison syndrome

82. Ans.— A. Hypoglycemia followed by hyperglycemia

83. Ans.— B. Substance-P

84. Ans.— B. Estrogen

85. Ans.— A. Follicle maturation and ovulation

86. Ans.— B. Pregnenolone

Cholesterol -> Pregnenolone->17 alpha-> hydroxyprogesterine

↓ ↓ ↓

Progesterone->17 alpha-hydroxy- >Progesterone ->Androstenedione

Dihydrotestosterone <——Testosterone

87. Ans.— C. 11-beta hydroxylase

88. Ans.— A. Adenohypophysis

89. Ans.— A. C3 and C17

90. Ans.— D. All

91. Ans.— B. Thyroxine

92. Ans.— A. Aldosterone

The existence of various natriuretic hormones has been postulated for some time. Two of these are secreted by the heart. The first natriuretic hormone isolated from heart was atrial natriuretic peptide (ANP) with a characteristic 17-amino acid ring. Second is brain natriuretic peptide (BNP) which contains 32 amino acids and there is C-type natriuretic peptide (CNP) which contains 22 amino acids.

93. Ans.— B. Progesterone

94. Ans.— A. Is independent on both (a viable fetus and a functioning placenta)

95. Ans.— B. Dopamine

96. Ans.— A. Substantia gelatinosa

97. Ans.— A. Angiotensin-II

98. Ans.— B. FSH

99. Ans.— D. Prolactin

100. Ans.— B. Increased plasma triglyceride concentration.

Triglycerides level may rise in thyroxine deficiency.

101 Ans.— A. Synthesis of thyroxine-binding globulin

102. Ans. — C. Lysosomal membranes to become unstable

103. Ans.— D. None of the above

104. Ans.— A. Cortisol

105. Ans.— B. Extracellular phosphate concentration

106. Ans.— B. 1, 25 dihydroxycholecalciferol

In liver 25 dihydroxycholecalciferol in formed whereas 1, 25 derivative is formed in kidney.

107. Ans.— D. Initiation of ejaculation

108. Ans.— A. LH

LH stimulates the Leydig cells which involves increased formation of cAMP via the serpentine LH receptor and G8. Cyclic AMP increases the formation of cholesterol from cholesteryl esters and the conversion of cholesterol to pregnenolone via the activation of protein kinase A. The testosterone secretion rate is 4-9 mg/d (13.9-31.33 mmol/d) in normal adult males.

109. Ans.— C. Decreasing the rate of glucose utilization by the cells.

110. Ans.— A. Estriol

Estriol is main hormone of pregnancy

111. Ans.— C. It increases cerebral metabolic oxygen consumption.

112. Ans.— A. They are formed by seminiferrous tubules of the testis.

113. Ans.— D. When present in excess, it commonly causes tetany.

114. Ans.— B. Heart

115. Ans.— B. Decreased calcium absorption by intestine

116. Ans.— C. Glucose

117. Ans.— C. Prevents early follicular growth

118. Ans.— B. Chronic Pancreatitis

119. Ans.— A. Thyroid

They secrete calcitonin.

120. Ans.— A. Anxiety

121. Ans.— B. A decrease in distal tubular permeability to water

122. Ans.— A. Hypothalamus

123. Ans.— A. Thyroid

Calcitonin is secreted by para follicular cells which are also known as clear or C-cells.

124. Ans.— A. First trimester

125. Ans.— C. Pineal gland

126. Ans.— C. Urine

127. Ans.— B. Leydig cells

128. Ans.— C. Sympathetic nerve activity

129. Ans.— A. Hydrocortisone

ACTH increases secretion of glucocorticoids. The morning plasma ACTH concentration in a healthy resting human is about 25 pg/mL (5.5 pmol/L).

130. Ans.— D. Secretion on progesterone

131. Ans.— D. None of the above

132. Ans.— C. Isomerisation product of T3 and inactive

133. Ans.— D. Gluconeogenesis

134. Ans.— A. Prolactin

135. Ans.— C. FSH

136. Ans.— C. Pituitary function state

It more active than T4

137. Ans.— C. Anterior pituitary

138. Ans.— D. All of these

139. Ans.— D. Aldosterone

140. Ans.— A. Calcium binding protein

141. Ans.— D. Shows all of these

142. Ans.— C. Increase in the number of lymphocytes

143. Ans.— B. It increases the excitability of myometrium

144. Ans.— D. Estrogen

Like other steroids, estrogens combine with protein receptors in the nucleus and the complex binds to DNA, promoting formation of new proteins which modify cell function.

145. Ans.— C. ↓ BMR

146 Ans.— C. Basophils

147. Ans.— B. Decreased Insulin

148. Ans.— A. Oestrogen

Osteoporosis is common after menopause

149. Ans.— A. Cachexia

150. Ans.— B. ACTH

151. Ans.— C. Pituitary

152. Ans.— C Cortisol

153. Ans.— B. Supraoptic nucleus

154. Ans.— B. Granulosa cell

155. Ans.— NONE

156. Ans.— C. Sertoli cells

157. Ans.— B. Small intestine

Some of the hormones produced are gastrin, cholecystokinin-pancreozymin, secretin, GIP, VIP, Motilin, Neurotensin, Substance-P, GRP, Bombesin, Somatostatin, Guanylin, Urogastrone etc.

158. Ans.— D. Adrenal Medulla

159. Ans.— D. Prolactin

Somatostatin inhibits secretion of GH, gastrin, VIP, GIP, secretion and motilin.

160. Ans.— C. Levels of thyroid hormones in blood

161. Ans.— C. Suprachiasmatic nucleus of hypothalamus

162. Ans.— D. Progesterone

163. Ans.— A. Proximal tubule

164. Ans.— B Thyroxine.

165. Ans.— B. Bound to neurophysin - II

- **The hormones of the post-pituitary gland (ADH and oxytocin) are synthesised in the cell bodies of magnocellular neurons in the supraoptic and para-ventricular nuclei.**
- **Vasopressin and oxytocin each have a characteristic neurophysin ass. with them in the granules in the neurons that secrete them, neurophysin-II in case of vasopressin and neurophysin-I in case of oxytocin.**
- **ADH secretion is enhanced by angiotensin-II, prostglandins, histamine, neuropeptide Y and Ach and is inhibited by GABA and ANP.**
- **ADH responsive water channel is collecting ducts of kidney is aquaporin-2.**

166. Ans.— D. Melatonin

Sertoli cells have receptors for FSH which stimulate by FSH and secrete the inhibin.

Sertoli :

- **Large, complex glycogen - containing cells.**
- **They provide nutrition to the developing sperm cells.**
- **They phagocytoze the injured or dead sperm cells.**

- They are the basis of blood testis barrier.
- They secrete *androgen-binding protein (ABP), inhibin and MIS.*
- They do not synthesize androgens, but they contain *aromatase*. The enzyme responsible for conversion of androgens to estrogens and they can produce estrogens.

Note:

- *ABP* probably functions to maintain a high, stable supply of androgen in tubular fluid.
- *Inhibin* inhibits FSH secretion.
- *MIS* causes regression of the mullerian ducts in males during fetal life.

167. Ans.— C. Gamma amino butyric acid (GABA)

Control of the onset of puberty :

- The factors that normally activate or restrain the hypothalamic neurons responsible for GnRH secretion are unknown.
- It is clear that GnRH is the major, if not the only, hormone responsible for the onset and progression of puberty.
- During the period from birth to puberty, a neural mechanism is operating to prevent the normal pulse release of GnRH. The nature of the mechanism inhibiting the GnRH pulse generator is unknown.
- Controversely, opioid peptide such as the enkephalins and β-endorphin reduce the frequency of GnRH pulses.
- The release of hypothalamic GnRH is also inhibited by melatonin (samson wright).
- Norepinephrine and possibly epinephrine in the hypothalamus increase GnRH pulse frequencies.

168. Ans.— C. Aromatase

169. Ans.— D. It inhibits secretion of FSH

INHIBIN :

- Factor of testicular origin that inhibits FSH secretion
- Source - Testes in Men

170. Ans.— B. Calcitonin

"Calcium lowers the circulating calcium and phosphate level. It exerts its calcium lowering effect by inhibiting bone resorption. This action is direct, and calcitonin inhibits the activity of osteoclast."

- Ovarian Follicles in women

171. Ans.— D. Thyroxine

"Thyroid hormones enter cells and binds to thyroid receptor in the nuclei. "The hormone receptor complex binds to DNA via zinc finger.

- Nuclear receptors for thyroid hormones are members of the superfamily of hormone sensitive nuclear transcription factor.

I. Hormones having intracellular receptors
1. Thyroid hormones
2. Glycocorticoids
3. Mineralocorticoids
4. Sex hormones

II. Hormones having cell membrane receptors :

a. Second messenger : cAMP

1. CRH	7. ADH
2. ACTH	8. Calcitonin
3. TSH	9. PTH
4. FSH	10. Catecholamines
5. LH	11. Glucagon
6. MSH	12. hCG

b. Second messenger : cGMP

1. ANF 2. No

c. Second messenger : Calcium/ Phosphatidylinositol (or both)

1. TRH	5. Catecholamines
2. GnRH	6. CCK
3. ADH	7. Gastrin
(Vasopressor action)	
4. Oxytocin	

d. Second messenger; Kinase/ Phosphatase

1. GH
2. Prolactin
3. Insulin

172. Ans.— A. ADH

173. Ans.— B. Acetylcholine

174. Ans.— A. Insulin

175. Ans.— A FSH

Sertoli cells are :

i. Form the blood-testis barrier
ii. Provide nutrition to the germ cells.
iii. Secrete androgen binding protein, inhibin (inhibits secretion of FSH), mullerian inhibiting substance (causes regression of the mullerian ducts in males during fetal life).

iv. Have receptors for FSH—FSH acts on the sertoli cells to facilitate the last stage of spermatid production. FSH also promotes production of ABP (the stages from spermatogonia to spermatids are androgen independent Maturation from spermatids to spermatozoa depends on androgens acting on sertoli cells in which the developing spermatozoa are embedded.

v. Sertoli cells contain aromatase (CYP19), which converts androgens to estrogens.

176. Ans.— A Raised parathyroid hormone levels

Circulating ionized calcium acts directly on the parathyroid glands in a negative feedback fashion to regulate the secretion of PTH.

177. Ans. — A Regulated by ADH

Free water is clearance represents the rate at which solute-free water is excreted in the absence of ADH) can be thought of as being made up of two fluid volumes:

1. A volume which contains the urine solutes at the same concentration as in plasma and called the Osmolar clearance.
2. Pure water excreted with no solutes, called positive free water clearance.

* A concentrated urine (produced in the presence of ADH) can be thought of as the difference between two volumes.

Cosm - V represents water free of solutes retained in the body due to the action of ADH. This called the negative free water clearane or tribular free water reabsorption

* Another way to define free water clearance (C820) - is the volume of blood plasma that is cleared of solute-free water per unit time.

178. Ans. — A Liver

The aldosterone receptor, also called mineralocorticoid receptor (or MR, MLR, MCR), is officially labelled nuclear receptor subfamily 3, group C, member 2, (NR3C2). It belongs to the steroid hormone receptor.

* MR is expressed in many tissues, such as the kidney, colon, heart, central nervous system (hippocampus), brown adipose tissue and sweat glands.

* The receptor is activated by mineralocorticoids such as aldosterone and deoxycorticosterone as well as glucocorticoids, like cortisol and cortison. It also responds to some progestins.

179. Ans.— C Increased inhibin levels

All options provided are examples of FSH Regulatory Peptides.

As the onset of puberty in males is delayed in comparison to females, the FSH Regulatory peptide levels which explains a delay in puberty will be the correct anser.

Amongst the options provided only increased inhibin levels can explain a delay in onset of puberty.

Inhibits suppress FSH secretions and hence increased Inhibin should delay puberty.

The increased production of inhibin in boys most probably results in greater negative feedback on FSH compared with girls, contributing to delayed onset of puberty in boys.

180. Ans.— B Straight tubules-rete-testis-efferent tubules

* The sperms are formed in the seminiferous tubules (spermatogenesis) and pass on to the straight tubules (tubuli recti).

* They then enter a network of tubules (rete testis), where they are exposed to high concentration of estrogen.

* The sperms get concentrated in the rete testis, and if they don't, infertility can result (due to diluted semen).

181. Ans. — C Requires temperature lower than core temperature

* Spermatogenesis requires a temperature considerably lower than that of the interior of the body.

182. Ans. — A Ionized calcium

The ionized calcium which is maintained at a concentration between 1.1 and 1.3 mmol/L is biologically the most active fraction.

183. Ans. A. Liver

* The mineralocorticoid receptor (or MR, MLR, MCR), also called aldosterone receptor, is officially labelled nuclear receptor subfamily 3, group C, member 2, (NR3C2) and is a receptor with high affinity for mineralocorticoids.

184. Ans. B. FSH and LH both normal

Both SH and LH are marker of testicular function, which tends to be normal in most cases of obstructive azoospermia so, the chances of finding normal FSH and LH levels are maximum.

185. Ans.— A & B. Zinc and Lysozyme

***Paneth cells*—endocrine cells located in the depths of the crypts of Lieberkuhn—secrete defensins, naturally occurring peptide antibiotics that are also secreted elsewhere in the body.**

186. Ans. D. Adipocytes

Insulin is required in adipose tissue and skeletal muscle for the transport of glucose inside the celsl via translocation of GLUT-4 transporters. The action of insulin on these tissues result in peripheral utilization of glucose. In brain, liver and RBC the glucose diffuses inside via GLUT again but does not require insulin. In case of fasting there is down regulationof insulin receptors in adipocytes which results in decrease uptake of glucose by adipose tissue thereby maintianign the blood glucose levels. This also explains the insulin resistance seen in starvation.

8.

IMPORTANT TEXT OF BLOOD

OSMOLAR SUBSTANCES IN EXTRACELLULAR AND INTRACELLULAR FLUIDS

	Plasma (mOsmol/L. of H_2O)	*Interstitial (mOsmol./L. of H_2O)*	*Intracellular (mOsmol./L. of H_2O)*
Na^+	144	137	10
K^+	5	4.7	141
Ca^{++}	2.5	2.4	0
Mg^{++}	1.5	1.4	31
Cl^-	107	112.7	4
HCO_3^-	27	28.3	10
HPO_4^{--} $H_2PO_4^-$	2	2	11
SO_4	0.5	0.5	1
Phosphocreatine			45
Carnosine			14
Amino acids	2	2	8
Creatine	0.2	0.2	9
Lactate	1.2	1.2	1.5
Adenosine triphosphate			5
Hexose monophosphate			3.7
Glucose	5.6	5.6	
Protein	1.2	0.2	4
Urea	4	4	4
Total mOsmol.	303.7	302.2	302.2
Corrected osomolar activity (mOsmol.)	282.6	281.3	281.3
Total osmotic pressure at 37° C. (mm. Hg)	5453	5430	5430

NORMAL VALUES FOR THE CELLULAR ELEMENTS IN HUMAN BLOOD

	Cells/μl (average)	*Approximate Normal Range*	*Percentage of Total White Cells*
Total WBC	9000	4000-11,000	....
Granulocytes			
Neutrophils	5400	3000-6000	50-70
Eosinophils	275	150-300	1-4
Basophils	35	0-100	0.4
Lymphocytes	2750	1500-4000	20-40
Monocytes	540	300-600	2-8
Erythrocytes			
Females	4.8×10^6	...	...
Males	5.4×10^6	...	...
Platelets	300,000	200,000-500,000	...

CHARACTERISTICS OF HUMAN RED CELLS

(Cells with MCVs > 95 are called macrocytes; cells with MCVs < 80 are called microcytes; cells with MCHs < 25 are called hypochromic

		Male	Female
Hematocrit (Hct) (%)		47	42
Red blood cells (RBC) (millions/µl)		5.4	4.8
Hemoglobin (Hb) (g/dl)		16	14
Mean corpuscular volume (MCV) (fl)	= Hct x 10 / RBC (10^6/µl)	87	87
Mean corpuscular hemoglobin (MCH) (pg)	= Hb x 10 / RBC (10^6/µl)	29	29
Mean corpuscuiar hemoglobin concentration (MCHC) (g/dl)	= Hb x 100 / Hct	34	34
Mean cell diameter (MCD) (µm)	= Mean diameter of 500 cells in smear	7.5	7.5

CLOTTING FACTORS IN THE BLOOD AND THEIR SYNONYMS

Clotting Factors	*Synonyms*
Fibrinogen	Factor-I
Platelets	Platelet factor-3
Prothrombin	Factor-II
Tissue thromboplastin	Factor-III
Calcium	Factor-IV
Factor-V	Proaccelerin; Labile factor; Ac-globulin; Ac-G
Factor-VII accelerator;	Serum prothrombin conversion SPCA; proconvertin; autoprothrombin-I
Factor-VIII	Antihemophilic factor; AHF; antihemophilic globulin; AHG
Factor-IX	Plasma thromboplastin component; PTC; Christmas factor; CF; autoprothrombin-II
Factor-X	Stuart factor; Stuart-Prower factor; Prower factor; autoprothrombin Ic
Factor-XI	Plasma thromboplastin antecedent; PTA
Factor-XII	Hageman factor
Factor-XIII	Fibrin stabilizing factor
Prothrombin activator	Thrombokinase; complete thromboplastin

MCQ's OF BLOOD

What is important in Blood

Production and function of important blood components, Haemostasis and Blood coagulation

1. Stuart Prower factor is factor : UPSC 1984, 94
A. VIII B. IX
C. X D. XII

2. MCHC (g/dl) is : AIIMS 1983; Delhi 1989, 99
A. 7.5 B. 29
C. 34 D. 87

3. Neutropenia is seen in all except : AIIMS 1984, 92
A. Pernicious anaemia
B. Severe bacterial infection
C. Trauma
D. Bone marrow depression

4. The most suitable anticoagulant for ESR determination by Wintrobe's method is : UPSC 1983, 86, 96
A. Sodium citrate B. EDTA
C. Heparin D. Double oxalation

5. What does facilitate the conversion of profibrinolysin to fibrinolysin : AIIMS 1987
A. Tissue enzymes B. Streptokinase
C. Urokinase D. All of the above

6. Haemoglobin first appears in : AMU 1985, 86, 97
A. Early normoblast
B. Intermediate normoblast
C. Late normoblast
D. Pronormoblast

7. Aggregation of platelets is inhibited by : Delhi 1984
A. Ca^{++} B. ADP
C. Thrombin D. None of the above

8. The life span of platelets is : UPSC 1984, 99
A. 4 days B. 9-12 days
C. 20-30 days D. 90 days

9. The cell membrane of human erythrocytes is more permeable to : AIIMS 1986, 97
A. Cl^+ than K^+ B. K^+ than Na^+
C. K^+ than urea D. Glucose than glycerol

10. Thrombosthenin is : AIIMS 1984, 86, 97
A. Coagulation factor
B. Contractile protein
C. A thrombosis promoting protein
D. A protein regulating platelet producting

11. Christmas disease results to lack of which of the following factor of coagulation : AMU 1986, 87
A. Factor-V B. Factor-VIII
C. Factor-IX D. Factor-X

12. Hb is a good buffer because of : Kerala 1994
A. Histidine residues B. Protein nature
C. Acidic nature D. Fe molecule

13. Thrombosthenin is present in : PGI 1988, 98
A. Plasma B. Platelets
C. Neutrophils D. RBC's

14. Haematocrit is ratio of : AMC 1983, 87, 99
A. WBC to plasma
B. Platelets to plasma
C. RBC's to plasma
D. Total blood cells to plasma

15. Hematocrit of venous blood is : DNB 1989, 99
A. 3% greater than arterial blood
B. 3 times greater than arterial blood
C. 3% less than arterial blood
D. 3 times less than arterial blood

16. H^+ is more bound to : AMU 1985, 98
A. Deoxygenated hemoglobin
B. Oxygenated hemoglobin
C. Both a+b equally
D. Not related to oxygenation

17. Myoglobin binds with : AP 1985, 95
A. 1 mol of oxygen per mol
B. 2 mol of oxygen per mol
C. 3 mol of oxygen per mol
D. 4 mol of oxygen per mol

18. Alkali resistant Hb is : Kerala 1994, 96
A. HbA B. HbA2
C. HbF D. HbS

Ans.	1. C	2. C	3. C	4. B	5. D	6. B	7. D	8. B	9. B	10. B
	11. C	12. A	13. B	14. C	15. A	16. A	17. A	18. C		

19. In anemia, the concentration of 2,3 DPG is : DNB 1988, 98

A. Decreased
B. Increased
C. a or b
D. Not changed

20. The commonest site of haemopoiesis in foetus is : Delhi 1989, 90

A. Liver
B. Spleen
C. Bone marrow
D. Gut

21. The no. of O2 molecules carried by on Hb molecule: AMU 1989, 94

A. 1
B. 2
C. 4
D. 8

22. A patient has a plasma concentration of HCO3 of 13 m M/L and a plasma PCO2 of 50 mm Hg. He has : AP 1990, 99

A. Compensated metabolic acidosis
B. Compensated respiratory acidosis
C. Respiratory acidosis and metabolic acidosis
D. Respiratory alkalosis and metabolic acidosis
E. Compensated respiratory alkalosis

23. Which one of the following statements concerning the monocyte is incorrect ? Kerala 1989, 99

A. More common in blood than eosinophil and basophil.
B. Produced in the adult by the bone marrow and lymph nodes.
C. Unlike neutrophil is rich in lipase.
D. Unlike neutrophil does not accumulate outside circulation in area of inflammation.

24. Which of the following statements about lymphocytes is incorrect ? Kerala 1989, 94

A. Produced by thymus, red bone marrow, spleen and lymph nodes.
B. Concentration falls in the blood abruptly and immune reaction is disturbed after removal of thymus in adult.
C. Probably change into plasma cells.
D. Constitute 20-40% of leukocytes.

25. The normal A/G ratio in blood is : AP 1989, 96

A. 5 : 1
B. 2 : 1
C. 1 : 2
D. 1 : 1

26. The life span of the average erythrocyte in a new born is : DNB 1992, 99

A. 100 days
B. 120 days
C. 160 days
D. 8 months

27. The absence of anti-A and anti-Rh agglunins in plasma means the subject is : AMU 1988, 98

A. A-positive or AP-positive
B. A-negative or AB-negative
C. A-positive, AP-positive
D. Type O

28. Which one of the following represents the most potentially dangerous situation ? PGI 1988

A. Rh positive mother with 2nd Rh-negative child
B. Rh negative mother with 2nd Rh-positive child
C. Rh positive mother with 1st Rh-negative child
D. Rh negative mother with 1st Rh-positive child

29. What does characterise function of platelets ? Orissa 1991, 95

A. Form thrombus and release serotonin
B. Initiate and accelerate clot formation
C. Contribute, possibly to integrity of capillary membrane
D. All of the above

30. Increased activity of delta-amino lavullinic synthetase results in : AMU 1986, 99

A. Thalasaemia
B. Sickle cell anaemia
C. Porphyria
D. Megaloblastic anaemia

31. In an adult man, there is about ——— g hemoglobin in circulating blood : DNB 1993, 95

A. 350
B. 500
C. 900
D. 1000

32. Half-life of transfused platelets is : AIIMS 1987, 97

A. 4 hours
B. 12 hours
C. 4 days
D. 17 days

33. Cyanosis is seen if the concentration of methaemoglobin is more than : AIIMS 1987; AI 1998

A. 1.5G%
B. 2.0G%
C. 3.0G%
D. 4.0G%

34. Erythropoietin is increased in : Delhi 1983, 85

A. Blood loss
B. High altitude
C. Exercise
D. All of the above

35. The need for Vitamin-B12 and folic acid in the formation of red blood cells is related primarily of their effects on : AIIMS 1984,94, 95

A. Synthesis and release of erythropoietin from the kidney
B. Absorption of iron from the gut
C. DNA synthesis in Bone marrow
D. Hemoglobin formation in the red blood cell

36. HbE is formed due to replacement of glutamic acid at 26th position by ——— : WB 1998, 99

A. Glycine
B. Lysine
C. Arginine
D. Valine

37. Which is wrong regarding factor-VIII and vWF : WB 1998, 99

A. Factor-VIII is produced by liver
B. vWF is produced by endothelial cell
C. vWF prevents platelet adhesion with collagen
D. Factor-VIII activates factor-X

Ans.									
19. B	20. A	21. C	22. C	23. D	24. B	25. B	26. A	27. C	28. B
29. D	30. C	31. C	32. C	33. A	34. D	35. C	36. D	37. C	

38. **Which one of the following statements regarding oxygenation and deoxygenation of haemoglobin (Hb) is correct ?** **CSE 1997, 98**
A. Oxygenated Hb is a stronger acid when compared to deoxygenated Hb.
B. Deoxygenated Hb is a stronger acid when compared to oxygenated Hb.
C. The acidic characters of the oxygenated Hb and deoxygenated Hb are of the same magnitude.
D. Since Hb is present inside the erythrocytes, its oxygenation or deoxygenation does not alter the acidic or basic character.

39. **Respiratory alkalosis may be produced by:** **CSE 1997, 98**
A. Chronic obstructive pulmonary disease
B. Drugs causing respiratory depression
C. Hyperpnoea
D. Excessive renal bicarbonate absorption

40. **Factor used in the extrinsic pathway of blood coagulation is :** **Delhi 1985, 98**
A. V B. VIII
C. Tissue factor-III D. X

41. **In polycythemia, the increase in blood pressure is due to increase in :** **PGI 1983, 95**
A. Blood volume B. Peripheral resistance
C. Thyroxin D. Renin

42. **Vitamin-K is required for the synthesis of factors :** **PGI 1982**
A. VII B. IX
C. X D. All of the above

43. **Carbonic anhydrase in RbC forms :** **AIIMS 1984; Delhi 1988**
A. Oxy hemoglobin
B. Carboxy hemoglobin
C. HCO_3- in blood
D. Carbamino hemoglobin

44. **When osmotic fragility is normal, RBC's begin to hemolyse when suspended in saline :** **DNB 1989, 99**
A. 0.33% B. 0.48%
C. 0.9% D. 1.2%

45. **Thromboxane A2 is released mainly by the :** **AIIMS 1982; AI 1990**
A. Platelets B. Vascular endothelium
C. Liver D. Muscles

46. **The best screening test for hemophilia is :** **Bihar 1991, 98**
A. BT B. PT
C. PTT D. CT

47. **The greatest amount of CO2 is transported in the blood as :** **Bihar 1991, 98**
A. RBC's B. HCO_3
C. Carbamino-Hb D. $H2CO_3$
E. Platelets

48. **Blood group antigens are :** **PGI 1987; AI 1988, 98**
A. Carried by sex chromosomes
B. Attached to plasma proteins
C. Attached to Hemoglobin molecule
D. Found in saliva

49. **A reliables screening test for platelet function is :** **Bihar 1991,94, 99**
A. CT B. PT
C. Thrombin time D. Clot retraction time

50. **In which of the following, bleeding time is characteristically increased :** **AIIMS 1988, 92**
A. Von Willebrand's disease
B. Hemophilia-A
C. Hereditary hemolytic telangiectasia
D. Henoch-Scholein purpura

51. **Freezing point of normal human plasma is :** **PGI 1984, 96**
A. 4°C B. 0°C
C. -0.54°C D. -1.54°C

52. **For cyanosis to be manifested, the amount of reduced hemoglobin in blood, should be :** **AIIMS 1982; 84; AMC 1987**
A. 1 gm% B. 3 gm%
C. 5 gm% D. 7 gm%

53. **Iron is stored in :** **PGI 1984; AMC 1986; AI 1990**
A. RBC
B. Reticulo endothelial system
C. Plasma
D. All of the above

54. **Adult hemoglobin has chains :** **Delhi 1983, 88, 99**
A. 2 α, 2 γ B. 2 α, 2β
C. 4α D. 2 α

55. **Endothelial cells synthesize :** **Delhi 1987, 93, 98**
A. Fibrinogen B. Factor VIII
C. Factor X D. Factor XII

56. **Life of R.B.C. is :** **Delhi 1992**
A. 30 days B. 90 days
C. 120 days D. 160 days

57. **The best method for estimation of Hb conc. in blood is :** **Delhi 1992, 99**
A. Acid heamatin method
B. Alkali haematin method
C. Cyammethaemoglobin method
D. Any of the above

58. **In vitro coagulation is initiated by factor :** **Delhi 1986, 92, 99**
A. XII B. XI
C. X D. VII

59. **Arneth Count is counting of :** **AIIMS 1988, 99**
A. Lymphocytes
B. Lobes in neutrophils
C. Granules in eosinophils
D. WBC in bone marrow

Ans.										
	38. B	39. C	40. C	41. B	42. D	43. C	44. B	45. A	46. C	47. B
	48. D	49. D	50. A	51. C	52. C	53. B	54. B	55. B	56. C	57. C
	58. A	59. B								

60. The no. of Fe atoms in one Hb molecule is : DNB 1992, 94
A. 1 B. 2
C. 4 D. 8

61. Vitamin-B12 is essential for what aspect of blood cell reproduction : PGI 1982, 94
A. Formation of hemoglobin
B. Extrusion of the nucleus from the normoblasts
C. Formation of DNA
D. Activation of erythropoietin

62. In a person with type O blood, what type or types of agglutinins does he has in plasma : AMC 1984; UPSC 1983, 84
A. None B. Alpha
C. Beta D. Alpha and beta

63. Reticulocytes are stained with : AIIMS 1988, 99
A. Methyl violet B. Brilliant Creasyl blue
C. Sudan black D. Indigo carmine

64. Cells with more than ——— MCV/(fl) are called macrocytes : AIIMS 1983, 94
A. 80 B. 87
C. 90 D. 95

65. Mean corpuscular diameter (nm) is : PGI 1984, 95
A. 4.1 B. 6.3
C. 7.2 D. 7.5

66. What is the maximum concentration of hemoglobin normally found in red blood cells : PGI 1986, 96
A. 5 per cent B. 10 per cent
C. 16 per cent D. 20 per cent
E. 34 per cent

67. When infection occurs a tissue, what type of white blood cells is first attracted from the blood into the tissue by the process of chemotaxis : PGI 1980, 98
A. Neutrophilis B. Monocytes
C. Eosinophilis D. Basophils

68. What is the first important event in hemostasis following severe tissue injury : AIIMS 1986, 95
A. Blood coagulation
B. Formation of a platelet plug
C. Vascular spasm
D. Formation of thromboplastin

69. The conversion of fibrinogen into fibrin occurs by : Delhi 1987, 89, 99
A. Prothrombin B. Thrombin
C. Thrombophlebitis D. Platelets

70. Eosinophilia is caused by all except : AIIMS 1993, 94
A. Stress B. Aspirin
C. PAN D. Ascariasis

71. Platelets growth factor are synthesized by : Delhi 1993, 95
A. Glial cells B. Endothelium
C. Fibroblasts D. All of the above

72. The theory of blood flow and lymph drainage is by: PGI 1995, 96
A. Starling B. Avagadro
C. Mitchell D. Bergili via vitalis

73. Complete erythropoisis occurs in ——— days : DNB 1994, 96
A. 3 B. 7
C. 14 D. 20

74. In a 30 years old man function of which bone marrow is not important for blood formation : Rajasthan 1994, 99
A. Vertebral B. Ribs
C. Sternum D. Shaft of humerus

75. Fetal RBC's differ from Adult RBC's by following except : AIIMS 1997, 99
A. Fetal RBC's bigger
B. More 2-3 DPG in foetal RBC's
C. Foetal RBC's have shorter life span
D. Less of carbonic anhydrase

76. The affinity of oxygen for Hb increased with fall in pH. This is called : Orissa 1999, 99
A. Bain bridge effect B. Bohr's effect
C. Haldane effect D. Hering effect

77. ↑ blood viscosity & slow circulation causes : TN 1999
A. RBC Rouleux formation
B. ↑ Plasma skimming
C. ↑ number of RBC is capillaries
D. ↑ WBC's count

78. Glycophorin is seen in : PGI 1999
A. Enterocyte B. Erythrocyte
C. Lymphocyte D. Hepatocyte

79. Clotting factor which is not formed by liver : PGI 1999
A. 10 B. 7
C. 8 D. 2

80. A haematocrit of 41% in the sample of blood analyzed means : TNPSC 1996
A. 41% of the blood volume is the plasma.
B. 41% of the total blood volume is made up of plasma.
C. 41% of the blood volume is the red blood cells.
D. 41% of the total blood volume is made up of red and white blood cells and platelets.

81. Increased osmotic fragility is found in all except : UP 1999
A. Spectrin deficiency
B. G-6PD deficiency
C. Hereditary homolytic anemia
D. Sickle cell disease

Ans. 60. C 61. C 62. D 63. B 64. D 65. D 66. E 67. A 68. C 69. B 70. A 71. D 72. A 73. B 74. D 75. B 76. B 77. A 78. B 79. C 80. C 81. D

82. **When a blood vessel wall is injured all of the following promote platelet activation except : Kerala 2000**
A. Prostacyclin B. Collagen
C. ADP D. Thrombin
E. von Willebrand factor

83. **Erythropoietin is secreted by A/E : PGI 2000**
A. Hemangioblastoma
B. Hepatoma
C. Renal cell carcinoma
D. Adrenocortical tumours

84. **Blood is non-newtonian fluid because : AI 2001**
A. Viscosity changes with velocity
B. Density changes with velocity
C. Density does not change with velocity
D. Viscosity does not change with velocity

85. **Cynosis is caused by : Rohtak 2001**
A. Reduced Hb above 7.5 gm/dl
B. Met Hb above 1.5 g/dl
C. Sulph. Hb above 0.5
D. All of the above

86. **Shape of RBC is maintained by : AIIMS 2002**
A. Integrin B. Spectrin
C. Globin D. Ankyrin

87. **A shift of posture from supine to upright posture is associated with cardiovascular adjustments. Which of the following is not true in this context : AIIMS 2003**
A. Rise in central venous pressure.
B. Rise in heart rate.
C. Decrease in cardiac output.
D. Decrease in stroke volume.

88. **All are correct about potassium balance except : AIIMS 2003**
A. Most of potassium is intracellular.
B. Three quarter of the total body potassium is found in skeletal muscle.
C. Intracellular potassium is released into extracellular space in response to severe injury or surgical stress.
D. Acidosis leads to movement of potassium from extracellular to intracellular fluid compartment.

89. **Which of the following is procoagulation protein? AI 2004**
A. Thrombomodulin B. Protein-C
C. Protein-S D Thrombin

90. **All endothelial cells produce thrombomodulin except those found in : AI 2005**
A. Hepatic circulation
B. Cutaneous circulation
C. Cerebral microcirculation
D. Renal circulation

91. **The type of hemoglobin that has least affinity for 2,3 - Diphosphoglycerate (2,3-DPG) or (2,3-BPG) is : AI 2005**
A. HgA B. HgF
C. HgB D. HgA2

92. **Heme is converted to bilirubin mainly in : AI 2005**
A. Kidney B. Liver
C. Spleen D. Bone marrow

93. **Hb is measured by all except : AIIMS 2007**
A. Drabkin's
B. Sahli's
C. Spectrophotometery
D. Wintrobe's

94. **The substance that is present in both serum and plasma is : AI 2007**
A. Fibrinogen B. Factor-VII
C. Factor-V D. Factor-II

95. **Site of RBC formation in 20 year old healthy male is : AI 2007**
A. Flat bones B. Long bones
C. Liver D. Yolk sac

96. **Which of the following helps in bridging the fibrin in a clot and stabilizing the clot? AI 2008**
A. Factor-III B. Factor-V
C. Factor-VIII D. Factor-XIII

97. **Cause of sigmoid shape of oxygen-hemoglobin dissociation curve (O2) is : AI 2009**
A. Binding of one O2 molecule increase the affinity of binding of other O2 molecules
B. Binding of one O2 molecule decrease the affinity of binding of other O2 molecules.
C. Bohr effect
D. Haldane effect

98. **Oxygen demand of heart : AI 2009**
A. Increases proportionately with heart rate
B. Depends upon duration of systole
C. Is negligible when heart is at rest
D. Is in constant relation with amount of work down

99. **Cyanosis doesn't occur in anemia because : AI 2009**
A. Certain min. amount of reduced Hb should be present
B. In anemia, O2 saturation increases
C. Hypoxia stimualtes erythropoieting production
D. O2 hemoglobin curve shifts to right

Ans.	82. A	83. D	84. A	85. D	86. B	87. A	88. D	89. D	90. C	91. B
	92. C	93. D	94. B	95. A	96. D	97. A	98. A	99. A		

EXPLANATIONS OF BLOOD

1. Ans.— C. X
2. Ans.— C. 34

MCHC (g/dL) is Hb x 100. It is 34 in both male and females. MCH is Hbx 10 ——— ——— (It is 29) and MCV is : Hematocrit

RBC count

$\frac{\text{Hct x 100}}{\text{RBC count}}$ (10^6 mL) (It is 87)

3. Ans.— C. Trauma
4. Ans.— B. EDTA
5. Ans.— D. All of the above
6. Ans.— B. Intermediate normoblast
7. Ans.— D. None of the above
8. Ans.— B. 9-12 days

Lifespan of tranfused platelets is only 4 days.

9. Ans.— B. K^+ than Na^+
10. Ans.— B. Contractile protein
11. Ans.— C. Factor-IX
12. Ans.— A. Histidine residues
13. Ans. B. Platelets
14. Ans.— C. RBC's to plasma

See Ques. 2

15. Ans.— A. 3% greater than arterial blood
16. Ans.— A. Deoxygenated hemoglobin
17. Ans.— A. 1 mol of oxygen per mol A. 1 mol of oxygen per mol
18. Ans.— C. HbF
19. Ans.— B. Increased

The concentration of 2,3 diphosphoglycerate (DPG or 2,3 DPG) is plentiful in red cells. It is formed from 3-phosphoglyceraldehyde, which is a product of glycolysis via Embden-Meyerhof pathway. One mole of deoxyhemoglobin binds 1 mol of 2,3 DPG. pH also affects concentration of 2,3 OPG in red cells. Acidosis inhibits red cell glycolysis and thus fall in 2,3 DPG whereas thyroid hormones, GH and androgens increase concentration of 2,3 DPG. High altitude also increases concentration of 2,3 DPG. Anemia and chronic hypoxia also increase 2,3 DPG.

20. Ans.— A. Liver
21. Ans.— C. 4

The number of oxygen molecules carried are four

22. Ans.— C. Respiratory acidosis and metabolic acidosis
23. Ans.— D. Unlike neutrophil does not accumulate outside circulation in area of inflammation
24. Ans.— B. Concentration falls in the blood abruptly and immune reaction is disturbed after removal of thymus in adult.
25. Ans.— B. 2 : 1

It is reversed in malnutrition

26. Ans.— A. 100 days

Lifespan of RBC's in adult is 120 days whereas that in tranfused blood is 90 days.

27. Ans.— C. A-positive, AP-positive
28. Ans.— B. Rh negative mother with 2nd Rh-positive child
29. Ans.— D. All of the above
30. Ans.— C. Porphyria

It is used in acute intermittent porphyria

31. Ans.— C. 900
32. Ans.— C. 4 days
33. Ans.— A. 1.5G%

Reduced hemoglobin concentration of blood in capillaries more than 5 gm/dL also causes cyanosis.

34. Ans.— D. All of the above
35. Ans.— C. DNA synthesis in Bone marrow
36. Ans.— D. Valine
37. Ans.— C. vWF prevents platelet adhesion with collagen

38. Ans.— B. Deoxygenated Hb is a stronger acid when compared to oxygenated Hb

39. Ans.— C. Hyperpnoea

40. Ans.— C. Tissue factor-ıII

41. Ans.— B. Peripheral resistance

42. Ans.— D. All of the above

43. Ans.— C. HCO_3- in blood

Carbonic anhydrase inhibitor is used as an ontacid, antiepileptic and as a diuretic.

44. Ans.— B. 0.48%

45. Ans.— A. Platelets

46. Ans.— C. PTT

PTT is best test whereas for platelet function, best is clot retraction time.

47. Ans.— B. HCO_3

48. Ans.— D. Found in saliva

49. Ans.— D. Clot retraction time

50. Ans.— A. Von Willebrand's disease

51. Ans.— C. -0.54°C

52. Ans.— C. 5 gm%

53. Ans.— B. Reticulo endothelial system

RES maximally stores cron

54. Ans. B. 2 α, 2β

55. Ans. B. Factor-VIII

Factors II, VII, IX and X are synthesized by Liver and serum or plasma concentration is 20 mg/dL.

56. Ans.— C. 120 days

57. Ans.— C. Cyammethhaemoglobin method

58. Ans.— A. XII

59. Ans.— B. Lobes in neutrophils

60. Ans.— C. 4

61. Ans.— C. Formation of DNA

62. Ans.— D. Alpha and beta

63. Ans.— B. Brilliant Creasyl blue

64. Ans.— D. 95

65. Ans.— D. 7.5

Mean corpuscular or cell diameter (mm) is Mean diameter of 500 cells in smear. In males and females, it is 7.5.

66. Ans.— E. 34 per cent

67. Ans.— A. Neutrophilis

68. Ans.— C. Vascular spasm

69. Ans.— B. Thrombin

70. Ans.— A. Stress

It is typically raised in filariasis and allergy.

71. Ans.— D. All of the above

72. Ans.— A. Starling

73. Ans.— B. 7

74. Ans.— D. Shaft of humerus

75. Ans.— B. More 2-3 DPG in foetal RBC's

76. Ans.— B. Bohr's effect

Bohr effect is closely related to the fact that deoxygenated hemoglobin binds H^+ more actively than does oxyhemoglobin. The pH of blood falls as its CO2 content increases.

77. Ans.— A. RBC Rouleux formation

78. Ans.— B. Erythrocyte

79. Ans.— C. 8

80. Ans.— C. 41% of the blood volume is the red blood cells

81. Ans.— D. Sickle cell disease

82. Ans.— A. Prostacyclin

83. Ans.— D. Adrenocortical tumours

Erythropoietin is a glycoprotein that contains 165 amino acid residues and four oligosaccharide chains that are necessary for its activity a vivo. Its blood level is markedly increased in anemia.

84. Ans.— A. Viscosity changes with velocity

85. Ans.— D. All of the above

86. Ans.— B. Spectrin

The membrane skeleton is formed by part of spectrin and is anchored is transmembrane protein band 3 by the protein ankyrin.

87. Ans.— A. Rise in central venous pressure.

88. Ans.— D. Acidosis leads to movement of potassium from extracellular to intracellular fluid compartment.

89. Ans.— D. Thrombin

- In the circulating blood, thrombin is a procoagulant that activates factors-V and VII.
- When thrombin kinds to thrombomodulin (thrombin-binding protein), it becomes an anticoagulant in that the thrombomodulin thrombin complex activates protein-C.

- Activated protein-C, along with its cofactor protein S, inactivates factor-V and VII and inactivates an inhibitor of tissue plaminogen activator, increasing the formation of plasmin (fibrinolysin).

90. Ans.— C. Cerebral microcirculation

"All endothelial cells except those in the cerebral microcirculation produce thrombomodulin a thrombin binding protein and express it on their surface."

* Thrombomodulin-thrombin complex activates protein-C.
* Activated protein-C along with its cofactor protein-S, inactivates factor V and VIII and inactivates an inhibitor of tissue plasminogen activator, increasing the formation of plasmin.

91. Ans.— B. HgF

"It is worth noting that does not combine with foetal haemoglobin (HbF).

- That is perhaps one reason why HbF has greater affinity for oxygen than adult Hb (HbA)
- The difference in affinity has great physiological significance because it is responsible for the transfer of oxygen from the mother to the foetus when their circulations come in intimate contact in the placenta.

92. Ans.— C. Spleen

Bilirubin (0.2 to 0.3 gm/day) production from here

Mononuclear phagocytic system

1. Spleen Bone marrow	1. Hepatic heme
2. Liver (premature destruction of cytochrome)	2. Hemoproteins (e.g. p-450 newly formed R.B.C.)

- Cells of the reticuloendothelial system degrades hemoglobin from wornout RBC. The porphyrin is converted into the yellow pigment bilirubin.
- The insoluble bilirubin is released in to the blood, where it is carried to the liver tightly bound to plasma albumin.
- Spleen is the primary site for extra-vascular hemolysis.

93. Ans.— D. Wintrobe's

In Drabkin's method hemoglobin is converted to cyanmethaemoglobin by Drabkin's reagent ($NaHCO_3$, potassium cyanide, potassium ferricyanide in distilled water) and the absorbance is measured in a photoelectric colorimeter. In Sahli's method the amount of hemoglobin can be estimated by conversion of known volume of blood into acid-hematin by addition of dilute HCl and subsequent comparison of the color of solution with a suitable standard. Spectrophotometery or photoelectric colorimetery—most common is the Drabkin's method. Wintrobe's method is used to determine PCV (or Hct) and ESR.

94. Ans. — B Factor-VII

Serum has essentially the same composition as plasma except that its fibrinogen and clotting factors-II, V and VIII have been removed and it has higher serotonin content because of the breakdown of platelets during clotting.

95. Ans.— A Flat bones

Beyond the age of 20 years most red cells continue to be produced in the marrow of membranous bones such as the vertebrae, sternum, ribs and ilia (Flat bones).

The marrow of long bones (except for proximal portions of humeri and tibia) becomes quite fatty & produces no more RBC after age of 20 years.

Flat bones is thus the single best site of erythropoesis after the age of 20 years.

96. Ans — D Factor-XIII

* The fibrin is initially a loose mesh of interlacing strands.
* It is converted by the formation of covalent cross-linkages to a dense tight aggregate (stabilization).
* This latter reaction is catalyzed by activated factor-XIII and requires Ca^{2+}.

97. Ans.— A. Binding of one O_2 molecule increase the affinity of binding of other O_2 molecules. This is also called relative affinity

98. Ans. — A. Increases proportionately with heart rate

The O2 consumption by the heart is determined primarily by the intramyocardial tension, the contractile state of the myocardium, and the heart rate.

99. Ans.— A. Certain minimum amount of reduced Hb should be present

Cyanosis is a blue coloration of skin and mucous membranes due to the presence of >5g/dl reduced hemoglobin in blood vessels near the skin surface.

9. IMPORTANT TEXT OF SPECIAL SENSES

COMPOSITION OF ENDOLYMPH, PERILYMPH, AND SPINAL FLUID

	Endolymph	*Perilymph*	*Spinal Fluid*
K^+	144.8	4.8	4.2
Na^+	15.8	150.3	150.0
Cl^-	107.1	121.5	122.4
Protein	15.0	50.0	21.0

TEMPERATURE REGULATING MECHANISMS

Mechanisms activated by cold: Post. hypo.

Shivering Hunger Increased voluntary activity Increased secretion of norepinephrine and epinephrine	Increase heat production
Cutaneous vasoconstriction Curling up Horripilation	Decrease heat loss

Mechanisms activated by heat: Ant. hypo.

Cutaneous vasodilatation Sweating Increased respiration	Increase heat loss
Anorexia Apathy and inertia ↓ed Secretion of TSH	Decrease heat production

SPECIAL SENSES IN OLD AGE

The Eyes

Besides graying of the hair, presbyopia or the loss of accommodation is the most well known and obvious sign of ageing. This change sets in rather early and by the age of 50 years. Most of the normal individuals, need reading glasses. After eighth decade, degenerative changes in the muscles of accommodation further accentuate the problem.

The pupillary responses to light and accommodation also decline with age.

The visual acuity gradually decreases in old age. Reduced secretion of the tears causes the dryness of cornea and conjunctiva.

The Ears

Degenerative changes in the organ of Corti (hair cells), ganglion cells as well as temporal cortex produce impairment of hearing (presbyacusis), especially for higher frequencies.

Taste and smell

The number of taste buds per papilla, decreases from an average of 250 in childhood to 90 by the age of 80 years. Hence the taste threshold is elevated in old age. The sensitivity of the sense of smell is also impaired.

9.2 PHYSIOLOGY

The Gastrointestinal Tract

Dryness of mouth is a common complaint in old age. The secretion of saliva under basal state and after reflex stimulation is only 1/3rd of normal adult values. Gastric secretion falls to **1/5th** the adult value by the age of 60 years.

The hepatic weight declines significantly after the age of 70 years.

Endocrines

The anterior pituitary hormone secretion is not reduced in old age. As compared to adult level, there is **15-fold** increase in secretion of FSH and 3-fold increase in LH. In males, the increase in FSH and LH secretion is not very significant. There is definite decrease in the secretion of thyroid hormones.

Basal plasma insulin levels seen to be unaffected but there is impairment of insulin response to a glucose load.

Blood

Total blood volume and total leucocyte count remain normal in old age. However, anaemia tends to be more common due to deficiency of iron and vitamin B12. Immune surveillance by T-lymphocytes is reduced. The function of coagulation of blood and platelet count remain normal in old age.

ESR value tends to be markedly elevated (upto 40 mm in 1st hour) without evidence of any disease.

Musculo skeletal system

Progressive loss of muscular power is a characteristic feature of ageing.

The physiological studies reveal a prolongation of latency, contraction period and relaxation period of a muscle twitch.

Degenerative changes in joints starts by the age of 30 years and becomes well marked by the age of 60-70 years.

Osteoporosis is an essential component of ageing.

Stature and Posture

In a longitudinal study of a group of people, the mean height decreased from **169 cm** at the age of 20 years to **164 cm** by the age to 80 years, and **161 cm** at the age of 90 years. After the age of 50-60 years osteoporotic changes cause a decreae in height of individual vertebra.

Skin and Hair

Wrinkling of skin and greying are hallmark of ageing. The greying of hair is due to loss of melanin pigment. In females, there is loss of axillary and pubic hair due to a decrease in the plasma level of adrenal androgens.

Sweat glands decrease in size and number. The thinning of epidermis, dermis and increased capillary fragility produce senile purpura.

Kidneys

By the age of 80 years, there is 30-40% decrease in the number of renal glomeruli, leading to a corresponding decrease in GFR. Maximum urinary osmolality is about **750 m** Osm/kg (specific gravity 1.024) at the age of 80 years.

MCQ's OF SPECIAL SENSES

What is important in Blood

Optics of vision, Receptor functions of the retina, Sense of hearing and smell

1. **Vanilloid receptors are activated by : AIIMS 2006, 2008**
   A. Pain B. Vibration
   C. Touch D. Pressure
2. **There is mutation of gene coding for the ryanodine receptors in malignant hyperthermia. Which of the following statements best explains the increased heat production in malignant hyperthermia ? AIIMS 2005**
   A. Increased muscle metabolism by excess of calcium ions
   B. Thermic effect of food
   C. Increased sympathetic discharge
   D. Mitochondrial thermogenesis
3. **The approximate refractive index of aqueous humour and vitreous humour is : PGI 1982; AIIMS 1984, 85**
   A. 1.21 B. 1.33
   C. 1.43 D. 1.56
4. **The sound become painful above decibel of : PGI 1986; Delhi 1987, 99**
   A. 70 B. 86
   C. 140 D. 160
5. **The semicircular canals contain hair cells which are stimulated by : PGI 1983, 93**
   A. Movement of perilymph
   B. Linear acceleration
   C. Cessation of rotation
   D. Rotation at constant velocity
6. **Rhodopsin is most sensitive and least sensitive to : PGI 1980, 94**
   A. Violet light, red light
   B. Red light, violet light
   C. Green light, red light
   D. Blue light, green light
7. **Which of the following is wrong : AIIMS 1986, 96**
   A. In the refracting eye, cornea causes more refraction than lens.
   B. Fovea lies on the temporal side of optic disc.
   C. Cones are more sensitive to light than rods.
   D. Squint may result due to damage to internal capsule.
8. **Kinesthetic sensations are detected mainly by what type of receptors : AMC 1984; Delhi 1984, 86, 99**
   A. Muscle spindles B. Golgi tendon apparati
   C. Skin receptors D. Joint receptors
9. **Normally, body temperature can be raised by : Delhi 1986, 89; UPSC 1984, 86, 93**
   A. Androgens B. Gonadotrophins
   C. Oestrogen D. Progesterone
10. **Receptors for touch is : AMU 1986, 98**
    A. Messner's B. Merkel's disc
    C. Free nerve terminal D. All of the above
11. **Which type of cone is it that has a peak absorbancy at a light wavelength of 430 milimicrons : AIIMS 1984, 98**
    A. Red cones B. Green cones
    C. Blue cones D. All of the above
12. **Taste buds are : Kerala 1994, 95**
    A. Surface epithelial cells
    B. Specialised nerve endings
    C. Modified epithelial cells
    D. Chemoreceptors
13. **Site where endolymph is seen : Kerala 1997, 99**
    A. Scala vestibuli B. Scala media
    C. Helicotrema D. All of the above
14. **Raised ECF K^+ levels seen in : TN 1999**
    A. Endolymph B. Ectolymph
    C. Aquous tumour D. Vitreous tumour
15. **Taste fibres relay in : TN 1999**
    A. Geniculate ganglion B. Gasserian ganglion
    C. Petrous ganglion D. Otic ganglion
16. **Pacinian corpuscles are the major receptors for : AIIMS 1989; JIPMER 1990, 92**
    A. Pain B. Touch
    C. Pressure D. Temperature

Ans.	1. A	2. A	3. C	4. C	5. C	6. C	7. C	8. D	9. D	10. D
	11. C	12. C	13. B	14. A	15. A	16. C				

17. Which of the following in the eye are pain sensitive : AMU 1988, JIPMER 1992
A. Iris B. Ciliary body
C. Choroid D. All of the above

18. The Helmholtz theory of colour vision states that : DNB 1991, 98
A. There are three kinds of cones in the retina responding to three primary colours.
B. There are two kinds of cones called dominators and modulators.
C. There is only one kind of cone and the colour is recognised only in area 17.
D. There are seven types of cones responding to the seven colours of the spectrum.

19. An aged violin player can get a correct pitch only by touching his teeth to the vibrating instrument. He is most likely to damage : AIIMS 1986, 98
A. Inner ear
B. Middle ear
C. Cochlear nuclei
D. Medial geniculate body

20. When light is thrown into one eye the pupil of other eye shows : AMU 1985, 96
A. Dilatation B. Consensual reaction
C. Unaffected D. None of the above

21. Which one of the following procedures is most likely to increase intraocular pressure of glaucoma patient? AIIMS 1986, 95
A. Use of atropine
B. Decreased pressure in jugular vein
C. High dose of vitamin-C
D. Dark environment
E. Carbonic anhydrase inhibitors

22. Most of the refraction that occurs in the eye occurs at the : UP 1992, 98
A. Anterior surface of cornea
B. Posterior surface of cornea
C. Anterior surface of lens
D. Posterior surface of lens

23. Red colour blindness is called : AMU 1992, 95
A. Deuteranopia B. Protanopia
C. Protanomaly D. Deuteranomaly

24. Crude touch sensations are carried by : Delhi 1984, 86, 99
A. Lateral spinothalamic tract
B. Ventral spinothalamic tract
C. Posterior columns
D. Pyramidal tract

25. The attenuation reflex is due to : AP 1991, 99
A. Contraction of tensor tympani
B. Contraction of stapedius
C. Contraction of tensor tympani and stapdius
D. Inward movement of the oval window

26. Which one of the following statement is most correct :
A. Taste buds are sensitive to all of the gustatory modalities.
B. There are over ten well defined distinct gustatory modalities.
C. Taste projection is at the foot of the post central gyrus.
D. None of the above

27. Meissner's corpuscles are believed to be sensitive to : AIIMS 1985, 99
A. pH of interstitial fluid
B. Histamine
C. Change of temperature
D. Mechanical deformation

28. The following are primary colours except : DNB 1991
A. Red B. Green
C. Blue D. Yellow

29. The receptors in retina for those of blue, green and red wavelengths are called : TN 1991
A. Modulators B. Trachomators
C. Dominators D. None of the above

30. The receptors in semicircular canals respond to : AP 1991
A. Linear acceleration
B. Angular acceleration
C. Both linear and angular accelerations
D. None of the above

31. Under resting conditions the ganglion cells of the retina discharge at approximately at what rate : Delhi 1980, 99
A. One per second B. Five per second
C. 25 per second D. 125 per second

32. Which of the following is not important in dark adaptation Delhi 1981, 99
A. Coversion of retinene into rhodopsin
B. Conversion of Vitamin-A into retinene
C. The pupillary reflex
D. Conversion of retinene into Iumirhodopsin

33. The portion of the vestibular system that is most important for preventing a person from suddenly falling. If he makes a sudden turn while moving forward is the : AIIMS 1982, 99
A. Saccule B. Utricle
C. Cochlea duct D. Semicircular canals

34. Ear is most sensitive to frequency (Hz) of : UPSC 1989; Delhi 1985, 99
A. 300-500 B. 1000-3000
C. 10000-2000 D. None of the above

Ans.										
	17. D	18. A	19. B	20. B	21. A	22. A	23. B	24. B	25. C	26. C
	27. D	28. D	29. A	30. B	31. C	32. D	33. D	34. B		

35. The visible range in electromagnetic spectrum for human eye is : Delhi 1984, 94
A. 200-300 nm B. 310-340 nm
C. 370-740 nm D. 740-870 nm

36. Stapes rests in : AIIMS 1984, 94
A. Round window B. Oval window
C. Tympanic membrane D. Basilar membrane

37. Ruffini end organ is associated with sensation of : Bihar 1989, 91, 92
A. Pressure B. Cold
C. Heat D. Touch
E. None of these

38. A light having a monochromate color stimulates the red cones about twice as much the green cones. What is the color of this monchromatic light : AIIMS 1988, 99
A. Green B. Orange
C. Red D. Yellow
E. Blue

39. Why sudden loud sound is more likely to damage the cochlea than a prolonged loud sound : AIIMS 1986, 97
A. The basilar fibres are sensitive to sudden sounds but adapt to prolonged sounds.
B. A sudden sound carries more energy.
C. The tympanic membrane becomes flaccid during prolonged loud sounds.
D. The fluid pressure in the scala tympani can decrease greatly during prolonged loud sound.

40. Which of the following taste buds help to protect against the ingestion of certain plant poisons : PGI 1986, 99
A. Sweet taste buds B. Bitter taste buds
C. Sour taste buds D. Salt taste buds

41. Movement of Malleus & Incus occurs at what sound frequency (Hz) : WB 1998, 99
A. 600 B. 1200
C. 1800 D. 2400

42. Kinetic receptors are : TN 1998, 99
A. Free nerve endings B. Pacinian corpuscles
C. Ruffini corpuscles D. Cortical cells

43. Eye gets totally adapted to darkness in ——— minutes : TN 1998, 99
A. 2 B. 5
C. 10 D. 20

44. Non-shivering thermogenesis done by following except : AI 1998, 99
A. Liver B. Spleen
C. Heart D. Small intestine

45. Consider the following receptors : CSE 1997, 99
1. Meissner's corpuscles
2. Merkel's disc
3. Pacinian corpuscles

Among these, rapidly adapting touch receptors would include :
A. 1,2 and 3 B. 1 and 2
C. 1 and 3 D. 2 and 3

46. The process of swallowing involves all of following except : AIIMS 1987, 97
A. Closure of the glotti.
B. Involuntary relaxation of the upper esophageal sphincter.
C. Involuntary movements of the tongue against the palate.
D. Esophageal peristalsis.

47. Sound waves in the ear travel in : AMU 1986, 88, 99
A. Air medium B. Solid medium
C. Liquid medium D. All of the above

48. When you look at a near object, the : Manipal 1995, 98
A. Depth of field decreases
B. Dioptric power of the lens decreases
C. Medial recti contract
D. Tension of the zonular fibres increases

49. The cones in the eye are : Manipal 1995, 99
A. Not responsible for colour vision.
B. More sensitive to light than the rods.
C. Associated with higher visual acuity than the rods.
D. Dependent on Vitamin-A for their function.

50. Cold (Shivering) is regulated by : Rajasthan 1998, 99
A. Ant. hypothalamus B. Post. hypothalamus
C. Thalamus D. Pons

51. Visual acuity is : Orissa 1999
A. A measure of sensitivity of retina to light
B. Better using one eye than using both eyes
C. Better with central than with peripheral vision
D. Reduced in colour blind persons

52. Itching is caused by stimulation of : Delhi 2001
A. A α fibres B. B fibres
C. C fibres D. Dorsal root ganglia

W.53. All are related to color vision except : Kerala 2001
A. Blobs B. General 3-6 layers
C. M ganglion cells D. Parvocellular pathway

54. Bitter taste is mediated by action of : Kerala 2001
A. Guanyl cyclase B. G-protein
C. Tyrosine kinase D. Epithelial Na+channels

55. Non-shivering thermogenesis in adults is due to : AI 2002
A. Thyroid hormone
B. Brown fat between the shoulders
C. Noradrenaline
D. Muscle metabolism

Ans.	35. C	36. B	37. B	38. B	39. D	40. B	41. A	42. B	43. D	44. D
	45. C	46. C	47. D	48. D	49. C	50. B	51. C	52. C	53. NONE	
54. B	55. A									

56. The optical power of the eye is : **Delhi 1983, 98**
A. 25 Diopters
B. 50 Diopters
C. 66 Diopters
D. 75 Diopters

57. For normal eye of an adult, near point is situated at : **AMC 1985, 99**
A. 9 cm
B. 14 cm
C. 20 cm
D. 25 cm

58. A travelling nerve impulse does not depolarize the area immediately behind it, because : **AIIMS 2002**
A. It is hyperpolarized
B. It is refractory
C. It is not self-propogating
D. The conduction is always orthodromic

59. The first physiological response to high environmental temperature is : **AI 2005**
A. Sweating
B. Vasodilatation
C. Decrease heat production
D. Non-shivering thermogenesis

Ans.	56. C	57. D	58. B	59. B

EXPLANATIONS OF SPECIAL SENSES

1. Ans.— A Pain
   * Vanilloid receptors or capsaicin receptors are activated by pain sensation.
   * The vanilloid receptor - 1 (VI) responds to capsaicin (the pungent component of chilli peppers), heat and extracellular acidification, and it is able to integrate simultaneous exposure to these stimuli.
   * Vanilloid receptor - 1 is essential for *inflammatory thermal hyperalgesia.*
2. Ans.— A Increased muscle metabolism by excess of calcium ions
   * Malignant hyperthermia is a life threatening event triggered by the administration of certain anaesthetics and neuromuscular blocking agents.
   * Clinical features
     — Severe hyperthermia due to heat production from the skeletal muscles
     — Contracture, rigidity
     — Metabolic acidosis.
     — Tachycardia
   * Drugs which trigger malignant hyperthermia.
     — Halogenated hydrocarbons anaesthetics (halothane, isoflurane and sevoflurane)
     — Succinylchlorine.
   * Mechanism
     — The event is triggered by uncontrolled release of Ca++ ions from the sarcoplasmic reticulum.
     — Association is seen with mutation in the gene Ry-R1 encoding for the skeletal muscle ryanodine receptors.
   * Treatment :
     — Malignant hyperthermia should be treated immediately with cessation of anaesthesia and intravenous administration of dantrolene. Procainamide should also be administered because of the possibility of ventricular fibrillation.
     — Rapid cooling, inhalation of 100% oxygen and control of acidosis should be considered adjunct therapy.
3. Ans.— C. 1.43
4. Ans.— C. 140
5. Ans.— C. Cessation of rotation
   They are life protective
6. Ans.— C. Green light, red light
7. Ans.— C. Cones are more sensitive to light than rods
8. Ans.— D. Joint receptors
   Serotonin plays a role in mechanisms activated by cold whereas norepinephrine plays a role in mechanisms activated by heat.
9. Ans.— D. Progesterone
10. Ans.— D. All of the above
11. Ans.— C. Blue cones
12. Ans.— C. Modified epithelial cells
13. Ans.— B. Scala media
14. Ans.— A. Endolymph
    Endolymph has high K+ concentration as compared to plasma.
15. Ans.— A. Geniculate ganglion
16. Ans.— C. Pressure
    Cutaneous sense organs include naked nerve endings expanded tips in sensory nerve terminals and encapsulated endings. The expanded endings include Merkel's disks and Ruffini endings whereas encapsulated endings are Pacinian corpuscles, Meissner's corpuscles and Krause's nerve endings.
17. Ans.— D. All of the above
18. Ans.— A. There are three kinds of cones in the retina responding to three primary colours.
19. Ans.— B. Middle ear
20. Ans.— B. Consensual reaction
21. Ans.— A. Use of atropine
    Atropine is a mydriatic and decreases aqueous flow resulting in precipitation of glaucoma.
22. Ans.— A. Anterior surface of cornea

23. Ans.— B. Protanopia

24. Ans.— B. Ventral spinothalamic tract

25. Ans.— C. Contraction of tensor tympani and stapdius

Both muscles contribute

26. Ans.— C. Taste projection is at the foot of the post central gyrus.

27. Ans.— D. Mechanical deformation

Meissner's and Pacinian corpuscles are rapidly adapting touch receptors whereas Markel's disks and Ruffini's endings are slowly adapting touch receptors.

28. Ans.— D. Yellow

29. Ans.— A. Modulators

30. Ans.— B. Angular acceleration

31. Ans.— C. 25 per second

32. Ans.— D. Conversion of retinene into Iumirhodop-sin

33. Ans.— B. Semicircular canals

Most common symptoms produced is dizziness. Cinnarizine is most common drug used to control it.

34. Ans.— B. 1000-3000

35. Ans.— C. 370-740 nm

36. Ans.— B. Oval window

37. Ans.— B. Cold

38. Ans.— B. Orange

39. Ans.— D. The fluid pressure in the scala tympani can decrease greatly during prolonged loud sound.

40. Ans.— B. Bitter taste buds

41. Ans.— A. 600

42. Ans.— B. Pacinian corpuscles

43. Ans.— D. 20

In contrast, light adaptation occurs in 5 minutes.

44. Ans.— D. Small intestine

45. Ans.— C. 1 and 3

46. Ans.— C. Involuntary movements of the tongue against the palate.

47. Ans.— D. All of the above

All the media are used

48. Ans.— D. Tension of the zonular fibres increases

49. Ans.— C. Associated with higher visual acuity than the rods

50. Ans.— B. Post. hypothalamus

51. Ans.— C. Better with central than with peripheral vision

Visual acquity is greatest at fovea centralis (rod free portion).

52. Ans.— C. C fibres

53. Ans.— NONE

Question is incorrectly framed

54. Ans.— B. G-protein

55. Ans.— A. It is hyperprolarized

55. Ans.— A Thyroid hormone

In adults, increased heat production due to increased thyroid hormone secretion (thyroid hormone thermogenesis) plays little role in response to cold. Dopamine and somatostatin and glucocorticoids inhibit TSH secretion.

56. Ans.— C. 66 Diopters

57. Ans.— D. 25 cm

58. Ans.— B. It is refractory

59. Ans.— B. Vasodilatation

Effects of Acute Heat :

I. Thermoregulatory Responses
   1. Cutaneous Vasodilatation
   2. Sweating

II Other effects :
   1. Metabolic rate
   2. Rate of Respiration
   3. Work of Breathing
   4. Anorexia
   5. Initial hypoglycaemia
   6. Pulse rate
   7. Stroke volume (Cardiac output doesn't change)
   8. Urinary volume

- First physiological response to high environment is vasodilatation
- Major thermoregulatory response in hot environment :

  Sweating
- Vasodilation is of the very limited value in extremely hot environment because it reaches its maximum at a very early stage of the exposure.

10.

IMPORTANT TEXT OF MISCELLANEOUS

METABOLIC DISTURBANCES

Condition	Arterial Plasma pH	HCO_3^- (mEq/liter)	PCO_2 (mm Hg)	Cause
NORMAL	7.40	24.1	40	
Metabolic	7.26	18.1	40	NH_4 Cl ingestion
acidosis	6.94	5.0	23	Diabetic acidosis
Metabolic	7.48	30.1	40	$NaHCO_3$ ingestion
alkalosis	7.54	49.8	58	Prolonged vomiting
Respiratory	7.35	25.0	48	Breathing 7% CO_2
acidosis	7.32	33.5	64	Emphysema
Respiratory	7.50	22.0	27	Voluntary hyperventilation
alkalosis	7.46	18.7	26	Three-week residence at 4000 maltitude

ANATOMICAL SITES OF VARIOUS ENDORPHINS

Endorphin	Site
ß - endorphin	Pituitary, Arcuate nucleus, hypothalamus, amygdala, Locus coeruleus, Locus accumbens
Met-encephalin Leu-encephalin	Substantia nigra (highest conc.) Globus pallidus Hypothalamus Hippocampus Amygdala Cortex
Dynorphins	Post. pituitary Spinal cord Hypothalamus Basal ganglia

MCQ's OF MISCELLANEOUS

What is important in Miscellaneous

Metabolism of carbohydrate, fat, protein and vitamins. Temperature regulation. All factual data, Named laws, principles, signs and tests

1. **What portion of cell membrane acts as a barrier to limit the movement of water and water-soluble substances through membrane? AMC 1984, 94; AIIMS 1990**
   A. Lipid
   B. Protein
   C. Mucopolysaccharide
   D. Pores
2. **The concentration of sodium on the first side of a membrane is two times as great as on the second side of the membrane. This concentration is now increased to five times as great on the first side as on the second side. How many times does the net rate of sodium diffusion through the membrane increase? AIIMS 1983, 93**
   A. Five times B. Four times
   C. 2.5 times D. Two times
3. **Percentage of body water is least in : Orissa 1998**
   A. Fatty man B. Fatty woman
   C. Normal build man D. Children
4. **All of the following statements about human plasma albumin are true except : Manipal 1995, 2000**
   A. It behaves as an anion at the pH of blood.
   B. It makes a greater contribution to the colloid oncotic pressure than does globulin.
   C. It is involved in the carriage of carbon dioxide in the blood.
   D. It is freely filtered at the renal glomeruli.
5. **All the following statements about the human intracellular fluid are true except : Manipal 1995, 99**
   A. It forms the major proportion of total body water
   B. Its principle cation is sodium
   C. Its principle anions are organic
   D. Its composition varies from tissue-to-tissue
6. **Potassium is maximum in : PGI 1982, 84, 99**
   A. Cell B. Plasma
   C. Interstitium D. Bone
7. **Sodium is maximum in : Delhi 1990, 98**
   A. Synovial fluid B. Extracellular spaces
   C. Interstitial spaces D. Bone
8. **Increased plasma potassium concentration causes all of the following except : PGI 1986, 97**
   A. Increased aldosterone release from the adrenal cortex
   B. Increased tubular secretion of potassium
   C. Increased tubular reabsorption of sodium
   D. Increased excretion of potassium in the urine
9. **Water molecule goes to interstitial fluid from plasma by : UP 1995, 2005**
   A. Active transport
   B. Facilitated diffusion
   C. With H+ exchange
   D. With Na+ exchange
10. **The resting membrane potential of a cell is established or maintained by all of the following except : AIIMS 1986, 98**
    A. The sodium-potassium pump
    B. Outward movement of sodium ions
    C. Inward movement of potassium ions
    D. A net inward movement of positive ions
11. **All of the following statements about muscle tone are true except : Manipal 1995, 99**
    A. It is the resistance offered by muscle to passive stretch.
    B. It is increased by the loss of function in the cerebellum.
    C. It is reduced by curare-like drugs.
    D. It is redistributed when the function of the semi-circular canals on one side is disturbed by disease.
12. **In potassium levels are 39 mg% calculate in meq/L: Delhi 1985, 95**
    A. 1 B. 3.9
    C. 10 D. 100

Ans. 1. A 2. B 3. B 4. D 5. B 6. A 7. D 8. D 9. B 10. D 11. B 12. C

13. **Smoking causes : Delhi 1985, 87, 97**
A. Increased Ciliary motility
B. Cellular hyperplasia
C. Decreased Mucous secretion
D. All of the above

14. **Profound hypothermic signs include all except : AIIMS 1983, 89**
A. Slow breathing B. Bradycardia
C. Hypotension D. Hyperactivity

15. **Weightlessness results in : Delhi 1985; DNB 1989, 99**
A. ↑ Cardiac output B. Hypotension
C. ↑ Gut motility D. Osteoporosis

16. **The non-ionic diffusion in body is seen in : AIIMS 1983, 92**
A. Gut B. Kidneys
C. Both D. None

17. **The emeiocytosis or reverse pinocytosis requires which ion : AIIMS 1983, 93**
A. Na+ B. K+
C. Ca++ D. Mg++

18. **Plasma K+ constitute what percentage of total body potassium : AIIMS 1986, 97**
A. 0.4% B. 7.6%
C. 10.4% D 89.6%

19. **All are steps in contraction of skeletal muscle except: AIIMS 1984, 85, 92**
A. Discharge of motor neurone
B. Ca+ release from sarcoplasmic reticulum
C. Binding of Ca+ to troponin-C
D. Release of Ca+ to troponin-C

20. **A child demonstrates irregular, spasmodic, involuntary movements of limbs and facial muscles. He is most likely to have a lesion in : AMC 1987, 97**
A. Caudate nucleus
B. Precentral gyrus of cortex
C. Postcentral gyrus of cortex
D. Rubrospinal tract

21. **Starling has made many epoch-making discoveries in physiology. They are the following except : AMU 1988, 98**
A. Discovery of the first hormone in the body
B. Eliciting law of the muscle
C. Discovery of the Vectocardiogram
D. Enunciating law of the intestines

22. **The normal serum calcium level is : AMC 1987, 97**
A. 4-6 mg/100 ml B 6-8 mg/100 ml
C. 9-11 mg/100 ml D. 14-16 mg/100 ml

23. **The quantity of water lost as sweat per day is : AMU 1991, 95**
A. 100 to 200 cc B. 600 to 800 cc
C. 1000 to 1200 cc D. Above 1200 cc

24. **α-interferon is produced by : WB 1998, 99**
A. Lymphocyte B. Monocyte
C. Macrophage D. Neutrophil

25. **In the female genital tract, the spermatozoa do not live for more than : Orissa 1991**
A. 12 hours B. 24 hours
C. 36 hours D. 72 hours

26. **The element that has been used as an intravascular dye : Bihar 1998, 99**
A. Sodium B. Iodine
C. Strontium D. Carbon

27. **In the days following ovulation are true except : PGI 1986, 97**
A. Plasma mucus more viscus and scanty
B. Cervical mucus more viscus and scanty
C. Plasma level for leutinizing hormone falls
D. Body temperature falls

28. **Entropy is the measure of : AIIMS 1987, 97**
A. Rate of enzymatic reaction
B. Energy which is unavailable for work
C. Reversibility of a reaction
D. Free energy of enzymatic reaction

29. **How many pKa values does orthophosphoric acid possess : Bihar 1991, 92**
A. One B. Two
C. Three D. Four

30. **The energy rich properties of ATP are related to which of its structural features : Bihar 1990, 92**
A. Heterocyclic ring
B. The N. glycoside linkage
C. Phosphate groups
D. Anhydride linkages

31. **Body fluid pH depends primarily on the renal control of : Kerala 1989, 99**
A. Reabsorption of sodium in exchange for potassium.
B. Secretion of H+ in exchange for ammonia.
C. Secretion of H+ in exchange for potassium.
D. Secretion of H+ in exchange for sodium.

32. **If a molecule has 5 asymmetric carbon atoms. It will have the following number of optical isomers : AMU 1989, 99**
A. 10 B. 16
C. 25 D. 32

33. **For bicarbonate buffer system the Henderson-Hasselbach equation is : AIIMS 1986, 87**
A. $pH = pK \dfrac{+HCO_3^-}{H_2CO_3}$
B. $pH = pK \dfrac{+H_2CO_3}{HCO_3}$
C. $pH = pK \dfrac{+\log HCO_3^-}{H2\ CO_3}$
D. $pH = pK \dfrac{+\log H_2CO_3}{HCO_3}$

Ans.	13. D	14. D	15. D	16. C	17. C	18. A	19. D	20. A	21. C	22. C
	23. B	24. A	25. D	26. C	27. D	28. B	29. C	30. D	31. D	32. B
	33. C									

34. If a lady presents with a very regular 29 days menstrual cycle, ovulation should occur on day : **Delhi 1987, 94**

A. 14 B. 15
C. 17 D. 19.

35. Which one of the following changes would not occur in blood after 7 days of storage? **AMC 1987, 92**

A. Decreased concentration of dextrose and increased concentration of lactic acid.
B. Decreased concentration of plasma potassium.
C. An increased prothrombin time.
D. A decreased concentration of platelets.

36. In excitable cells, repolarization is closely associated with one of the following events : **PGI 1989, 95**

A. Na efflux B. Na influx
C. K efflux D. K influx

37. 'g' is the acceleration which a mass exhibits due to gravitational force. Numerically this value is : **AMU 1985, 98**

A. 760 cms/sec2 B. 760 mm Hg
C. 981 cms/sec2 D. 380 cm/sec2

38. Reynold's number is a ratio which is an index in estimating whether turbulance will occur. Laminar flow will occur in conditions in which Reynold's number is less than : **AIIMS 1985, 93**

A. 1000 B. 2000
C. 500 D. 100

39. The velocity of propagation of an electromagnetic radiation is : **AIIMS 1985, 92**

A. 4 x10^{10} cms/sec B. 3 x 10^{10} cms/sec.
C. 3 x10^{8} cms/sec. D. 3 x10^{6} cms/sec.

40. The following are electromagnetic radiations except : **AIIMS 1987, 97**

A. X rays B. g-rays
C. Visible light D. Ultrasound

41. The frequency of current used in short wave diathermy is : **AIIMS 1987, 99**

A. 27.12 MHz B. 1000 Hz
C. 2450 MHz D. 24.5 MHz

42. The frequency of current used in Microwave diathermy is : **DNB 1992, 99**

A. 27.12 MHz B. 1000 Hz
C. 2450 MHz D. 1.75 MHz

43. The frequency of current used in surgical diathermy is : **DNB 1990, 94**

A. 1-3 MHz B. 1000 Hz
C. 3000 Hz D. 27.12 MHz

44. The length-tension diagram in a skeletal muscle shows a peak of maximum tension occurring with sarcomere length (in microns) of : **AIIMS 1985**

A. 0.1-1.1 B. 3.0-3.5
C. 1.1-2.0 D. 2.0-2.2

45. Hyperosmolarity of ECF leads to : **Rajasthan 1990, 98**

A. Volume receptor increased, ADH decreased
B. Volume receptor increased, ADH increased
C. Volume receptor decreased, ADH increased
D. Volume receptor decreased, ADH decreased

46. The effect of heavy exercise is : **Bihar 1998, 99**

A. Shift of O2 diffusion curve to left
B. Shift of O2 diffusion curve to right
C. Decrease in oxygen diffusing capacity
D. Decrease in residual capacity of lung

47. Foetal death is the typical result of absence of foetal : **DNB 1990, 94**

A. Brain function B. Kidney function
C. Liver function D. Cardiac function

48. Which does not change in the old age : **AIIMS 1986; AI 1993**

A. Haematocrit B. GFR
C. Glucose tolerance D. Blood pressure

49. Spermatozoa mature in which of the following organs : **AI 1993, 95**

A. Epidydimis B. Vas-deferens
C. Rete-testes D. Prostate

50. Which of the following organ does not utilise FA/ketones as a means of energy : **Delhi 1992, 98, 99**

A. Kidney B. Skeletal muscles
C. Heart D. Liver

51. Anaphylaxis is mediated by all except : **AP 1990, JIPMER 1992, 99**

A. Serotonin B. Prostaglandins
C. Bradykinin D. Anaphylatoxins

52. Nernest equation deals with : **JIPMER 1992, 95**

A. Chloride shift
B. Oxygen uptake
C. Cellular ATP levels
D. Plasma bicarbonate level

53. Which of the following diffuses freely from plasma to extracellular space : **JIPMER 1993, 95**

A. Water B. CO_2
C. Proteins D. Glucose

54. Chemical gradient across cell membrane is maintained mainly by : **JIPMER 1993, 98**

A. K^+ B. Na^+
C. Cl^- D. Ca^{++}

55. Yellapragada Subba Rao was a great Indian Scientist. He discovered : **AP 1990, 98**

A. Cyanocobalamine
B. Ureastibamine
C. Streptomycin
D. Cardiac Catheterization

Ans.	34. B	35. B	36. D	37. C	38. A	39. B	40. D	41. A	42. C	43. A
	44. D	45. B	46. B	47. D	48. A	49. A	50. D	51. B	52. A	53. C
	54. A	55. A								

56. **The value of resting membrane potential in a nerve fibre is : AIIMS 1985, 95**
A. -50 mV B. -70 mV
C. -110 mV D. -130 mV

57. **Red body in red body myopathy is : Kerala 1998, 99**
A. Z-fibrils B. I-band
C. H-band D. Actinmyosin junction

58. **The ionic channels in excitable membrane are lined by : AIIMS 1984, 94**
A. Cephalins B. Proteins
C. Lipids D. Carbohydrates

59. **Resting nerve membrane is more permeable to K+ than to Na+ by : AIIMS 1983, 93**
A. 1-5 times B. 1-5 times
C. 20-50 times D. 50-100 times

60. **N_2 has a role in body as it : AMC 1985, 96**
A. Decreases rate of combustion
B. Delays alveolar collapse
C. Prevents atelectesis
D. All of the above

61. **O_2 toxicity may lead to : AIIMS 1984, 98**
A. Nasal congestion and resp. tract irritation
B. Coughing
C. Decreased surfactant production
D. Convulsions, acidosis and coma

62. **The average number of muscle fibres attached to one golgi tendon organ are : AIIMS 1984, 92**
A. 0-3 B. 3-25
C. 25-42 D. 52-68

63. **Isotonic contraction differs from an isometric contraction in that in isotonic contraction : AIIMS 1988, 95**
A. Heat of activation is greater
B. Muscle is less efficient
C. Muscle uses more high energy phosphate
D. Recovery heat is reduced

64. **The band which appears on muscular contraction is : AIIMS 1984, 96**
A. A B. H
C. I D. M or CM

65. **A decrease in extracellular calcium causes : PGI 1983, 92**
A. Decreased membrane stability
B. Hyperpolarization
C. Decreased excitability
D. All of the above

66. **The band which disappears on muscular contraction is : Delhi 1982, 92**
A. H B. I
C. A D. Z

67. **D_2O (Deuterium oxide) is used to measure volume of : Delhi 1988, 94**
A. Blood B. Total body water
C. Extracellular fluid D. Intracellular fluid

68. **Semen contains all except : AIIMS 1983, 98**
A. Fructose B. Thromboplastin
C. Fibrinogen D. Prothrombin

69. **The sperms are normally motile at the rate of : AIIMS 1984, 98**
A. 0-1 cm/min B. 1-3 cm/min
C. 3-10 cm/min D. 10-15 cm/min

70. **Besides Cl- the most abundant extracellular anion is : AI 1993, Delhi 1986**
A. HCO_3^- B. Phosphate
C. Potassium D. Calcium

71. **All of the following endocrines are enlarged during pregnancy except : UPSC 1983**
A. Thyroid B. Thymus
C. Parathyroid D. Adrenal cortex

72. **Ferestration are seen in : JIPMER 1997, 99**
A. Brain B. Lungs
C. Intestinal villi D. Skeletal muscle

73. **Average pH of semen is : PGI 1987; DNB 1989,95, 99**
A. 6.2 B. 7.0
C. 7.5 D. 7.9

74. **In which of the following, the carbonic anhydrase concentration is the highest : Rohtak 1986, 95**
A. Blood B. RBC's
C. Skeletal muscle D. Neutrophils

75. **The retention of phosphate and calcium body is caused by : AMC 1983, 86; AIIMS 1987**
A. Vitamin-A B. Biotin
C. Thiamine D. Vitamin-D

76. **The average value of total body water in a young man is —— % of body weight : AMC 1984**
A. 20-40 B. 30-50
C. 60-65 D. 90-96

77. **Arginine lysine ratio in total serum proteins is : AIIMS 1983, 87**
A. 10 :14 B. 10:18
C. 10:24 D. 10:36

78. **When skeletal muscle shortens in response to stimulation there is : Delhi 1986, 97**
A. Decreased Width of I and H-bands
B. Decreased Width of A-band
C. Decreased Width of A and I-bands
D. Increased Width of H-zone

79. **Troponin is a : JIPMER 1997, 98**
A. Produces sliding movement of microtubules
B. Contains globular head
C. Binds to Ca++ produces skeletal muscle contraction
D. Beating of cilia and flagella

Ans.									
56. B	57. A	58. B	59. C	60. C	61. D	62. B	63. C	64. C	65. A
66. A	67. B	68. D	69. B	70. A	71. B	72. C	73. C	74. B	75. D
76. C	77. B	78. A	79. C						

80. In a man weighing 70 kg, water content of body is : AMC 1983, 93

A. 20-30 L B. 30-40 L
C. 40-45 L D. 50-60 L

81. All of the following vitamins play important role in development and growth of bone except : AMC 1983, 93

A. A B. B
C. C D. D

82. Stimulus is : Rajasthan 1998, 99

A. Proportional to log of intensity
B. Inversally proportional to log of intensity
C. Proportional to duration
D. Any of the above

83. Cell-to-cell conduction is not possible in : AIIMS 1985, 90

A. Skeletal muscle B. Cardiac muscle
C. Smooth muscle D. All of the above

84. Total body sodium in meq/kg is : AMC 1982, 89

A. 41 B. 58
C. 70.7 D. 91.0

85. Total blood volume (% of body weight) is : AIIMS 1982, 92

A. 8 B. 20
C. 40 D. 80

86. Normal range of serum magnesium in blood (in meq/L) : Delhi 1981, 91

A. 0.5-2 B. 1.5-2.5
C. 3-4.5 D. 4.5-6

87. Normal iron binding capacity in mcq/100 ml is : Rohtak 1985, 88

A. 65-175 B. 200-250
C. 250-350 D. 350-450

88. The equilibrium potential of which ion is equal to that of resting membrane potential (i.e -70 mv) : AIIMS 1983, 93

A. Na+ B. K+
C. Cl- D. None

89. In an average male which of the following age group has the maximum total body water : AIIMS 1984

A. 10-18 years B. 18-40 years
C. 40-60 years D. Above 60 years

90. When solvent is moving in one direction, the solvent tends to drag along some molecules of solute. This is called : PGI 1981, AMU 1986, 89

A. Filtration B. Osmosis
C. Donnan effect D. Solvent drag

91. Donnan effect is seen on the distribution of : AIIMS 1980, 90

A. Diffusible ions B. Lipids
C. Non-diffusible ions D. Only proteins

92. Which of the following formula is useful in evaluating and asessing the contribution of the various components to normal plasma osmolality : AIIMS 1980, 99

	Osmolality= (MOsm/L	Na+ (meq/L)	+	Glucose (mg/dl)	+	BUN (mg/dl)
A.		2	+	0.33	+	0.05
B.		2	+	0.05	+	0.33
C.		0.05	+	2	+	0.33
D.		0.05	+	0.033	+	2

93. Which of the following is true about percentage of total non-exchangeable body sodium in body : Delhi 1987, 97

A. 6.8 B. 14.8
C. 29.3 D. 70.7

94. Which of the following has the maximum exchange able sodium : AMU 1985, 92

A. Plasma B. Interstitial fluid
C. Bone D. Transcellular

95. Bound K+ is mainly found in following except : AMU 1985, 86

A. Brain B. Bone
C. RBC's D. Platelets

96. Total exchangeable K+ is measured by using : Delhi 1989, 92

A. I^{131} B. Phosphorus
C. D_2O D. K42

97. The principle buffers in the ECF are the following except : AMC 1986, 94

A. Haemoglobin B. Protein
C. Phosphate D. H_2CO_3

98. The pH of venous plasma as compared to arterial pH (7.40) is : Rohtak 1986

A. Lower B. Higher
C. Equal D. A or B

99. Alkalosis occurs whenever pH is above : UPSC 1981, 94

A. 7.00 B. 7.24
C. 7.36 D. 7.40

100. If the resting membrane potential of a nerve cell falls, there is a net : AIIMS 1980, 90

A. Gain of Na^+ into the cells
B. Loss of K^+ from cells
C. No loss of K^+ from cells
D. Gain of Cl^- into cells
E. All of the above

Ans.									
80. C	81. B	82. A	83. A	84. B	85. A	86. B	87. C	88. C	89. B
90. D	91. A	92. B	93. C	94. B	95. D	96. D	97. C	98. A	99. D
100. E									

101. In excitable cells, repolarization is most closely associated with which of the following events : AIIMS 1979, 89

A. Sodium ion efflux
B. Sodium ion influx
C. Potassium ion efflux
D. Potassium ion influx
E. Decreased excitability

102. Body temperature increases due to : Rajasthan 1995, 99

A. Vasoconstriction of skin
B. Vasodilatation of skin & sweating
C. Vasoconstriction & decreased BMR
D. Vasodilatation & increased BMR

103. Age related changes include the changes in following except : AIIMS 1997, 99

A. GFR B. Haematocrit
C. Brain atrophy D. ECG

104. Extracellular fluid pH is : UP 1995

A. 7.4 B. 6.5
C. 6.0 D. 5.0

105. Energy release which is determined not only by the activation process but also by the work load imposed on the muscle is : PGI 1980, 89

A. Dick principle B. Mary's Law
C. Fenn effect D. Fick principle

106. One of the following does not stimulate peripheral chemoreceptors : AI 1995, 97

A. Hypoxia B. Hypercarbia
C. Acidosis D. Alkalosis

107. A sprinter utilises in the first 3 to 4 minutes of a race: AIIMS 1997, 99

A. Creatinine phosphate
B. Muscle glycogen
C. Blood glucose
D. None of the above

108. Resting nerve membrane is more permeable to K+ than to Na+ AIIMS 1982, 92, 99

A. 5-10 times B. 10-50 times
C. 50-100 times D. 200-300 times

109. Normal plasma membrane resistance (in Ohms) is : AIIMS 1984; 87; PGI 1983, 88

A. 7 B. 10
C. 50 D. 100

110. The maximum force that can be applied on a muscle without producing injury is : AIIMS 1982, 84, 88

A. 1 G B. 4 G
C. 100 G D. 1000 G

111. The membrance potential is negative because of : AIIMS 1993, 84; AMC 1985, 88, 89

A. Anions B. Cations
C. Protein molecules D. All of the above

112. Molarity is because of : AIIMS 1984, 87; Delhi 1985, 87

A. Anions B. Cations
C. Protein molecules D. All of the above

113. Total body sodium is : AIIMS 1983; AMC 1986, 92

A. 7500 m mol B. 5000 m mol
C. 10000 m mol D. 500 m mol

114. Metastatic calcification occurs when calcium is in : PGI 1984; AMC 1988

A. Acidic pH B. Alkaline pH
C. Neutral pH D. Ionic equilibrium

115. Which is true about serum albumin : AI 1990

A. Contribute maximally to plasma oncotic pressure
B. It is anionic
C. Freely permeable in kidney
D. Not synthesised in liver

116. Which is not found in biological membrane : AI 1993, 99

A. Cytochrome 450 B. Steroid Receptors
C. Lipids D. Proteins

117. The bicarbonate buffer system is important in regulating extracellular fluid H+ concentration because : AIIMS 1984, 92

A. The concentration of CO2 and HCO3- in the extracellular fluid relatively high.
B. The pH of the bicarbonate buffer system is very close to the pH of the extracellular fluid.
C. The two elements of the bicarbonate buffer systems (CO2) and HCO2-) are regulated by renal and respiratory mechanisms.
D. B and C.

118. Which of the following changes would not occur as a result of dehydration (loss of water, but not solute) : AIIMS 1986, 98

A. Increased secretion of antidiuretic hormone.
B. Increased plasma sodium concentration.
C. Increased permeability of the collecting duct to water.
D. Increased solute concentration in the renal medulla.

119. Energy source for muscle contraction is : AIIMS 1985, 95

A. Actin-tropomyosin B. ATP
C. Lactic acid D. Nicotinamide

120. In a healthy person, metabolic requirements of tissue may exceed circulatory capacity in order to increase perfusion in : Delhi 1984, 95

A. Heart B. Brain
C. Lungs D. Muscles

Ans.										
	101. C	102. D	103. B	104. A	105. C	106. A	107. B	108. C	109. B	110. C
	111. B	112. D	113. B	114. B	115. A	116. B	117. D	118. C	119. B	120. D

121. At normal room temperature most body heat loss is by : AMC 1984

A. Convection B. Direct conduction
C. Radiation D. Sweating

122. The role of chromium in the body is : AIIMS 1983; AI 1988

A. Facilitates action of insulin
B. Erythropoiesis
C. Growth
D. Spermatogenesis

123. Highest concentration of potassium is seen in : UPSC 1986; AMC 1989, 92

A. Saliva B. Gastric juice
C. Bile D. Pancreatic secretion

124. Highest concentration of Vitamin-C in the body is found in the : AIIMS 1986

A. Liver B. Kidney
C. Adrenal cortex D. Spleen

125. Testes does not produce : AI 1989, 99

A. Estradiol B Testesterone
C. Fructose D. Inhibin

126. Penile erection is caused primarily by : AIIMS 1982, 84, 89, 94

A. Reflex sympathetic constriction of the arterioles.
B. Parasympathetically induced dilatation of the arterioles.
C. Contraction of the bulbocavernous muscle.
D. Reflex-parasympathetic constriction of the venules.
E. Sympathetic-induced constriction of the veins.

127. An adolescent desire of increasing his muscle mass is advised to : Manipal 1998, 99

A. Increase protein intake
B. Exercise the muscle
C. Take steroids
D. Take fatty food

128. The following physiological changes appear when a person is suddenly transported to an altitude of 3000 m (nearly 10,000 feet) : CSE 1998, 99

1. Hyperventilation
2. Decrease in arterial pO2
3. Stimulation of aortic and carotid bodies
4. Increase in arterial pO2

A. 2,3,4,1 B. 2,3,1,4
C. 3,2,1,4 D. 3,2,4,1

129. Daily loss of water from skin in absence of visible sweating is : AIIMS 1994, 98

A. 200-300 ml B. 500-700 ml
C. 1 Litre D. 1.5 Liter

130. What probably causes stimulation of the thermal receptors? AIIMS 1985

A. Change in the membrane structure caused by heat or cold.
B. Change in the metabolic rate of the nerve ending.
C. Change in the viscosity of the fluid surrounding the neuron.
D. Change in the concentration of sodium ions outside the neuron caused by changes in temperature.

131. The energy levels on two differ from each other by 10,000 times; how much difference in this in decibels? AIIMS 1983, 93

A. 4 B. 40
C. 20 D. 80

132. The maximum number of ribosomes that a messenger RNA molecule can be attached to at any one time is : AIIMS 1983, 93

A. Zero B. One
C. Two D. More than two

133. Metabolic alkalosis associated with prolonged vomiting is primarily due to loss of : AI 1989, 92

A. Sodium B. Pottasium
C. Chloride D. Hydrogen ion

134. Which of the following is correct about the energy required to cause diffusion through a cell membrane? AIIMS 1988, 98

A. No energy is required.
B. The energy that causes the diffusion comes from chemical reaction in the cell membrane.
C. Energy for diffusion is required only when a net rate of diffusion must occur against a concentration gradient.
D. The energy that causes the diffusion comes from the kinetic energy of the particles of the solution.

135. The mean span of the corpus luteum is lengthened in the event of pregnancy by : AMU 1988, 94

A. Placental hormone B. Ovarian hormone
C. Pituitary hormone D. Calcitonin

136. Plasma sodium concentration is : Kerala 1994, 98

A. 120 meq/l B. 3.5 meq/l
C. 140 meq/l D. 110 meq/l

137. Na+ content of gastric juice is : PGI 1994, 96

A. 30-40 meq/L B. 50-60 meq/L
C. 60-80 meq/L D. 100 meq/L

138. Atrial natriuretic peptide (ANP) causes : PGI 1993, 99

A. ↓ Cardiac output B. ↑ Blood volume
C. ↑Urine output D. ↑ Renin secretion

Match the following (139-142) AIIMS 1984, 94

A. D_2O
B. Thiocyanate
C. I^{131} fibrinogen
D. Thiocyanate and sucrose
E. Antipyrine and bromide

139. Total body water :

140. Intra cellular fluid volume :

Ans.	121. C	122. A	123. A	124. C	125. C	126. B	127. B	128. B	129. A	130. C
	131. D	132. D	133. C	134.	135. C	136. C	137. C	138. A	139. A	140. C

141. **Total extracellular fluid volume :**

142. **Plasma volume :**

143. **Charles's law states that : Karnataka 1989, 99**
A. Temperature is inversely proportional to volume.
B. The volume of a gas is directly proportional to the absolute temperature, pressure constant.
C. The pressure of a gas is inversely proportinal to the volume.
D. The pressure of a gas is inversely proportinal to the volume, temperature constant.

144. **Most of the proteins loss after injury comes from : Karnataka 1994**
A. Plasma proteins B. Liver and other organs
C. Bone D. Muscle proteins

145. **All of the following statements of the post-traumatic state are true except : Karnataka 1994**
A. There is rise in blood lymphocytes
B. There is rise in neutrophils
C. There is a rise in platelet count
D. There is suppression of the reticuloendothelial system

146. **One nanometer is equal to : Karnataka 1994**
A. One-millionth of a millimeter
B. One-tenth of a millimeter
C. One-hundredth of millimeter
D. One-thousandth of a millimeter

147. **Gene transmitted but not translated : AIIMS 1994**
A. Histone B. Keratin
C. t-RNA D. Glycosyl transferase

148. **In the typical reaction of 'fright' or 'flight' there is : AMU 1991**
A. Slowing of the heart rate
B. Fall of blood pressure
C. Dilatation of the pupils
D. Relaxation of anal and urethral sphincters

149. **In the clinical determination of B.M.R. it is necessary, according to common practice, to measure the patients' : AMU 1992**
A. Surface area B. Lean body mass
C. Specific gravity D. Somatotype
E. Height and weight

150. **Major intracellular anion, excluding K^+ is : PGI 1995**
A. HCO3- B. Cl-
C. Serum protein D. HPO4

151. **DNA fragment separation is done by : AIIMS 1996**
A. Paper chromatography
B. Agaros gel
C. Thin layer chromatography
D. Electrophorosis

152. **Sperm motility is caused by : AIIMS 1996**
A. Epididymis B. Vas deferens
C. Testis D. Prostatic secretion

153. **Complete in younger individuals than in older ones is —— law : DNB 1995**
A. Rubner's B. Pajot's
C. Spallanzani's D. Sherrington's

154. **Cushing's reflex helps in maintaining : AMC 1994**
A. Coronary blood flow
B. Cerebral blood flow
C. Hepatic blood flow
D. Pancreatic secretion

155. **All are in higher concentration in ICF than ECF except : Rajasthan 1994**
A. Mg B. K
C. PO4 D. HCO3

156. **All are true about lysosomes except : Rajasthan 1994**
A. They are formed by Golgi apparatus
B. Contain oxidases
C. Have a bilipid layer
D. Function is autolysis

157. **If Na+ conc in ECF is 140 mEq & in ICF is 14 m EQ. the Nernst potential is : Rajasthan 1994**
A. +61 mv B. -61 mv
C. +10 mv D. +14 mv

158. **For each mole of ATP hydrolysed, 3 Na+ are extruded from cell for each ------K+ into the cell : DNB 1997**
A. 1 B. 2
C. 3 D. 6

159. **Primary increase in CO_2 in the body is seen in : PGI 1999**
A. Respiratory acidosis
B. Metabolic alkalosis
C. Respiratory alkalosis
D. Metabolic acidosis

160. **Mechanism of reperfusion injury is : PGI 1999**
A. Vitamin-E B. Ca2
C. Mg2+ D. Superoxide

161. **Intensity and amplitude are proportional to : TN 1999**
A. Weber Fechner law B. Starlings law
C. Pouille's law D. Laplace's law

162. **In a control system, negative feedback : MAHE 1999**
A. Is the only mechanism occurring in a biological system.
B. Brings back the variable to operational level.
C. Maintains the variable to a fixed level.
D. All of the above.

Ans.									
141. B	142. C	143. B	144. D	145. B	146. A	147. A	148. C	149. A	150. D
151. B	152. A	153. C	154. B	155. D	156. B	157. A	158. B	159. A	160. D
161. A	162. B								

163. Consider the following statements : CSE 1999
'Flare' in 'Triple response' can appear
1. With intact nerves
2. After the division but before the degeneration of nerves
3. After the division and degeneration of nerves

Which of the statements is/are correct?
A. 1 and 2 B. 3 alone
C. 2 alone D. 1 and 3

164. Which of the following does not dilate arterioles in the skin ? Karnataka 1999
A. Epinephrine B. Vasopressin
C. Bradykinin D. Substance-P

165. Calmodulin activates : TN 1999
A. Muscle phosphorylase
B. Protein kinase
C. Tyrosine kinase
D. Pyruvate synthetase

166. In flight reaction, blood flow to muscles is due to : AI-2000
A. Sympathetic cholinergic
B. Parasympathetic
C. Local metabolites
D. Endothelin

167. Nitric O2 acts by : MAHE 2000; AI 2000
A. cGMP B. cAMP
C. Tyrosine kinase D. NADP

168. Cross-linkage in sarcomere is by: JIPMER 2000
A. Action B. Myosin
C. Tropomyosin D. Callmodulin

169. Muscle strength is increased by : IAM 2000
A. Isometric exercise B. Isotonic exercise
C. Electric stimulation D. Chemical stimulation

170. Which receptor complex has 7 members : Delhi 2000
A. 5 HT B. LH
C. ACTH D. GABA

171. Which of the following is not primarily a function of the plasma ? TNPSC 1996
A. Transport of hormones
B. Maintenance of red cell size
C. Transport of antibodies
D. None of the above

172. Operon is composed of : TNPSC 1998
A. Regulator elements and 1 gene
B. Regulator elements and structural gene
C. 1 gene and structural gene
D. None of the above

173. Oxygen toxicity involves the following except : TNPSC 1998
A. Disturbance in sleep
B. Retrolental fibroplasia
C. Lung cysts in infants
D. Irritation of respiratory tract

174. Calcium binding sites are following except : UP 1999
A. Troponin B. Tropomyosin
C. Calmodulin D. Calbindin

175. EDRF simulates action of : UP 1999
A. CAMP B. NO
C. Halothane D. Ether

176. Spectrin, true is all except : UP 1999
A. Protein in nature
B. Functions similar to ankyrin
C. Deficiency causes spherocytosis
D. Responsible for primary structure of cell

177. During exercise following physiological changes occurs to increase oxygen demand by muscles except : UP 2000
A. Increased oxygen extraction
B. Shift to left of oxygen dissociation curve
C. Increased stroke volume
D. Shift of blood supply to muscle

178. Creatine is : UP 2000
A. Muscle protein
B. Release from acetylcholine in the muscle
C. Provide energy in the muscle
D. Synthesized in the muscle

179. Tetrododoxin blocks : UP 2000, 2002
A. Increase gNa+ during action potential
B. Increase gK+ during action potential
C. gNa+ during resting state
D. gK+ during resting state

180. Hypomagnesemia is seen in : TNPSC 2000, 2002
A. Dehydration B. Uremia
C. Addison's disease D. Chronic alcoholism

181. If the membrane conductances for sodium and potassium are equal the membrane potential is close to : TNPSC 2000
A. —90 mV B. —70 mV
C. —15 mV D. 0 mV

182. All are increased during exercise except : TNPSC 2000
A. Cardiac output
B. Venous return
C. Coronary blood flow
D. Peripheral vascular resistance

183. Moderate muscular exercise causes : MAHE 2000
A. ↓ in blood flow to the brain
B. ↓ in blood flow to the heart
C. ↓ in blood flow to the skeletal muscle
D. ↓ in total peripheral resistance

184. Core temperature is closest to : MAHE 2000
A. Esophageal temp. B. Rectal temp.
C. Axillary temp. D. Oral temp.

Ans.									
163. A	164. B	165. A	166. C	167. A	168. B	169. A	170. A	171. D	172. B
173. A	174. B	175. B	176. D	177. B	178. C	179. A	180. D	181. D	182. D
183. D	184. B								

185. Exocytosis : PGI 2000
A. Extrusion of cell bound vesicles
B. Intrusion of liquid particles
C. Intrusion of solid particles
D. All of the above

186. O2 consumption is minimal when temp. gradient between skin and ext. temp. is : PGI 2000
A. < 0.5° B. > 2.5°
C. <1.5° D. > 3.5 °

187. Phospholamban is an intracellular protein with the following function : AIIMS 2000
A. Transporting calcium out of the mitochondria
B. Ca/Na pump
C. For sequestration of calcium into the sarcoplasma
D. Binds actin myosin

188. Force generating proteins are : AI 2001
A. Myosin and myoglobin
B. Dynein and kinesin
C. Calmodelin and G-protein
D. Troponin

189. Protein involved in intercellular connections : AI 2001
A. Connexin B. Integrin
C. Adhesin D. Dystrophin

190. Nitrogen washout test is used to measure : Delhi 2001, 2002
A. Residual volume
B. Inspiratory reserve volume
C. Expiratory reserve volume
D. Vital capacity

191. Earliest change in high altitude is : Kerala 2001, 2002
A. Hyperventilation
B. Decrease in work capacity
C. Drowsiness
D. Polycythemia

192. Which of the following is true regarding a system which favors oscillatory responses : AI 2002
A. Proportional component
B. Has a greater gain
C. Has a lesser gain
D. Positive feedback system

193. Normal anion gap in humans is (in meq) : SGPGI 2002, 2004
A. 5-10 B. 8-14
C. 14-20 D. 20-30

194. Which of the following has strongest affinity for calcium : Maharashtra 2000, 2005
A. Tropomyosin B. Troponin-T
C. Troponin-I D. Troponin-C

195. Decrease in plasma oncotic pressure will cause : Maharashtra 2000, 2004
A. Shift of fluid to ICF
B. Shift to fluid to ECF
C. Shift of fluid from capillaries to interstitium
D. None

196. Sweating is seen in : CMC 2001, 2002
A. Exercise B. Vomiting
C. Spicy foods D. All of the above

197. Transport mechanisms requiring carrier protein are all except : Maharashtra 2002
A. Simple diffusion B. Passive diffusion
C. Active transport D. Facilitated diffusion

198. Sodium-potassium ATPase pump transfers : BHU 2002
A. 3 potassium out & 2 sodium inside the cell
B. 3 sodium out & 2 potassium inside the cell
C. 3 potassium out & 3 sodium inside the cell
D. 2 sodium out & 2 potassium inside the cell

199. Teratozoospermia denotes : BHU 2002
A. Decreased life span of the sperms
B. Increased sperm viability
C. Decreased sperm count
D. Deformed & abnormally shaped sperms

200. The figure below represents the pH of the digestive juices aspirated from the alimentary tract as a function of position along the alimentary tract during digestion of a meal : AI 2003
A. A typical value for Y2 is 9.0
B. A typical value for Y3 is 10.0
C. The segment-C represents the pylorus
D. The digestive enzymes active in segment A are inactivated in segment-B

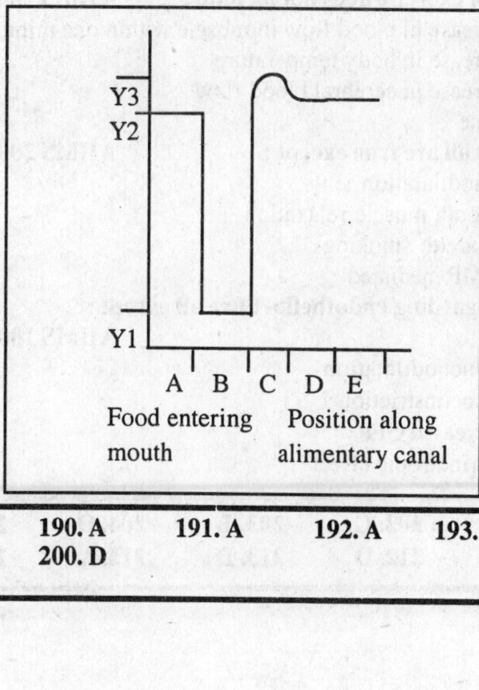

Ans.	185. A	186. A	187. C	188. B	189. A	190. A	191. A	192. A	193. B	194. D
	195. B	196. D	197. A	198. B	199. D	200. D				

201. The cells belonging to the following type of epithelium are provided with extra reserve of cell membrane : **AI 2003**

A. Transitional B. Stratified squamous
C. Stratified cuboidal D. Stratified columnar

202. The buffering capacity of a buffer is maximum at pH equal to : **AI 2003**

A. 0.5 pKa B. pKa
C. pKa + 1 D. 2 pKa

203. Which of the following is present intracellularly in muscle cells : **AI 2003**

A. Insulin B. Corticosteroid
C. Epinephrine D. Glucagon

204. All the statements about lactoferrin are true except : **AI 2003**

A. It is present in secondary granules of neutrophils
B. It is present in exocrine secretions of body
C. It has great affinity for iron
D. It transports iron for erythropoiesis

205. During acclimatization to high altitude all of the following take place except: **AI 2004, 2005**

A. Increase in minute ventilation
B. Increase in the sensitivity of central chemoreceptors
C. Increase in the sensitivity of carotid body to hypoxia
D. Shift in the oxygen dissociation curve to the left

206. The membrane protein, clathrin is involved in : **AI 2005**

A. Cell motility
B. Receptor mediated endocytosis
C. Exocytosis
D. Cell shape

207. Cellular and flageliar movement is carried out by all of the following except : **AI 2005**

A. Intermediate filaments
B. Actin
C. Tubulin
D. Myosin

208. Effect of exercise does not include : **AIIMS 2007**

A. Increase in blood flow in muscle within one minute
B. Increase in body temperature
C. Increase in cerebral blood flow
D. None

209. For NO all are true except : **AIIMS 2007**

A. Vasodilatation
B. Smooth muscle relaxation
C. Cigarette smoking
D. cAMP mediated

210. True regarding endothelin-1 are all except : **AIIMS 2007**

A. Bronchodilatation
B. Vasoconstriction
C. Decreased GFR
D. Has inotropic effect

211. In isometric exercise all are increased except : **AIIMS 2007**

A. Heart rate
B. Cardiac output
C. Mean arterial pressure
D. Systemic vascular resistance

212. For PCR which of the following is not required : **AIIMS 2007**

A. Taq polymerase B. d-NTP
C. Primer D. Radiolabelled DNA probe

213. Which of the following is not true regarding p53? **AIIMS 2007, 2008**

A. Controls the production and encodes 53 KD
B. Present on chromosome 17
C. Arrests cell cycle in G1 phase
D. Is required for normal cell development

214. Transport of neutral substances across the cell membrane occurs via : **AI 2008**

A. Porins
B. Ionophore
C. Lipopolysaccharides
D. Diffusion

215. The blood pressure measured by sphygmomanometer is : **AI 2008**

A. Lower than the intra-arterial pressure
B. Higher than the intra-arterial pressure
C. Same as the intra-arterial pressure
D. The same with different cuff sizes

216. Histamine is formed by ——————of histidine : **AI 2008**

A. Methylation B. Reduction
C. Oxidation D. Carboxylation

217. Equilibrium potential for an ion is calculated using : **AIIMS 2008**

A. Gibbs-Donnan equation
B. Nernst equation
C. Goldmann equation
D. Any of the above

218. Sorting of proteins occurs in which of the following organelles? **AI 2008**

A. Golgi bodies B. Ribosome
C. Lysosome D. Endoplasmic reticulum

219. Pertussis toxin does not lead to : **AIIMS 2008**

A. ADA ribosylation of GI alpha subunit
B. Blocks adenylyl cyclase
C. Increased calcium release from sarcoplasmic reticulum
D. Persistent activation of GS alpha subunit.

Ans.	201. C	202. C	203. B	204. D	205. D	206. B	207. A	208. C	209. D	210. A
	211. D	212. D	213. D	214. A	215. B	216. D	217. B	218. A	219. B	

220. Facillitated diffusion : **AIIMS 2008**
A. Requires carrier protein
B. Is a form of active transport
C. Along concentration gradient
D. Requires creatinine phosphate

221. Cell-cell interaction occurs by all of the following mechanism except : **AI 2009**
A. Hormones
B. Gap junctions
C. G-protein receptors
D. Neurotransmitters released at synapse

222. Muscle's blood supply increases during exercise due to : **AI 2009**
A. Increased blood pressure
B. Accumulation of active metabolites
C. Increase vasodilatation
D. Increase heart rate

223. Rise in 2-3 bisphosphoglycerate is seen in all of the following except : **AI 2009**
A. Chronic anemia B. Chronic hypoxia
C. Inosine D. Hypoxanthine

Ans. 220. A 221. C 222. B 223. D

EXPLANATIONS OF MISCELLANEOUS

1. Ans.— A. Lipid
2. Ans.— B. Four times
3. Ans.— B. Fatty woman

   Total body water in 10-18 years (59% in males, 57% in females), 18-40 years (61% in males, 51% in females), 40-60 years (55% in males, 47% in females) and over 60 (52% in males and 46% in females).
4. Ans.— D. It is freely filtered at the renal glomeruli
5. Ans.— B. Its principle cation is sodium

   Ultrasound is not a electromagnetic radiation but a sound wave
6. Ans.— A. Cell
7. Ans.— D. Bone

   Sodium content intracellular is 9% and extracellular is 91% (bone 36.5%, interstitial fluid is 29%, dense contractile tissue and cartilage is 11.7%, plasma 11.2% and transcellular 2.6%).
8. Ans.— D. Increased excretion of potassium in the urine
9. Ans.— B. Facilitated diffusion

   Both volume receptor and ADH are increased.
10. Ans.— D. A net inward movement of positive ions
11. Ans.— B. It is increased by the loss of function in the cerebellum
12. Ans.— C. 10
13. Ans.— D. All of the above
14. Ans.— D. Hyperactivity
15. Ans.— D. Osteoporosis
16. Ans.— C. Both
17. Ans.— C. Ca++
18. Ans.— A. 0.4%

    Total intracellular potassium is 89.6% and extracellular is 10.4% (bone-7.6%, Transcellular 1.0% interstitial fluid 1.0% plasma 0.4% and dense connective tissue and cartilage 0.4%).
19. Ans.— D. Release of Ca+ to troponin-C

    Potassium is the main ion involved
20. Ans.— A. Caudate nucleus
21. Ans.— C. Discovery of the Vectocardiogram
22. Ans.— C. 9-11 mg/100 ml

    Total diffusible calcium in human plasma is 1.34 mmol/L. Ionized calcium is 1.18 and complexed to HCO3-, citrate etc. is 0.16, total non-diffusible protein bound iodine is 1.16 mmol/L (bound to albumin 0.92 and bound to globulin 0.24). Total plasma calcium is 2.50 mmol/L.
23. Ans.— B. 600 to 800 cc
24. Ans.— A. Lymphocyte
25. Ans.— D. 72 hours
26. Ans.— C. Strontium
27. Ans.— D. Body temperature falls

    Cervical mucus is plenty and less viscus following ovulation
28. Ans.— B. Energy which is unavailable for work
29. Ans.— C. Three
30. Ans.— D. Anhydride linkages
31. Ans.— D. Secretion of H+ in exchange for sodium
32. Ans.— B. 16
33. Ans.— C. $pH = pK + \log \frac{H_2CO_3}{H2\ CO_3}$
34. Ans.— B. 15

    The day of ovulation is calculated by substracting 14 from duration of menstrual cycle.
35. Ans.— B. Decreased concentration of plasma potassium
36. Ans.— D. K influx
37. Ans.— C. 981 cms/sec2
38. Ans.— A. 1000
39. Ans.— B. 3 x 10^{10} cms/sec.
40. Ans.— D. Ultrasound
41. Ans.— A. 27.12 MHz

42. Ans.— C. 2450 MHz

43. Ans.— A. 1-3 MHz

44. Ans.— D. 2.0-2.2

45. Ans.— B. Volume receptor increased ADH, increased

46. Ans.— B. Shift of O2 diffusion curve to right

Exercise has been reported to produce an increase in 2,3 DPG within 60 minutes, although the rise may not occur in trained athletes. P50 is also increased during exercise, because the temperature rises in active tissues and CO_2 and metabolites accumulate lowering the pH.

47. Ans.— D. Cardiac function

48. Ans.— A. Haematocrit

In old age, BP rises, GFR decreases and glucose tolerance also decreases.

49. Ans.— A. Epidydimis

There is underactivity

50. Ans.— D. Liver

51. Ans.— B. Prostaglandins

52. Ans.— A. Chloride shift

53. Ans.— C. Proteins

54. Ans.— A. K^+

55. Ans.— A. Cyanocobalamine

56. Ans.— B. -70 mV

57. Ans.— A. Z-fibrils

58. Ans.— B. Proteins

59. Ans.— C. 20-50 times

60. Ans.— C. Prevents atelectesis

61. Ans.— D. Convulsions, acidosis and coma

Death may occur

62. Ans.— B. 3-25

63. Ans.— C. Muscle uses more high energy phosphate

64. Ans.— C. I

65. Ans.— A. Decreased membrane stability

66. Ans.— A. H

67. Ans.— B. Total body water

68. Ans.— D. Prothrombin

69. Ans.— B. 1-3 cm/min

70. Ans.— A. HCO_3

71. Ans.— B. Thymus

Thymus does not show any change

72. Ans.— C. Intestinal villi

73. Ans.— C. 7.5

An average volume per ejaculate is 2.5 to 3.5 ml after several days of continence. Normal count is about 100 million sperms/ml of semen. Human sperms move at a speed of about 3 mm/min through female genital tract and reach uterine tubes 30-60 min after copulation.

74. Ans.— B. RBC's

75. Ans.— D. Vitamin-D

76. Ans.— C. 60-65

77. Ans.— B. 10:18

78. Ans.— A. Decreased Width of I and H-bands

79. Ans.— C. Binds to Ca++ produces skeletal muscle contraction

It is important for muscle contraction

80. Ans.— C. 40-45 L

81. Ans.— B. B

82. Ans.— A. Proportional to log of intensity

83. Ans.— A. Skeletal muscle

Cell-to-cell conduction is not seen in skeletal muscle.

84. Ans.— B. 58

85. Ans.— A. 8

86. Ans.— B. 1.5-2.5

87. Ans.— C. 250-350

88. Ans.— C. Cl-

89. Ans.— C. 18-40 years

90. Ans.— D. Solvent drag

91. Ans.— A. Diffusible ions

When there is an ion on one side of membrane that cannot diffuse through membrane, the distribution of other ions in which membrane is permeable is affected in a predictable way Gibbs Donnan equation holds for any pair of cations and anions of the same valance.

92. Ans.— B. 2 + 0.05 + 0.33

93. Ans.— C. 29.3

94. Ans.— B. Interstitial fluid

In interstitial fluid, sodium content is 29.0%. In bone sodium content is 36.5% (11.0% exchangeable whereas 25.5% is nonexchangeable).

95. Ans.— D. Platelets

96. Ans.— D. K42

97. Ans.— C. Phosphate

98. Ans.— A. Lower

99. Ans.— D. 7.40

100. Ans.— E. All of the above

101. Ans.— C. Potassium ion efflux

102. Ans.— D. Vasodilatation & increased BMR

103. Ans.— B. Haematocrit

Haematocrit is not affected

104. Ans.— A. 7.4

105. Ans.— C. Fenn effect

106. Ans.— A. Hypoxia

107. Ans.— B. Muscle glycogen

108. Ans.— C. 50-100 times

109. Ans.— B. 10

110. Ans.— C. 100 G

111. Ans.— B. Cations

When depolarization exceeds 7 mV, the voltage gated Na+ channels start to open at an increased rate (Na+ channel activation).

112. Ans.— D. All of the above

113. Ans.— B. 5000 m mol

114. Ans.— B. Alkaline pH

115. Ans.— A. Contribute maximally to plasma oncotic pressure

116. Ans.— B. Steroid Receptors

117. Ans.— D. B and C

118. Ans.— C. Increased permeability of the collecting duct to water

119. Ans.— B. ATP

ATP is main source of energy

120. Ans.— D. Muscles

121. Ans.— C. Radiation

122. Ans.— A. Facilitates action of insulin

123. Ans.— A. Saliva

Duodenal fluid is also rich

124. Ans.— C. Adrenal cortex

125. Ans.— C. Fructose

126. Ans.— B. Parasympathetically induced dilatation of the arterioles.

127. Ans.— B. Exercise the muscle

128. Ans.— B. 2,3,1,4

129. Ans.— A. 200-300 ml

Insensible water loss amounts to 50 mL/hour in humans. During muscular exertion in a hot environment sweat secretion reaches values as high as 1600 mL/h. Heat loss by vaporization of water varies from 30 to over 900 kcal/h.

130. Ans.— C. Change in the viscosity of the fluid surrounding the neuron.

131. Ans.— D. 80

132. Ans.— D. More than two

133. Ans.— C. Chloride

There is also loss of Na+

134. Ans.—

135. Ans.— C. Pituitary hormone

136. Ans.— C. 140 meq/l

Plasma sodium constitutes 11.2% of extracellular sodium.

137. Ans.— C. 60-80 meq/L

138. Ans.— A. ↓ Cardiac output

139. Ans.— A. D_2O

140. Ans.— C. I^{131} fibrinogen

141. Ans.— B. Thiocyanate

142. Ans.— C. I^{131} fibrinogen

143. Ans.— B. The volume of a gas is directly proportional to the absolute temperature, pressure constant.

144. Ans.— D. Muscle Proteins

145. Ans.— B. There is rise in neutrophils

146 Ans.— A. One-millionth of a millimeter

147. Ans.— A. Histone

148. Ans.— C. Dilatation of the pupils

149. Ans.— A. Surface area

150. Ans.— D. HPO4

151. Ans.— B. Agaros gel

152. Ans.— A. Epididymis

153. Ans.— C. Spallanzani's

154. Ans.— B. Cerebral blood flow

When intracranial pressure is increased, the blood supply to vasomotor area is compromised and local hypoxia and hypercapnia increases its discharge. The resultant rise in systemic arterial pressure (Cushing's reflex) tends to restore the blood flow to medulla.

155. Ans.— D. HCO3

156. Ans.— B. Contain oxidases

157. Ans.— A. +61 mv

158. Ans.— B. 2

159. Ans.— A. Respiratory acidosis

160. Ans.— D. Superoxide

Antioxidants are used as scavengers

161. Ans.— A. Weber Fechner law

162. Ans.— B. Brings back the variable to operational level

163. Ans.— A. 1 and 2

164. Ans.— B. Vasopressin

165. Ans.— A. Muscle phosphorylase

166. Ans.— C. Local metabolites

167. Ans.— A. cGMP

Nitric oxide is a compound released by endothelium of blood vessels as endothelium derived relaxing factor (EDRF) a reaction catalyzed in brain by one of the 3 forms of NO synthase. It activates guanylyl cyclase.

168. Ans.— B. Myosin

169. Ans.— A. Isometric exercise

170. Ans.— A. 5 HT

171. Ans.— D. None of the above

172. Ans.— B. Regulator elements and structural gene

173. Ans.— A. Disturbance in sleep

174. Ans.— B. Tropomyosin

175. Ans.— B. NO

It is important for action of sildenafil (viagra)

176. Ans.— D. Responsible for primary structure of cell

177. Ans.— B. Shift to left of oxygen dissociation curve

178. Ans.— C. Provide energy in the muscle

179. Ans.— A. Increase gNa+ during action potential

180. Ans.— D. Chronic alcoholism

181. Ans.— D. 0 mV

182. Ans.— D. Peripheral vascular resistance

183. Ans.— D. ↓ in total peripheral resistance

Peripheral resistance is markedly decreased.

184. Ans.— B. Rectal temp.

185. Ans.— A. Extrusion of cell bound vesicles

186. Ans.— A. $<0.5°$

187. Ans.— C. For sequestration of calcium into the sarcoplasma

188. Ans.— B. Dynein and kinesin

Molecular motors are — microtubule based (kinesins and Dyneins) and actin based (myosins). Kinesin is a double headed molecule that moves its cargo toward the '+' ends of microtubules. Some kinesins are associated with mitosis and meiosis. Dyneins have two heads with their neck pieces embedded in a complex of proteins. Cytoplasmic dynein is like kines in except it moves particles and membranes dynein oscillates and is responsible for beating of flagella and cilia.

189. Ans.— A. Connexin

190. Ans.— A. Residual volume

191. Ans.— A. Hyperventilation

192. Ans.— A. Proportional component

Proportional component is most important for oscillatory responses.

193. Ans.— B. 8-14

194. Ans.— D. Troponin -C

195. Ans.— B. Shift to fluid to ECF

196. Ans.— D. All of the above

197. Ans.— A. Simple diffusion

198. Ans.— B. 3 sodium out & 2 potassium inside the cell

199. Ans.— D. Deformed & abnormally shaped sperms

200. Ans.— D. The digestive enzymes active in segment A are inactivated in segment-B

As the pH of segment-A is high (Basic) & pH of segment-B is low (acidic). So it is not possible for digestive enzymes of segment-A to function at the pH of segment B & vice versa so the answer is surely D.

201. Ans.— C. Stratified cuboidal

IBS Histology states that. "In stratified squamous epithelium superficial layers are constantly being removed and replaced by proliferation of cells from the basal (germinal) layer. This layer therefore shows frequent mitosis".

202. Ans.— C. pKa + 1

Maximum Buffering capacity occurs at (PKa ± 1 pH)

203. Ans.— B. Corticosteroid

"Out of given four choices only corticosteroids are having intracellular (Nuclear) recepters". Hence it will be present intracellularly.

204. Ans.— D. It transports iron for erythropoiesis

Lactoferrin—Iron Binding Protein

It inhibits growth of certain bacteria by binding iron & may be involved in regulation of proliferation of myeloid cells.

It is found in secondary granules of Neutrophilis

It is also found in breast milk "Hence it is an exocrine secretion," (Ghai's Paediatrics clearly mentioned it).

205. Ans.— D. Shift in the oxygen dissociation curve to the left

206. Ans.— B. Receptor mediated endocytosis

"Endocytosis can be constitutive or clathrin mediated". Constitutive endocytosis is not a specialized process, whereas clathrin mediated endocytosis occurs at membrane endentation where the protein clathrin accumulates."

207. Ans.— A. Intermediate filaments

Cytoskeleton

Microtubules	*Intermediate Filaments*	*Microfilaments*
Composed of Tubulin	**- Connect the nuclear membrane to the cell**	**- Actin polymerize to form F-actin**
Cilia and Flagellum are made up of actin Microtubules	**- Form flexible scaffolding for the cell and help it to resist extenal pressure**	**_ Made up of actin**
	No role in movement	**- Release of Ca2+ triggers the process.**
		Myosin present in the cell acts on the ATPase and also engages mechanically to make actin slide part one another

Functions of Microtubular and Microfilaments :

1. **Locomotion by means by pseudopodia**
2. **Movement of cilia and Flagella**
3. **Movement of intestinal microvilli**
4. **Changes in cell shape during phagocytosis, pinocytosis or exocytosis**
5. **Formation of mitotic spindle (Tubulin)**

208. Ans.— C Increase in cerebral blood flow

Blood flow increase at or even before the start of exercise. The cerebral blood flow remains unchanged during exercise. Blood flow increases in heart and active skeletal muscles; decreases in inactive skeletal muscles, kidney, liver, GIT.

209. Ans.— D cAMP mediated

NO or endothelium derived relaxing factor (EDRF) has the following functions:

- **i. Relaxation of vascular smooth muscle via stimulation of soluble guanylyl cyclase and generation of cGMP.**
- **ii. Role in maintenance of normal blood pressure.**
- **iii. GI smooth muscle dilatation.**
- **iv. Necessary for the cytotoxic activities of macrophages.**
- **v. Penile erection**
- **vi. No acting via cGMP is important in brain function.**
- **vii. Involved in vascular remodelling and angiogenesis.**
- **viii. No involved in pathogenesis of atherosclerosis.**

210. Ans.— A Bronchodilatation

* Endothelin-1 causes bronchoconstriction
* Endothelin-1 (ET-1) is a 21 amino acid peptide that is produced by vascular endothelium.
* Actions of ET-1 are :
  - Vasoconstriction
  - Cardiac stimulation (inotropic)
  - Stimulates aldosterone secretion
  - Decreases renal blood flow and glomerular filteration rate
  - Releases atrial natriuretic peptide
* Diseases and conditions associated with elevated endothelin-1.

  Because of its powerful vasoconstrictor properties, and its effects on intracellular calcium, ET-1 has been implicated in the pathogenesis of :
  - hypertension
  - coronary vasospasm
  - heart failure

211. Ans.— D Systemic vascular resistance

* CVS changes in isometric exercise :
  - Heart rate rises
  - Systolic and diastolic blood pressure rises sharply
  - Stroke volume changes relatively little.
  - Cardiac output increases
* CVS changes in isotonic exercise :
  - Heart rate rises
  - Stroke volume increases markedly
  - Peripheral resistance decreases d/t vasodilation in exercising muscle.
  - Systolic B.P. rises only moderately, whereas diastolic pressure usually remains unchanged or falls.
  - Cardiac output increases

212. Ans.— D Radiolabelled DNA probe

* DNA polymerase (e.g. Taq polymerase) which can sustain high temperature (> 60°C). (Heat stable Taq polymerase is obtained from *Thermus aquaticus* (or other the thermophilic bacteria) an organism found in hot springs.)
* A large number of free deoxynucleotides (dNTPs).
* The target DNA fragment

213. Ans.— D Is required for normal cell development

* p53 is not required for normal cell development but its absence greatly increases the occurrence of tumors and is associated with genome instability.
* The protein p53 binds to the DNA and acts as a transcriptional regulator. It regulates the genes that govern the cell cycle.
* The levels of p53 increase whenever the DNA is damaged. p53 causes arrest of cycle in G1 so that damaged DNA is not replicated and there is time for DNA repair to occur. That's why p53 is called guardian of the genome.

214. Ans.— A Porins

* Uncharged or neutral molecule passes freely through lipid bilayer. But some uncharged molecules, and chared ones require specific carrier protein to transfer them.
* These channels or porins are beta barrel proteins that cross cellular membrane and act as pores through which molecules can diffuse.
* Unlike other membrane transport proteins, pores are large enough to allow passive diffusion, i.e. they act as channels that are specific to different types of molecules.
* They typically control diffusion of small molecules like sugar, amino acid and some ions.

215. Ans.— B Higher than the intra-arterial pressure

* Since the cuff pressure gets dissipated between the cuff and the artery by the interspersed tissues, the blood pressure measured by the sphygmomanometer is always higher than the intraarterial pressure.

216. Ans.— D. Carboxylation

* Histamine is also found in cells in the gastric mucosa and in heparin-containing cells called mast cells that are plentiful in the anterior and posterior lobes of the pituitary gland.
* Histamine is formed by decarboxylation of the amino acid histidine.
* Histamine has been related to arousal, sexual behaviour, regulation of the secretion of some anterior pituitary hormones, blood pressure, drinking, and pain thresholds.

217. Ans.— B. Nernst Equation

* **The equilibrium potential for Na+ in mammalian neurons, calculated by using the Nernst equation, is about +60 mV."**

218. Ans.— A Golgi bodies

The Golgi apparatus plays two important roles in the membrane synthesis; first, it is responsible for processing of oligosaccharide chain of membrane glycoprotein and also contains enzymes for glycosylation.

219. Ans. B. Blocks adenyly cyclase

Two bacterial toxins have important effects on adenylyl cyclase that are mediated by G proteins. The A subunit of cholera toxin catgalyzes the transfer of ADP-ribose to an arginine residue in the middle of the subunit of Gs. This inhibits its GTPase activity, producing prolonged stimulation of adenylyl cyclase. Pertussis toxin catalyze ADP-ribosylation of a cysteine residue near the crboxyl terminal of the subunit of GI. This inhibits the function of GI.

220. Ans. A. Requires carrier protein

Diffusion through the cell membrane is divided into two subtypes called simple diffusion and facillated diffusion.

* ***Simple diffusion* means that kinetic movement of molecules or ions occurs through a membrane opening or through intermolecular spaces without any interaction with carrier proteins in the membrane. The rate of diffusion is determined by the amount substance available, and sizes of openings in the membrane through which the molecules or ions can move.**

* ***Facillated diffusion* requires interactin of a carrier protein. The carrier proten aids passage of the molecules or ions through the membrane by binding chemically with them and shutting them through the membrane in this form.**

221. Ans. C. G-protein receptors

A common way to translate a signal to a biologic effect inside cells in by way of nucleotide regulatory proteins G-proteins) that bind GTP. They act as 2nd messenger system for signal transduction. When the signal reaches a G-protein, the protein exchanges GDP for GTP. The GTP-protein complex brings about the effect. The inherent GTPase activity of the protein then converts GTP to GDP, restoring the resting state. So G-protein receptors are responsible for taking the information inside the cell after the primary messenger, i.e. the ligand binds to them.

222. Ans. B. Accumulation of active metabolites

The most important factor responsible for the increased blood flow in the exercising muscles is local, there is accumulation of metabolites which open up the precapillary sphincters, thereby recruiting more capillaries into circulation.

223. Ans. D. Hypoxanthine

Factors affecting the concentration of 2,3 BPG in the red cells include pH. Because acidosis inhibits red cell glycolysis, the 2,3 BPG concentration falls when the pH is low. Thyroid hormones, growth hormone, and androgens increae the concentration fo 2,3-BPG and the P50.

REVIEW PAPERS

(Based on Difficult & Important MCQ's)

CVS

1. **Ratio of cardiac index to cardiac output is about :**
A. 4 : 5 B. 3 : 5
C. 2 : 5 D. 1 : 3
2. **Cardiac reserve in a normal person is slightly more than —— %**
A. 100 B. 200
C. 300 D. 500
3. **Rhythmicity of ventricular muscle is —— per min :**
A. 20—40 B. 40—60
C. 60—80 D. 90—120
4. **Action potential of normal cardiac muscle is :**
A. 60 B. 85
C. 105 D. 120
5. **Cardiac output in young females is about —— that of young males :**
A. 5% less B. 15% less
C. 20% less D. 10% more
6. **The average cardiac output of a young male under resting conditions would be about (in L/min) :**
A. 4.2 B. 5.6
C. 7.5 D. 9.0
7. **R-wave in healthy subjects denote a dipole with an electrical axis of — degree :**
A. 30 B. 45
C. 60 D. 90
8. **The duration of S3 is — sec :**
A. 0.10 B. 0.16
C. 0.20 D. 0.24
9. **Pressure in left ventricle in diastole is —— mm Hg :**
A. 0 B. 60
C. 80 D. 120
10. **Hypertrophic cardiomyopathy is likely when the LV wall is thicker than —— mm :**
A. 7 B. 9
C. 11 D. 13
11. **There is decline in maximum cardiac output in response to exercise at the rate of —— % per year after the age of 40 years :**
A. 0.5 B. 1.0
C. 2.0 D. 2.5
12. **The combined output of two ventricles at birth is —— ml/kg as compared to 140 ml/kg/BW in adults :**
A. 210 B. 280
C. 360 D. 420
13. **When one is standing absolutely still, pressure of veins of feet is — mm Hg :**
A. 0 B. 30
C. 90 D. 120
14. **SA node is approximately —— mm wide :**
A. 1 B. 2
C. 3 D. 5
15. **Cardiac reserve of heart is —— beats per min :**
A. 60-90 B. 100-120
C. 130-140 D. 170-180
16. **The body water is relatively —— % smaller in females than in males :**
A. 3% B. 5%
C. 7% D. 13%
17. **In fetal life, the ratio of left ventricle to right ventricle is :**
A. 0.5 B. 1.0
C. 2.0 D. 3.0
18. **Cardiac contractility (inotropic state) may vary in re-sponse to physiologic needs. Which of the following changing conditions will not produce an alteration in contractility?**
A. Increasing heart rate.
B. Increasing catecholamine secretion and/or sympathetic stimulation.
C. Depressed stroke work without a change in diastolic filling.
D. Decreasing diastolic filling.
19. **Vasoconstrictor tone is decreased in response to increased activity of :**
A. Carotid sinus pressoreceptors
B. Medullary chemoreceptors
C. Pain receptors
D. Carotid body chemoreceptors

Ans. 1. B 2. C 3. A 4. C 5. B 6. B 7. C 8. A 9. A 10. D 11. B 12. C 13. C 14. C 15. C 16. C 17. B 18. D 19. D

LUNGS

20. **There are about——— million alveoli in man :**
A. 100 B. 200
C. 300 D. 500

21. **The binding of myoglobin to oxygen in comparison to that of haemoglobin is :**
A. 1/5 B. 1/4
C. 1/2 D. Twice

22. **The difference between venous and arterial blood pCO_2 is about —— mm Hg :**
A. 5 B. 10
C. 20 D. 25

23. **If the value of dyspnoeic index usually falls below —— %, dyspnoea is generally present :**
A. 40 B. 50
C. 60 D. 70

\24. **An increase in pCO_2 from normal level of 40 mm Hg to 63 mmHg causes a ——— fold increase in alveolar ventilation :**
A. 2 B. 5
C. 10 D. 20

25. **Carbon dioxide excreted per minute is —— ml :**
A. 100 B. 200
C. 350 D. 500

26. **In a healthy adult, daily production of CO_2 is — litres :**
A. 110 B. 220
C. 330 D. 410

27. **In sternous exercise, PO_2 falls from 40 to —— mm Hg :**
A. 36 B. 25
C. 15 D. 10

28. **At 3000 m above sea level, PO_2 is about —— mmHg**
A. 9 B. 80
C. 60 D. 40

29. **Maximum work of breathing is —— Kgm/breath :**
A. 5 B. 10
C. 20 D. 30

30. **Total area of alveolar walls in contact with capillaries in both lungs in about — sq. m :**
A. 30 B. 70
C. 110 D. 170

31. **Functional residual capacity in females is —— % less than that in males :**
A. 5 B. 10
C. 25 D. 40

32. **About ——% of heat is lost by evaporation from body including lungs :**
A. 5 B. 10
C. 25 D. 40

33. **The diffusion of CO2 across the alveolar membrane is faster than that of O2 because :**
A. CO2 is actively transferred.
B. The alveolar area available for CO2 diffusion is larger.
C. CO2 is more soluble in H2O (than is O2), which enables it to pass through the membrane with greater readiness.
D. The CO2 pressure gradient is larger.

34. **The earliest effect of acute hypoxia is :**
A. Muscular incoordination
B. Hyperpnea
C. Headache and lassitude
D. Euphoria initially; then, hyperpnea, incoordination, and lack of concentrating capability

35. **Pressure across a pulmonary capillary bed is approximately ——— mm Hg :**
A. 8 B. 12
C. 16 D. 25

36. **100% inspired O2 increases the alveolar PaO2 to about ——— mmHg :**
A. 200 B. 400
C. 600 D. 800

37. **Following lung functions are decreased in aged except :**
A. Vital capacity
B. Pulm. compliance
C. Diffusion capacity
D. FEV1

38. **The most potent stimulant of respiration would be :**
A. A twofold increase in the PCO2 of inspired air
B. A twofold increase in the PO2 of inspired air
C. A 50% decrease in the PCO2 of inspired air
D. A 50% decrease in the PO2 of inspired air

KIDNEY

39. **Transport maximum for plasma protein is —— mg/ml:**
A. 0 B. 30
C. 60 D. 180

40. **Nephron was first experimentally demonstrated by :**
A. Ludwig B. Heidanhain
C. Bowman D. Malpighi

41. **Normal filtration pressure in glomerulus is :**
A. 18 B. 24
C. 28 D. 32

42. **Average renal fraction is —— %**
A. 12 B. 21
C. 62 D. 80

Ans. 20. C 21. B 22. A 23. C 24. C 25. B 26. C 27. B 28. C 29. B 30. B 31. C 32. C 33. C 34. D 35. A 36. C 37. B 38. A 39. B 40. C 41. B 42. B

43. Optimum capacity upto which the inhibition of emptying the bladder can be exerted by voluntary effort is ——— ml :
A. 250 B. 500
C. 700 D. 900

44. Total area of glomerular capillary endothelium across which filteration occurs in humans is —— sq. m :
A. 0.2 B. 0.8
C. 1.4 D. 2.4

45. Which of the following has minimum concentration in human bile :
A. Cholic acid B. Lithocholic acid
C. Deoxycholic acid D. Chenodeoxycholic acid

46. Which of the following is least reabsorbed in kidney :
A. K+ B. Total solute
C. Urea D. Uric acid

47. Rate of tubular reabsorption is maximum for :
A. Glucose B. Alanine
C. Na+ D. K+

48. Glucose and ——— are 100% reabsorbed by kidney :
A. Na+ B. Water
C. Cl- D. HCO_3

49. During first year of life, bladder capacity increases by —— times :
A. 2 B. 3
C. 4 D. 5

50. Most NH_3 in kidney is formed in :
A. PCT B. DCT
C. PCT + DCT D. CT

51. PO2 of renal medulla is between ——- mm Hg :
A. 1-10 B. 10-20
C. 20-30 D. 30-40

52. About ———% of renal plasma flow is filtered :
A. 10 B. 20
C. 40 D. 60

53. Glycine and alanine contributes to about —— % of renal ammonia :
A. 10 B. 20
C. 40 D. 60

54. In dialysate, following electrolyses are in approximately equal concentration to uraemic plasma except :
A. Na+ B. K+
C. Mg++ D. Cl-

55. In urinary dilution test for tubular function, the patient can excrete at least —— % of volume ingested within 4 years :
A. 40 B. 50
C. 75 D. 90

56. In fasting states, obligatory urine volume is reduced to —— ml per day :
A. 450 B. 550
C. 750 D. 850

57. Current evidence indicated that renin secretion is regulated by :
A. Left atrial volume receptors.
B. Plasma potassium concentration.
C. The rate of delivery of sodium and/or chloride to the macula densa segment of the renal tubule.
D. Baroreceptors in the carotid sinus.

58. Active secretion by the renal tubules is important in the metabolism of :
A. Sodium B. Potassium
C. Bicarbonate D. Chloride

59. Saliva contains highest concentration of :
A. Na B. K
C. Cl D. HCO3

60. If the volume of gastric residue is atleast —— ml or more, it is suggestive of pyloric obstruction :
A. 50 B. 100
C. 250 D. 500

61. Alkalosis occurs when pH of blood is above :
A. 7.34 B. 7.36
C. 7.38 D. 7.40

62. Normal individuals secrete —— mEq. of HCl in one hour in response to histamine :
A. 4—8 B. 8—12
C. 12—16 D. 16—20

63. Hepatic venous pressure is —— mm Hg :
A. 3 B. 5
C. 10 D. 70

64. Trebutyrase is secreted by :
A. Stomach B. Gall bladder
C. Liver D. Pancreas

65. An adult pancreas contains —— lac islets :
A. 1—5 B. 2.5—7.5
C. 7.5—12.5 D. 10—15

CIRCULATION

66. Transport maximum for hemoglobin is ——— mg/min :
A. 0 B. 1
C. 60 D. 180

67. Blood flow in each 2 mg carotid body is —— ml/min :
A. 0.01 B. 0.04
C. 0.08 D. 0.16

68. Normally, plasma load for glucose is —— mg/min :
A. 125 B. 300
C. 600 D. 750

69. Reynold's number is increased by decrease in :
A. Velocity of flow B. Density of fluid
C. Diameter of tube D. Viscosity of fluid

Ans. 43. C 44. B 45. B 46. C 47. C 48. D 49. C 50. A 51. B 52. B 53. C 54. B 55. C 56. B 57. C 58. B 59. B 60. C 61. D 62. B 63. B 64. A 65. B 66. B 67. B 68. C 69. D

70. Which of the following promotes the Rouleaux formation :

A. Albumin B. Globulin
C. Fibrinogen D. Prothrombin

71. The volume of blood flow in the aorta is, under constant conditons :

A. Greater than the pulse wave velocity.
B. Approximately equal to the pulse wave velocity.
C. Inversely proportional to aortic diameter.
D. Directly proportional to the square of the aortic radius.

72. ——c.c% O2 unsaturation is the least amount which must be present in the capillary blood to produce cyanosis :

A. 3.7 B. 5.0
C. 6.7 D. 7.2

73. Linear velocity of blood at normal cardiac output aorta is —— cm/sec :

A. 20 B. 25
C. 32 D. 40

74. The most important renal defense against respiratory alkalosis is :

A. Increased secretion of K+
B. Decreased production of NH_3
C. Increased excretion of Na HCO_3
D. Increased excretion of H+

75. The conversion of the intermittent blood flow in the aortic arch to a smooth blood flow is ——— effect :

A. Hallberg B. Haldane
C. Russel D. Wind Kessel

76. Capillaries have a surface area of approximately ——— sq. m. :

A. 200 B. 250
C. 300 D. 350

77. Transmural pressure in a vessel (PT) equals :

A. Wall tension in vessel (T) x radius (R) of vessel
B. $T \times R^2$
C. $T \div R$
D. $T X R^2$

78. The percentage oxygen saturation of mixed venous blood (PvO2 40 mm Hg) is about ———% :

A. 50 B. 60
C. 75 D. 85

79. Normal anion gap is ——— mmol/L :

A. 0—8 B. 8—16
C. 16—24 D. 24—32

80. Normally, the greater portion of the circulating blood is located in the :

A. Heart
B. Large arteries
C. Capillaries
D. Large veins and main venous branches

ENDOCRINOLOGY

81. Following amino acids are stimulants of glucagon secretion except :

A. Alanine B. Glycine
C. Serine D. Lysine

82. Testosterone secretion begins in —— th week of intrauterine life :

A. 5 B. 6
C. 7 D. 8

83. ACTH secretion is minimum at about :

A. 4 pm B. 6 pm
C. 8 pm D. 1 hour after sleep

84. In body, heparin is secreted by :

A. Lymphocytes B. Neutrophils
C. Basophils D. RBC's

85. Pituitary cells absent in children under 10 years of age and disappears after first trimester of pregnancy :

A. Alpha B. Beta
C. Gamma D. Delta

86. Growth hormone has the half life of ——— minutes :

A. 10-20 B. 20-30
C. 40-60 D. 60-90

87. Term, "Prostaglandin" was suggested by :

A. Von Euler B. Goldblatt
C. Wilson D. Benting

88. Calcitonin has a strong effect on :

A. Osteocyte B. Osteoblast
C. Osteoclast D. All of the above

89. Which of the following is most efficacious in stimulating sodium ATPase pump :

A. Catecholamines B. Insulin
C. Thyroxine D. Aldosterone

90. The ratio of T3 to T4 in circulation is :

A. 1 : 50 B. 1 : 100
C. 1 : 150 D. 1 : 250

91. The peak and trough of Corticosteroid secretion is at :

A. 0600, 2400 B. 0600, 1800
C. 0400, 1600 D. 0400, 1800

92. The half life of catecholamines in circulation is —— min :

A. 1 B. 2
C. 6 D. 10

93. Aldosterone secretion in response to extracellular volume depletion of 500-1000 ml will peak at ——— hours :

A. 1 B. 2
C. 4 D. 6

Ans. 70. C 71. D 72. C 73. C 74. C 75. D 76. C 77. C 78. C 79. B 80. D 81. D 82. C 83. D 84. C 85. D 86. B 87. A 88. C 89. C 90. B 91. A 92. B 93. C

94. **The catecholamines, which are converted to VMA, are ——— %:**
A. 10 B. 30
C. 50 D. 70

95. **Among the following which stimulates the sodium ATPase pump the least :**
A. Thyroxine B. Catecholamines
C. Insulin D. Aldosteron

96. **Among current concepts, the most important factor in the moment-to-moment control of antidiuretic hormone (ADH) secretion is :**
A. Glomerular filtration rate (GFR)
B. Left atrial volume
C. Mean systemic arterial blood pressure
D. Plasma osmolality

97. **Increased rate of respiration resulting from moderate and heavy exercise is due to :**
A. Increased body temperature
B. Joint movement
C. Lowered serum pH
D. All of the above

BLOOD

98. **Fletcher factor is factor :**
A. XII B. XIII
C. XIV D. XV

99. **Under physiological conditions, diurunal variation in RBC count occurs as ——% in 24 hours :**
A. 1 B. 2
C. 5 D. 10

100. **Colony stimulating factor increases production of :**
A. Lymphocytes B. Neutrophils
C. Eosinophils D. Macrophages

101. **Marrow stores —— days supply of granulocytes :**
A. 3 B. 6
C. 12 D. 30

102. **Bone marrow of all bones produces RBC's till the age of ——— years :**
A. 1 B. 3
C. 5 D. 12

103. **Average life of transfused blood is ——— of normal blood :**
A. 1/2 B. 1/3
C. 2/3 D. 3/4

104. **The exact role of which of the following factor is not known :**
A. IV B. V
C. VI D. VII

105. **Diameter of platelet in about — of RBC :**
A. 1/3 B. 1/4
C. 1/5 D. 1/6

106. **Lysine : Arginine ratio in blood is :**
A. 0.8 B. 1.8
C. 2.4 D. 4.2

107. **Which of the following platelet factor helps in neutralizing heparin :**
A. I B. III
C. IV D. VII

108. **The presence of Hemoglobin increases the oxygen carrying capacity of the blood by —— fold :**
A. 20 B. .40
C. 78 D. 100

109. **Maximum concentration of hemoglobin normally found in RBC's is ——% :**
A. 24 B. 28
C. 34 D. 36

110. **Antifibrinolysin is platelet factor :**
A. IV B. V
C. VI D. VII

111. **Half life of transfused platelets is about —— of normal platelets :**
A. 1/5—1/6 B. 1/4—1/5
C. 1/2—1/3 D. Same

112. **In vitro, coagulation is initiated by factor —— :**
A. VIII B. X
C. XI D. XII

113. **Orthophosphoric acid possesses —— pKA value :**
A. 1.5 B. 3.0
C. 4.5 D. .6.0

114. **The longest living WBC is :**
A. Lymphocytes B. Eosinophils
C. Neutrophils D. Monocytes

115. **"Fresh" blood refers to blood which is administered :**
A. Immediately B. Within 12 hours
C. Within 24 hours D. Within 72 hours

116. **Major loss of RBC's in stored blood occurs in :**
A. First 24 hours B. 48-72 hours
C. 3-7 days D. 14-21 days

117. **Which of the following shows little change in stored blood :**
A. Na+ B. K+
C. Lactic acid D. Ammonia

118. **Hemolytic anemia of exercise is mainly due to :**
A. ↑ Blood volume B. ↓ Synthesis of Hb
C. Damage to RBC's D. ↓ RBC production

119. **With a plasma pH of 7.4, the Red blood cell has a pH of :**
A. 7.0 B. 7.2
C. 7.3 D. 7.4

Ans. 94. B 95. D 96. D 97. D 98. C 99. C 100. B 101. B 102. C 103. D 104. B 105. A 106. B 107. C 108. C 109. C 110. C 111. C 112. D 113. B 114. C 115. C 116. A 117. A 118. C 119. B

120. Fitzgerald factor is coagulation factor :
A. XII B. XIII
C. XIV D. XV

121. Erythroid cell maturation normally takes ——— days :
A. 3—5 B. 6—8
C. 12—14 D. 16—20

122. Alpha thalassemia contains more of :
A. HbH B. HbC
C. HbS D. HbA2

123. The risk of microalbuminuria increases logarithmically when HbA Ic exceeds :
A. 4.2% B. 5.7%
C. 6.2% D. 8.1%

SPECIAL SENSES

124. Bitter taste is felt at following part of tongue :
A. Tip B. Back
C. Middorsal D. Sides

125. Shivering can increase the rate of heat production upto —— times :
A. 2 B. 5
C. 8 D. 12

126. Tract of Lissauer is mainly associated with :
A. Pain B. Crude Touch
C. Pressure D. Proprioceptors

127. Inter-neurons are not functioning in ——— reflex :
A. Stretch B. Visual
C. Swallowing D. Flexion

128. Frequencies of upto ——— Hz will not produce tetany in fast twitch muscles :
A. 100 B. 150
C. 200 D. 250

129. An after-sensation of colour is ——— effect :
A. Doppler B. Danysz
C. Compton D. Mc Collough

130. The relation between intensity and area of illumination i.e. intensity times area equals constant is —— law :
A. Raoult's B. Ricco's
C. Stokes D. Talbot

131. When complete fusion occurs and the sensation is uniform, the intensity is same as would occur were the same amount of light spread uniformly over the disc is ——— law :
A. Rubner B. Ricco's
C. Talbot's D. Wolff's

MISCELLANEOUS

132. Somatomedin - C is synthesized in the following except :
A. Liver B. Kidney
C. Muscle D. Lungs

133. The amount of iron lost from body per day is —— mg :
A. 0.01-0.05 B. 0.5-1.0
C. 5-10 D. 20-25

134. Yellowish tint of skin in myxoedema is due to :
A. ↓ RBC B. ↓ Hemoglobin
C. ↑ Cholesterol D. Carotinemia

135. First plasma protein to appear in embryonic life is :
A. Prothrombin B. Globulin
C. Albumin D. Fibrinogen

136. Dysbarism is due to :
A. Sudden fall in pressure of ambient gases in body
B. Gradual fall in pressure of ambient gases in body
C. Gradual rise in pressure of ambient gases in body
D. Sudden rise in pressure of ambient gases in body

137. Bence Jones proteins in urine are found in :
A. Leukemia
B. Hodgkin's disease
C. Multiple myeloma
D. All of the above

138. For every 10 m of depth in sea water, the ambient pressure increases by —— atmosphere :
A. 0.5 B. 1.0
C. 1.5 D. 2.0

139. Sperms are normally motile at a rate of ——cm/min :
A. 0.1—1 B. 1—3
C. 3—6 D. 7—10

140. The maximum rate of transfer of glucose is —— mg/min :
A. 180 B. 240
C. 300 D. 375

141. Following immunoglobulins are monomers except :
A. IgG B. IgM
C. IgD D. IgE

142. IgG levels in infants reaches the adult level by —— years of age group :
A. Half to one B. 1-2
C. 3-5 D. 5-7

143. Hemming bodies are found in :
A. Pituitary B. Thalammus
C. Medulla D. Pons

144. Secretin may be found in the following except :
A. Hypothalamus B. Hippocampus
C. Cerebral cortex D. Spinal cord

Ans. 120. D 121. B 122. A 123. D 124. B 125. B 126. A 127. A 128. A 129. D 130. B 131. C 132. D 133. B 134. D 135. C 136. A 137. D 138. B 139. B 140. D 141. B 142. B 143. A 144. D

145. Keshan disease results when ——— is deficient :

A. Chromium B. Selenium
C. Cobalt D. Molybdenum

146. The muscle ruptures when it is stretched atleast —— times its equilibrium length :

A. 2 B. 3
C. 5 D. 10

147. Normal base output is —— mmol/hour :

A. 1-5 B. 5-10
C. 10-15 D. 15-20

148. Zona occludens is found in :

A. Pancreas B. Liver
C. Kidney D. Spinal cord

149. Ratchet theory is for :

A. Maintenance of cardiac output
B. Maintaining respiratory drive
C. Muscle contraction
D. Nerve conduction

150. Pudic nerve controls :

A. Ext. sphincter of rectum
B. Ext. sphincter of bladder
C. Size of pupil
D. Gastroesophageal junction

151. Hartman's solution is ringer except that —— mmol Cl- is replaced by lactate :

A. 12 B. 22
C. 28 D. 32

152. In ORS, a carbohydrate : sodium ratio, of about —— is ideal for maximum H2O and electrolyte absorption :

A. 1 : 1 B. 2 : 1
C. 3 : 1 D. 4 : 1

153. Which of the following does not change with exercise :

A. CVP B. End diastolic volume
C. Coronary blood flow D. Skin blood flow

154. Total peripheral resistance falls about —— % in moderate exercise :

A. 10 B. 25
C. 50 D. 75

155. Skin blood flow rises by —— % with exercise :

A. 0 B. 0.5
C. 2 D. 5.0

156. Exercise produces :

A. ↑ HDL cholesterol B. ↓ HDL cholesterol
C. ↓ LDL D. ↓ HDL : LDL ratio

157. Assume ICF 25 litres, ECF - 15 L, osmolality 30 mosmol/Kg, if 2 L of 4.4% NaCl is infused, both ECF and ICF will be ——— L :

A. 17 B. 21
C. 25 D. 27

158. In the above question, if ECF is expanded by 10 L of water, osmolality of both compartments will be ——— mosm/Kg :

A. 220 B. 240
C. 260 D. 280

159. Absence of gravity causes following except :

A. ↑ muscle mass
B. ↓ Blood volume
C. Osteoporosis
D. ↓ circulating T-cells

160. Increased perfusion pressure and subsequent stretch of vascular smooth muscle contraction and increased resistance, which returns to normal inspite of elevated perfusion pressure is ——— effect :

A. Russell B. Bruce
C. Bayliss D. Whitten

161. The ideal systolic pressure for an adult is the figure represented by 100 plus half the age in years is called ——— rule :

A. McDonald B. Jackson
C. Rolleston D. Young

162. The body weight of an adult ought to be as many kilograms as his body length in centimetres exceeds 100 is —— rule :

A. Octet B. Quetelet's
C. Weinberg D. Fried

163. In hemophilia, only women transmit the condition, only men inherit is —— rule :

A. Allen B. Arey
C. Lossen D. Octet

164. pCO2 is maximum in :

A. Umbilical artery B. Umbilical vein
C. Uterine artery D. Uterine vein

165. The decrease in measured viscosity observed when a flow of blood or other liquid suspension of particles is measured in tubes of small diameter, usually below 0.5 mm is called :

A. Edison effect
B. Hering effect
C. Fahraeus-Lindquist effect
D. Mierzejewki effect

166. The converse of Bohr's effect is :

A. Donnan effect B. Haldane effect
C. Crab tree effect D. Deelman effect

167. The disproportionate development of gray and white matter in the brain, the gray being excessive is called :

A. Pasteur effect B. Orbeli effect
C. Donnan effect D. Mierzejewki effect

Ans. **145. B 146. B 147. D 148. C 149. C 150. B 151. C 152. C 153. C 154. C 155. C 156. A 157. B 158. B 159. A 160. C 161. C 162. B 163. C 164. A 165. C 166. B 167. D**

168. The phenomenon wherein the response of a fatigued nerve muscle preparation can be enhanced by electrical sympathetic nerve stimulation is called :
A. Purkinje effect B. Stiles Crawford effect
C. Orbeli effect D. Deelman effect

169. Oxygenation of hemoglobin lowers its affinity for carbon dioxide is called :
A. Bainbridge effect B. Haldane effect
C. Bohr's effect D. Pasteur effect

170. The generation of new impulses following the arrival of a synchronized potential at the artificial synapse formed at the cut end of a nerve is —— effect :
A. Cotton B. Pasteur
C. Crab tree D. Hering

171. In infants, body water constitutes about —— %
A. 60 B. 70
C. 80 D. 90

172. Sodium exerts osmotic pressure of approximately ——% of total :
A. 30 B. 40
C. 50 D. 70

173. Ryanodine receptor controls uptake of ————— :
A. Calcium by sarcoplasmic reticulum
B. K+ by sarcoplasmic reticulum
C. Na+ by mitochondria
D. Mg by nucleus

174. Double Bohr's effect is seen in :
A. Fetus B. Infants
C. Elderly D. Chronic asthmatic

175. The extended body parts of warm -blooded species are relatively shorter in the colder regions of a species range than in the warmer is called ——— rule :
A. Allen B. Arey
C. Bastedo D. Budin

176. The law that regeneration is more complete in younger individuals than in older ones is —— law :
A. Ricco's B. Rubner's
C. Spallanzani's D. Talbot's

177. The loss or destruction of elements in the organic world is apt to be followed by over production of such elements in the reparative process is ——— law :
A. Walton's B. Weigert's
C. Wolff's D. Wundt-Lamansky

178. A granular layer of each transparent lateral disk of a muscle fibril is ——— layer :
A. Cheivitz B. Floegels
C. Haller's D. Huxley's

179. A muscle situated above an imflamed membrane is often affected with paralysis is —— law :
A. Raoult B. Proust's
C. Rosa's D. Stokes

180. Zeissels layer is found in :
A. Stomach B. Colon
C. Pancreas D. Adrenal

181. An aluminium band for temporarily occluding large blood vessel in order to check condition of the collateral circulation is called ——— band :
A. Lane's B. Matas
C. Flarris D. Henle

182. Brodel's white line is found in :
A. Liver B. Pancreas
C. Kidney D. Gums

183. Microscopic broken or scalariform lines at the junction of cardiac muscle cells are ——— lines :
A. Eberth B. Ellis
C. Kaes D. Kilian's

184. A line of junction between the ectoderm and endoderm is :
A. Frommann's B. Feiss
C. Ectental D. Gottinge

185. Konio cortex refers to :
A. Agranular cortex
B. Granular cortex
C. Cortex of spinal cord
D. Cortex with long vertical columns

Ans. 168. C 169. B 170. D 171. C 172. C 173. A 174. A 175. A 176. C 177. B 178. B 179. D 180. A 181. B 182. C 183. A 184. C 185. A

PHYSIOLOGY

References Quoted

S.No.	Books
1.	W.F. Ganongs **Review of Medical Physiology**. Prentice-Hall International Inc., USA.
2.	R.K. Marya's **Medical Physiology.** CBS Publishers & Distributors Pvt. Ltd., Delhi.
3.	Harrison's **Principles of Internal Medicine.** McGraw Hill, New York.
4.	Bhatia's **Quick Medical Text Review Series.** CBS Publishers & Distributors Pvt. Ltd., Delhi.

Unforgetable Supplement

Bhatia's **Quick Medical Text Review Series** (Quick revision of all the subjects in shorttime. No need to underline the books (read important points). CBS Publishers & Distributors Pvt. Ltd., Delhi.